The Cancer Syndrome

RALPH W. MOSS

Grove Press, Inc./New York

First Edition 1980
First Printing 1980
ISBN: 0-394-50859-9
Grove Press ISBN: 0-8021-0187-9
Library of Congress Catalog Card Number: 79-2300

Library of Congress Cataloging in Publication Data

Moss, Ralph. The Cancer Syndrome.

    Bibliography: p.
    Includes index.
    1. Cancer.   2. Cancer—Political aspects.
3. Cancer—Economic aspects.   I. Title.
RC263.M64   338.4'7'362196994   79-2300
ISBN 0-394-50859-9

Manufactured in the United States of America

Distributed by Random House, Inc., New York

GROVE PRESS, INC., 196 West Houston Street, New York, N.Y. 10014

TO MARTHA

There is nothing more admirable than when two people who see eye to eye keep house as husband and wife, confounding their enemies and delighting their friends, as they themselves know best.

HOMER
The Odyssey, Book VI

ACKNOWLEDGMENTS

Many individuals contributed to the making of this book.

The following read the text, or portions of it, and offered valuable comments at various stages: Irwin D. J. Bross, Ph.D., Alan Gaby, M.D., Joseph Gold, M.D., Virginia Livingston-Wheeler, M.D., Linus Pauling, Ph.D., Alec Pruchnicki, Charles Russell, Ph.D., Barbara Solomon, M.D., and Jonathan Wright, M.D.

Needless to say, any remaining errors are solely my responsibility.

My friends and family members contributed their help and support, especially my parents, Nat and Irene Moss, and my children, Melissa and Benjamin. My agent, Ruth Hagy Brod, and editor, Kent Carroll, performed above and beyond what was required of them. I wish to express my appreciation to those who worked on the production of this book, including Claudia Menza, Reginald Gay, and Diane Root.

Many workers and scientists in the cancer field, especially former colleagues at Memorial Sloan-Kettering Cancer Center, shared their knowledge, ideas, and theories freely. Among those colleagues was a friend and teacher, Dr. Kanematsu Sugiura, who died while this book was going to press. I am also indebted to the hundreds of cancer patients I have known. Esther Moore, who died tragically at forty-four, embodied the courage of these patients: "If death is coming, then death, come on with it, but let me meet you at the door, dammit, on my feet!"

Chapter 8, "The Laetrile Controversy," was first prepared for Louis Lasagna (ed.), *Controversies in Therapeutics*, Philadelphia: W. B. Saunders and Co., 1980. My thanks to Dr. Lasagna and his publisher for permission to reprint it here.

"Do Not Go Gentle into That Good Night" is from Dylan Thomas, *Poems*. Copyright 1952 by Dylan Thomas. Reprinted by permission of New Directions.

The Publisher wishes to thank Herman Goodman for bringing this manuscript to his attention.

Contents

DO NOT GO GENTLE INTO THAT GOOD NIGHT

by Dylan Thomas

Do not go gentle into that good night,
Old age should burn and rave at close of day;
Rage, rage against the dying of the light.

Though wise men at their end know dark is right,
Because their words have forked no lightning they
Do not go gentle into that good night.

Good men, the last wave by, crying how bright
Their frail deeds might have danced in a green bay,
Rage, rage against the dying of the light.

Wild men who caught and sang the sun in flight,
And learn, too late, they grieved it on its way,
Do not go gentle into that good night.

Grave men, near death, who see with blinding sight
Blind eyes could blaze like meteors and be gay,
Rage, rage against the dying of the light.

And you, my father, there on the sad height,
Curse, bless, me now with your fierce tears, I pray.
Do not go gentle into that good night.
Rage, rage against the dying of the light.

(Written in 1946 to the poet's father, dying of cancer.)

PART ONE
Proven Methods
(That Often Don't Work)

1

The Crisis of Credibility

A decade ago, there was tremendous optimism about cancer. America had put a man on the moon, and it was natural to ask whether the nation which could achieve that once-proverbial impossibility couldn't also conquer mankind's most dreaded disease.

Congress had appointed a blue-ribbon "National Panel of Consultants on the Conquest of Cancer" whose purpose, in the words of Senator Ralph Yarborough (D.-Tex.), was to "recommend to Congress and to the American people what must be done to achieve cures for the major forms of cancer by 1976. . . ."

In his foreword to the consultants' final report, Senator Yarborough put the case for an all-out "war on cancer" bluntly:

> Cancer is a disease which can be conquered. Our advances in the field of cancer research have brought us to the verge of important and exciting developments in the early detection and control of this dread disease . . . (Yarborough, 1970).

At the same time, forces close to the American Cancer Society, calling themselves the "Citizens' Committee for the Conquest of Cancer," began a skillful public-relations campaign aimed at passage of a "war on cancer" act. In full-page ads, the "Citizens' Committee" cried out:

MR. NIXON: YOU CAN CURE CANCER

> If prayers are heard in Heaven, this prayer is heard the most: "Dear God, please. Not cancer."
> Still, more than 318,000 Americans died of cancer last year.
> This year, Mr. President, you have it in your power to begin to end this curse (*New York Times*, December 9, 1969).

R. Lee Clark of Houston's M. D. Anderson Hospital declared unequivocally that "with a billion dollars a year for ten years we could lick cancer" (quoted in Edson, 1974).

On December 23, 1971, after much political jockeying, President Nixon signed into law the National Cancer Act, thus launching a full-scale assault on the dread disease. Congress had designated the act "a national crusade to be accomplished by 1976 in commemoration of the 200th anniversary of our country. . . ." (Rosenbaum, 1977). Nixon called for "the same kind of concentrated effort that split the atom and took man to the moon." This was Richard Nixon's Christmas present to the nation.

From the start, all this talk about curing cancer in time for the Bicentennial was good public relations, but terrible science. Curing cancer was just not like sending a man to the moon. Landing on the moon—or sending a rocket to Jupiter—is basically an engineering feat. Not enough was known about cancer to be able to predict its cure.

Writing for a business audience in 1970, Jerry E. Bishop, the *Wall Street Journal*'s science writer, spelled out the dilemma and the reason for the deception:

It is highly unlikely that any group of experts can promise that cures for major forms of cancer will be achieved within five years even if appropriations for cancer research were unlimited. To do so could raise high hopes among the public and result in a disenchantment, as 1976 rolled around, that might do considerable harm to public support of cancer research in the long run. Yet without such dramatic promises, public enthusiasm for a major "assault" on cancer that the researchers have longed for may be more difficult to arouse (August 26, 1970).

Thus, in Bishop's view, the war on cancer, with its inflated rhetoric and promises, was a clever way to prime the public for a "war" it might not otherwise support.

Not surprisingly, soon after the "war" was launched, it was in trouble. "Will the war ever get started?" *Science* magazine asked two years later (September 7, 1973).

"President Nixon's war on cancer . . . appears to be stalled in low gear, plagued by an increasingly bitter three-way battle for control of the $500 million of federal funds . . ." wrote the *Wall Street Journal* (July 28, 1973).

The administrators of the war drew up incredibly complicated 1,000-page battle plans including a "National Cancer Program Strategy" that will undoubtedly live on as a classic example of bureaucratic obscurity (Figure 1).

No sooner had the plan been drafted than it came under sharp

Figure 1
The National Cancer Program Strategy
(from National Cancer Institute, *1975 Fact Book*)

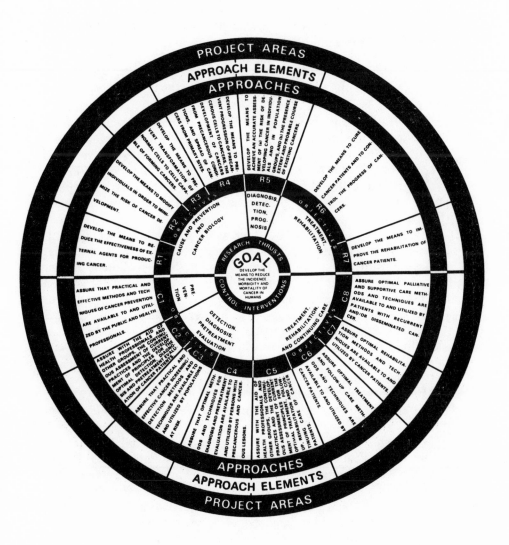

criticism from scientists within the cancer field itself. The basic assumption of the plan seemed to be that cancer could, in fact, be controlled by existing means. This corresponded to the political needs of President Nixon and the American Cancer Society, but simply didn't correspond to the scientific reality.

"There are many types of cancer for which today's technologies simply do not work," said a National Academy of Sciences panel headed by the president of Memorial Sloan-Kettering Cancer Center (*Wall Street Journal,* July 23, 1973). "What is most urgently needed for problems of this kind is an abundance of new ideas, and these are most likely to emerge from the imagination and intuition of individual scientists. It is much less likely that the administrators of large programs . . . at the center of a highly centralized bureaucracy can generate the kinds of ideas that are needed" (ibid.).

By 1974 the public, which had enthusiastically hoped a cure for cancer was in the offing, was beginning to feel it had been betrayed. The cancer war was Nixon's "other war," and when Nixon resigned over Watergate, this only fueled public suspicion of a double-cross.

"The Cancer Rip-Off" was science writer Lee Edson's summary of the situation, less than three years after the war was launched (Edson, 1974).

"We don't know how to attack cancer, much less conquer it, because we don't understand enough about how it works and what causes it," said Rockefeller University's Dr. Norton Zinder. Zinder was asked by the National Cancer Advisory Board (a body of laymen and professionals established by Nixon) to look into the special virus program, upon which most hopes were then pitched.

Zinder's committee found that the virologists had made the assumption that human cancer was indeed caused by a virus. But, said the review committee (which included top scientists from Sloan-Kettering, the National Cancer Institute, New York University, and the University of Colorado), "these assumptions were wrong. There wasn't enough knowledge to mount such a narrowly targeted program" (ibid.).

The committee also found some peculiar financial transactions within the multimillion-dollar program. They wrote: ". . . it is in large part an in-house operation and those who run it are also often recipients of large amounts of the money they dispense" (ibid.).

Private companies clustered around the National Institutes of Health in Bethesda, Maryland, were charging the government 144 percent overhead, plus a nine percent profit to perform virus research.

In early 1975 criticism of the program began to make headlines. Nobel Prize–laureate James Watson declared at a cancer symposium at the Massachusetts Institute of Technology that the American public had been sold a "nasty bill of goods about cancer" *(New York Times,* March 9, 1975). It was a "soporific orgy," which produced no "promising leads," as it claimed, but "only delaying actions" (Rosenbaum, 1977). He reputedly summed up the entire situation in four well-chosen words: "A bunch of shit!" (ibid.).

A few weeks later, Dr. Charles C. Edwards, who had resigned in January 1975 as Secretary of Health of the U.S. Department of Health, Education and Welfare, wrote in an article that the war on cancer was politically motivated and based on the dubious premise that cancer could, "like the surface of the moon, be conquered if we will simply spend enough money to get the job done" *(New York Times,* March 22, 1975).

As the Bicentennial approached, the leaders of the cancer war frantically attempted to come up with some bona fide achievements that would placate an increasingly restless public. "All of us receive a multitude of inquiries on what the National Cancer Program is doing to help people," wrote Frank J. Rauscher, Jr., Ph.D., director of the program (and of the National Cancer Institute). "In short, 'What are we doing with the taxpayer's money?'"

To answer that question, Rauscher issued a list of accomplishments. With no false modesty, the young virologist, who had been called "Nixon's protégé" *(Medical World News,* May 26, 1972), declared, "In every sense, these advances are remarkable and have already saved many lives" (National Cancer Institute, 1976a).

First on the list was a combination of drugs used after surgery to decrease the recurrence rate of breast cancer. The method was brand new at the time, and virtually unproven, but Rauscher called it "a great and justifiable cause for optimism."

Several months before, however, this treatment method had been sharply criticized in *Science* magazine as one whose "significance has been greatly exaggerated" *(Science,* March 12, 1976). And Mary E. Costanza, a doctor at Tufts-New England Medical Center Hospitals in Boston, has warned that "all in all, there is reason to be skeptical as well as optimistic about the effects of long-term chemoprophylaxis against breast cancer" *(New England Journal of Medicine,* November 20, 1975).

Second on Rauscher's list was "a study of the treatment of breast cancer with less radical surgery" which had shown that "it may be as effective as radical surgery."

Far from being an accomplishment of the war on cancer, the use of limited surgery in breast cancer had long been the position of mavericks in the cancer field, who had had to buck the establishment to get their position heard (see Chapter 3).

The report went on to repeat many of the claims that had been made for surgery, radiation, and chemotherapy over the years. It included such inspired achievements as "a communication network [that] has been developed . . . to provide cancer information to health professionals" and "toll-free telephone services . . . established at each Center." It also stated that "scientists within and outside the National Cancer Program have found again that fluoridation of drinking water does not contribute to a cancer burden for people"—a claim which was sharply contested by unorthodox scientists such as Dean Burk, Ph.D., and John Yiamouyiannis, Ph.D. (Congressional Record, December 16, 1975).

What the report didn't say was what millions of people had been led to expect: that the National Cancer Program had found a cure for even one major type of human cancer.

Not long after this, Dr. Rauscher stepped down as head of the cancer program.

By 1979—ten years after the promised quick cure—the beginning of the end still did not appear to be in sight. "A medical Vietnam" is how Food and Drug Administrator Donald Kennedy, Ph.D., succinctly described the war on cancer. In June 1979 Kennedy resigned his post to return to academe. His inability to ban saccharin and the unorthodox cancer therapy laetrile were two of the main reasons given for his rather sudden departure (New York Times, October 6, 1979).

"We have been simplistic," said Dr. Arthur Upton, who succeeded Rauscher as head of the National Cancer Institute. "I think we're wrong to expect a cure to come soon" (Wall Street Journal, October 24, 1978).

There's a "crisis of credibility," said Dr. Theodore Cooper, the former assistant director of the Department of Health, Education and Welfare (ibid.).

The reason for this crisis is the tremendous gap between the promises and claims of cancer orthodoxy and the grim reality. No amount of cheerful optimism has been able to obscure the obvious fact that we are not winning the war on cancer.

Every day more than 1,000 people die of cancer in the United States. Almost 400,000 a year. One every 80 seconds.

Over 765,000 Americans a year discover that they have a malignancy. These are the most serious cases. If we add to this 300,000 to 600,000 cases of skin cancer, and about 40,000 cases of carcinoma-in-situ (limited to one small site) of the uterine cervix, over one million of us will be treated for cancer each year (ACS, 1979).*

* Skin cancer (basal cell carcinoma) and carcinoma of the uterine cervix are generally so readily curable through surgery and radiation that they are not included in the cancer statistics.

If the present trend continues, at least one in four of us will contract cancer. One in five will die of the disease.

While public spokesmen speak with assurance about cancer, it is obvious that very little is really known about the disease in any fundamental sense. What exactly is cancer? Scientists can describe certain features common to cancer cells. For example, they are strangely misshapen and immature. They can invade neighboring tissues. They can break free from a tumorous growth, float through the blood or lymph system, and set up new colonies (called metastases) in other vital organs.

According to the American Cancer Society (ACS), "Cancer is a large group of diseases characterized by uncontrolled growth and spread of abnormal cells" (ibid.). Yet even so basic a summation does not find universal acceptance. Not only do many unorthodox doctors contest this definition, but even the president of Memorial Sloan-Kettering Cancer Center has said that he believes cancer to be a single disease and that some "as yet unidentified pathological mechanism is involved in all varieties of cancer" (MSKCC *Center News*, March 1975). In fact, an ACS-published textbook states that, "To date no single definition [of cancer] is universally acceptable" (Rubin, 1971:18).

There is clearly no unanimity among scientists on even the most basic facts of cancer. But if cancer is a biological puzzle, it is even more a social, economic, and political one. The newspapers, magazines, radio, and television are daily filled with a welter of confusing and conflicting stories about cancer.

We are told that great strides are being made in the conquest of the disease—and then we are told that the incidence of cancer is on the rise. We are told that chemicals cause cancer—but then that animal tests prove nothing and human data are inconclusive. We are told to examine our bodies for changes in every wart, mole, and growth—and then we are told that we are suffering from "cancerphobia." We are told that we must be protected from cancer quackery—and then we learn that twenty states have legalized a supposedly quack remedy.

Why is there such confusion, controversy, emotion, and bitterness associated with the question of cancer? The main reason appears to be that cancer exacts an enormous toll from the American people, yet no one seems to know how to go about ridding the country or the world of this plague.

The emotional toll of cancer is incalculable. Most cancer victims suffer the agony of a painful, disabling, and socially stigmatized disease (Sontag, 1977). They live in fear of the disease, an unknown terror, and of death. They live in fear of the orthodox treatment, surgery, irradiation, and poisonous chemotherapy. Men fear castration, physical or chemical. Women fear the loss of their sexuality, their breasts, and their womb. These are the bitter facts about cancer.

Despite much easy talk about cures, victims are rarely free of the fear that someday the cancer will return. "Five-year survival" is a conventional milestone for cancer patients, and a realistic goal for doctors. Anyone who survives this long after diagnosis may well be in the clear. But the doubts and fears remain in the back of a cancer patient's mind—often for a lifetime.

This emotional background lends all disputes in cancer a particular urgency. Each side in such a controversy believes the other side is raising false hopes, causing needless despair, or even performing "murder by proxy."

Equally important is the financial burden of the disease, which has become truly staggering in recent years.

A few years ago, *Consumer Reports* estimated that the average cost of cancer was $20,000 for the medical services alone (cited in ACS, 1979). Samuel S. Epstein estimates a cost range of $5,000–30,000 (Epstein, 1978).°

Such figures, although considerable, seem to understate the true economic impact of cancer in today's inflationary times. A survey of cancer patients in the New York Metropolitan area in 1971–72 showed that the range of total costs was $5,000–50,000. The average at that time was $21,718. Twenty percent spent over $30,000 (Cancer Care, Inc., 1973:21). As the authors of this study indicated, however, "the point regarding costs is that they exceed family income" (ibid.). The median cost of the illness ($19,054) was *two-and-one-third times* the family's median income.

This situation has only worsened in recent years. A day in a cancer hospital can now cost up to $600, according to Robert M. Heyssel, executive vice-president and director of Johns Hopkins Hospital. He adds an important point: "Each new medical or scientific breakthrough improves the quality and the outcome of care, but in most instances the cost of care rises proportionately" *(New York Times,* July 16, 1979).

In the late 1970s, medical inflation outstripped the overall rate of price rises. In fact, according to some economists, medical costs are *doubling* every five years *(Time,* May 28, 1979).

Direct treatment costs for cancer are currently about $20 billion a year. At the current rate of inflation, however, this will be $40

° "There is surprisingly little information in detail about the costs of long-term illness," according to Cancer Care, Inc. (1973). The American Cancer Society adds that "the cost of cancer treatment varies so widely from case to case that it is difficult to cite any typical figure" (ACS, 1979).

billion by 1984 and around $80 billion by the end of the 1980s. Short of some simple, economical cure, any "breakthroughs" could greatly increase the cost. What would happen, for instance, if an experimental drug treatment currently priced at $50,000 per patient turned out to be an effective anticancer agent? Who can put a lid on such expenditures, without being accused of cruelty?

But the direct expenses of cancer are only about half of the total cost to society. If we add the *indirect* costs, such as loss of earning power due to premature disability, the expense to society of research into the disease, or the billions spent on regulating industry, the total already comes to around $40 billion a year (Epstein, 1978).

The logical corollary of this massive expenditure, however, is that *someone* is receiving much of the money that the cancer victim disburses. Cancer care is not a charity: it is a business—big business.

To begin with, cancer patients are said to pay 50 million visits to their physicians each year (Applezweig, 1978). In his frantic search for help, a cancer patient may bounce from one specialist to another, from an internist to a surgeon to a radiologist and finally to a practitioner of "fringe" medicine. Although no one consciously planned it that way, cancer generates a great deal of business for the medical profession.

If each new cancer patient undergoes only one surgical operation (the average at Memorial Sloan-Kettering Cancer Center) this means that America's surgeons perform 750,000 cancer operations each year. This does not include the many thousands of operations for skin cancer or benign growths, nor the biopsies, which exceed the number of large-scale operations.

Another source of revenue for doctors and hospitals is the use of radiation in the diagnosis and treatment of cancer. There are 270,000 X-ray units in the United States, 120,000 of them in the hands of medical doctors or related health professionals—the rest mainly belong to dentists (*New York Times,* July 4, 1979). In 1973 it was estimated that there were 3,000 telecobalt units, 300–400 linear accelerators, and 35–50 cyclotrons treating cancer patients throughout the world) (Richards, 1972).

According to some experts, 70 percent of all cancer patients, or more than 500,000 individuals, receive X-ray therapy each year (*New York Times,* July 4, 1979).

It is impossible to give an accurate cost figure for these treatments, which vary widely from hospital to hospital. Since each patient usually receives a *series* of X-ray treatments, the financial impact of this form of therapy is apparent.

Hospitals find radiation equipment to be a worthwhile investment. Memorial Sloan-Kettering, for example, recently spent $4.5

million to replace all its radiation machinery (MSKCC *Center News*, July/August 1977).

Over 1,000 hospitals have rushed to install new, sophisticated X-ray devices called CAT scanners, at a cost of $700,000 or more per machine (*Time*, October 29, 1979). Each CAT scan cost the patient between $220 and $400, according to a survey of New York hospitals (see also *Medical World News*, June 14, 1976).

Cancer diagnosis is a huge medical business, fanned by the public's fear of the disease and thirty years of publicity by the American Cancer Society. In 1974, the latest year for which data are available, more than 56 million women over the age of seventeen had Pap smears in the United States—and this for only one, relatively minor type of cancer (*Science*, July 13, 1979).

Drugs have begun to assume importance in the cancer field, as well. Although still modest by Wall Street standards, their sales are climbing steadily and form an important part of the cost of cancer for many patients (see Chapter 5).

So great has fear of cancer's economic cost become that a new industry has sprung into existence: cancer insurance.

"Insurance salesmen are now marketing cancer insurance door-to-door in the vicinity of Three Mile Island," according to Sam Allalouf, public-relations director for Cancer Care, Inc. (*New York Times*, July 16, 1979).

Such insurance often provides coverage which simply duplicates that of Blue Cross or the other major plans—or fails to provide needed coverage. In 1978, the attorney general of Ohio conducted an investigation of an insurance company which billed itself a "pioneer and world's leader in the field of cancer expense insurance." The policies, he said, paid the cancer victim only while he was hospitalized ($100 per day). This appears to be a liberal payment; however, most patients spend an average of only fourteen days a year in the hospital. Most treatment today is provided on an outpatient basis.°

As one indication of the profit to be made in this field: this insurance company paid out only 40 percent of the premiums it collected in Ohio, compared to 90 percent paid out by Blue Cross.

The current crisis in cancer cries out for radical solutions. The public is confused, frightened, restless, and on the point of rebellion against the old, inadequate ways of treating the disease. The growing personal and national cost of cancer—the incredible tragedy and suffering, plus the staggering financial waste of it all—make new directions not just a dream, but a necessity.

° In 1977, for example, Memorial Sloan-Kettering Cancer Center had 14,440 inpatient admissions and 127,936 visits to the outpatient clinics (MSKCC, 1977a).

2

The "Proven" Methods

Officially, however, all is well with the cancer war. Publications of the American Cancer Society (ACS) continue to exude optimism about the current ways of managing the disease.

Cancer is not just treatable, but *curable*. In fact, it is "one of the most curable of the major diseases in the country" (ACS publication cited in Daniel Greenberg, 1975). "Many cancers can be cured," we are assured, "if detected early and treated promptly" (ACS, 1979).

What exactly does the American Cancer Society mean by "cure"? In general parlance, as in the dictionary, a cure is a restoration to health or a sound condition—the elimination of a disease.

For years, however, the American Cancer Society maintained a peculiar definition of a cancer cure as a five-year survival after diagnosis. Asked by a *New York Times* reporter for his definition of the word, a baffled ACS vice-president admitted, "I've never gone to a dictionary to look up a definition of cure. We really do not know what we mean by cure because there is a great difference between cure and long-term survival" *(New York Times, April 17, 1979)*. The president of Memorial Sloan-Kettering Cancer Center, Lewis Thomas, M.D., agreed: he "rarely hears the term 'cure' when doctors talk among themselves," he told the same reporter.

In recent years, however, the ACS definition of cure has become even hazier. For example, among the 2 million cured cancer victims in the United States are included individuals who "still have evidence of cancer" (ACS, 1979). And while most people can be considered cured after five years, some patients can be declared cured after only *one* or perhaps three years (ibid.).

This peculiar bookkeeping of cure rates has led to some bizarre situations. Thus, a person who is treated for cancer and survives five years is entered in the record books as a "cure." What happens, however, if he has a recurrence of this cancer sometime later? What happens if he dies? He will then be in the paradoxical situation of having been officially cured of cancer, and dying of it at the same time.

This Alice-in-Wonderland logic may actually help to overstate the number of people being permanently freed of the disease, and to exaggerate the benefit of the so-called proven methods of treatment.

The bottom line for a cancer therapy is how many people it actually saves. By the ACS's own statistics, only "about one-third of all people who get cancer this year will be alive at least five years after treatment" (ibid.).

This does not speak very well for the current, officially approved methods of treating the disease: a one-third "cure" rate by a very questionable definition of cure.

Two interpretations of this anomaly are possible. First, one might say that there is something wrong with the currently employed "proven" methods of treatment. This the American Cancer Society will not say, since it has helped to promote these methods for many years and is committed to them.

The difficulty, says the Society, lies with the people themselves. They need "education" to trust in these methods; and in the fight against cancer the best weapons are an annual checkup and a check, according to the famous slogan.

If people would avail themselves of the current methods of treatment through earlier diagnosis and treatment, the Society claims, 128,000 cancer victims could be saved each year.

There are serious questions about the safety and efficacy of some of these diagnostic techniques. At this time, there is still no chemical test which can detect the presence of cancer in the body and "it will apparently be many years before a biochemical assay for cancer will be in use" (Maugh and Marx, 1975:94). The establishment must therefore rely on less certain methods for detection, whose value is in doubt.

For over thirty years, the Society has been associated with the Pap smear test for cancer, a prime means of diagnosing cervical and uterine cancer.

The rate of death from this type of cancer has, indeed, plummeted since the 1940s. For years the ACS lauded the Pap test as the *cause* of this decline. However, some students now claim that the Pap test had little to do with this trend:

> The mortality rate from cervical cancer was already dropping in this country in the late 1940s, before screening became popular, and the critics suggest that Pap smears have made little or no contribution to the continuing decline (*Science,* July 13, 1979).

In 1979 the ACS quietly dropped its recommendation that women receive an *annual* Pap test, and insists only on a *regular* one (ibid.). It has also demoted the Pap test from the sole cause of the decline in mortality for this disease to one of three, including better education and hygiene (ACS, 1978).

Despite four decades of Pap tests and 56 million tests a year, more than one out of five women with cancer of the uterus still dies of the disease—11,000 out of 53,000 (ACS, 1979).

Why then is the Pap test so widely utilized in the United States? According to two scientists from New York University and Yale University School of Medicine, the answer is primarily economic. As they told *Science:*

> . . . the annual Pap smear has become so entrenched in this country partly because it has been so heavily promoted and partly because so much of the cost is borne by the private individual. In England and Canada, where the governments bear practically all the costs, annual tests are not recommended, at least for low-risk women *(Science,* July 13, 1979).

The Pap smear may indeed be, as the magazine suggests, "an idea whose time has gone."

No less questionable—and controversial—is the use of X rays to detect breast cancer: mammography. The American Cancer Society promoted the procedure as a safe and simple way to detect breast tumors early, and thus allow women to undergo mastectomies before their cancers had metastasized.

Three hundred thousand women were enrolled in a joint ACS–National Cancer Institute (NCI) program at twenty-seven breast cancer detection centers in 1972 and given an average of two rads of radiation per examination *(New York Times,* March 28, 1976).

Criticism of this project started almost immediately within the NCI. Dr. John Bailar III, editor of the *Journal* of the National Cancer Institute, went public with these criticisms in January 1976 when he wrote:

> There is a body of information that the benefits to women under the age of fifty may not be as great as was thought when the project was started (ibid.).

There is a possibility, Bailar added, that the procedure would cause as many deaths through the carcinogenic effect of radiation as it would save through early diagnosis.

As the controversy heated up in 1976, it was revealed that the hundreds of thousands of women enrolled in the program were never told the risk they faced from the procedure (ibid.). Young women faced the greatest danger. In the thirty-five- to fifty-year-old age group, each mammogram increased the subject's chance of contracting breast cancer by 1 percent, according to Dr. Rauscher, director of the National Cancer Institute (*New York Times,* August 23, 1976).

The NCI appointed a committee of experts, headed by Dr. Lester Breslow of UCLA, to recommend a way out of the dilemma. The Breslow report recommended that the agency discontinue the routine use of X-ray screening for breast cancer in symptom-free women under the age of fifty (*New York Times,* July 15, 1976). An "extremely reluctant" American Cancer Society deferred to this decision, which was a direct slap in the face to their early-detection strategy.°

At the present time, the NCI recommends mammography in symptom-free women only when they are (1) age fifty or over, (2) age thirty-five to forty-nine and have had cancer in one breast, and (3) age forty to forty-nine whose mother and/or sister have had the disease (Cancer Information Service, 1977).

In other cases, the benefits of mammography are simply not worth the risk.°°

Clearly, then, no current method of cancer detection is likely to dramatically decrease the death rate from the disease. In fact, there are many instances in which patients have followed the ACS's advice, gotten checkups, received approved therapy early in the course of their illness, and still died.

From 1976 to 1978, the public had a dramatic illustration of the unpredictability of the "proven" methods of diagnosis and treatment. Senator Hubert H. Humphrey (D.-Minn.) was treated for bladder cancer and died in full view of the media.

Humphrey did not die because he lacked knowledge about the disease. He was, in fact, one of the staunchest supporters of orthodox cancer research on Capitol Hill (Prescott, 1976).

Nor did he fail to get early diagnosis. Doctors found tiny, apparently nonmalignant growths, no bigger than pinheads, on his bladder in 1966.

By 1973, however, Senator Humphrey had cancer of the bladder. This was treated, with apparent success, by X-ray therapy. He then underwent urologic examinations every six months. In May 1976 Humphrey's physician, Dr. Dabney Jarman, declared that he found no reason to prescribe further treatment for the condition (*New York*

° In the midst of the debate, Kodak took out full-page ads in scientific journals entitled "About breast cancer and X rays: A hopeful message from industry on a sober topic" (see *Science,* July 2, 1976). Kodak is a major manufacturer of mammography film.

°° This is so despite the fact that the amount of radiation has decreased from an average of 2 to 1.5 rads per procedure (*U.S. News and World Report,* May 14, 1979). Some hospitals now claim to use less than 0.5 rad per procedure through the use of new films and screens.

Times, May 6, 1976). A few months later the cancer was back with a vengeance.

On October 6, 1976, Senator Humphrey was operated on by a team of doctors at Memorial Hospital, the treatment wing of Memorial Sloan-Kettering. His surgeon, Willard Whitmore, appeared before the press and television cameras at a crowded news conference and declared, "As far as we are concerned, the Senator is cured" *(New York Times,* October 8, 1976). He added that 70 percent of patients who undergo this operation have no recurrence of their cancer (ibid.). Merely as a preventive measure, to "wipe out any microscopic colonies of cancer cells that may be hidden somewhere in the body" (ibid.), his doctors began treatment with experimental drugs. Within about a year, Senator Humphrey was dead. In that short time he had withered from a vigorous middle-aged man to an old, balding, and feeble cancer victim. Humphrey himself blamed chemotherapy for at least contributing to his demise, calling it "bottled death" and refusing in the end to return to Memorial Hospital for more drug treatments *(New York Daily News,* January 14, 1978).

Humphrey was certainly not alone in his experience with orthodox therapy.

In Humphrey's case, as in many others, the orthodox strategy of early detection and early treatment with surgery, radiation, and chemotherapy proved ineffective. Many cancer patients have their cancers detected in an early stage, receive proper treatment and skillful care—and yet they still die.

Years of cultivating the press had made the American Cancer Society virtually sacrosanct. From 1945 to 1975 one could search in vain for an incisive, critical article on the Society or its methods. Then, in the mid-1970s, criticism suddenly burst into the open about the whole topic of cancer. The "war on cancer" had made the leading organizations visible and vulnerable.

In 1975, as part of the trend, Daniel S. Greenberg, a well-known Washington reporter, published an article titled "A Critical Look at Cancer Coverage" (Daniel Greenberg, 1975). The piece, which appeared in the respected *Columbia Journalism Review,* was widely reprinted and quoted.

Studying government figures and talking to cancer therapists and researchers, Greenberg found that the cancer picture was in fact very discouraging: it is "a far gloomier picture than has been generally conveyed to a hopeful public by our leading cancer research institutions and by the American Cancer Society." Greenberg noted that

Today's patient, who is supposedly the beneficiary of the burgeoning of cancer research that began in the early 1950s, has approximately the same chance of surviving for at least five years as a patient whose illness was diagnosed before any of that research took place (ibid.).

By surveying the then most recent National Cancer Institute (NCI) figures, published in 1972, Greenberg found that the cancer survival rates for most types of cancer had largely remained static from the 1950s on. And what improvement was noted from 1930 to 1950 was probably the result of better support systems and nursing care in the hospitals surveyed, rather than true improvements in cancer therapy.

By adding some more recent data supplied by NCI, Greenberg contended that the survival rates for some kinds of cancer had actually *declined* in recent years. The one-year survival for cancer of the colon, for example, had been 68 percent in the period 1965–69; it fell to 65 percent in 1970–71, according to government figures. Why the decline? Some experts told Greenberg it was because of the more vigorous application of "proven" methods, like toxic chemotherapy, which sometimes kills those patients on whom it is used.

Orthodox cancer literature has stressed the dramatic breakthroughs in the treatment of leukemia and other childhood diseases. Undoubtedly, dramatic improvement has been made in this area. But Greenberg found that "the official statistics do not support the optimistic claims" emanating from cancer center public-relations offices. The survival rates for all kinds of leukemia, for example, although "apparently improving as a result of new chemotherapies, remain tragically low." The median survival time in government statistics on leukemia victims is still measured in *months*, not years (see Chapter 5).

A cancer statistician cautioned Greenberg to take all "cure" statistics on relatively rare diseases, such as leukemia, with a dose of skepticism:

When you're dealing with such small numbers [he said] it is easy for a small amount of misdiagnosis to produce a big change in the survival statistics. I wouldn't be surprised if they're curing a lot of leukemia that never existed (ibid.).

Another scientist told him that the high cure rates in general are based on inept diagnoses. Some regional hospitals, he said, list people with undiagnosed lumps and bumps as "cancer cases." These often turn out noncancerous. Nonetheless, such cases go into the records as cancer patients, and when they survive five years they are officially "cured" of a disease they never had.

"Actually," this researcher told Greenberg, "there has been little improvement since 1945."

There are many ways to arrange statistics to make them look favorable to a particular method.

Clinicians can select their cases, for example, and choose only those patients whom they feel have the best chances of survival. In *The Savage Cell*, Pat McGrady, Sr., remarked on this phenomenon:

If one examines closely enough the cases operated upon by a surgeon enjoying an extraordinarily high cure rate, he is almost certain to find that the surgeon has refused to operate on many patients with only a fair-to-middling chance of cure. The cure rates by other surgeons of equal skill may be low because of the number of long-shot gambles they take in trying to cure patients of doubtful curability (McGrady, Sr., 1964:310).

Most clinicians would like to have a high cure rate: such statistics can be instrumental in determining the allocation of federal grants, promotions, or the procurement of future patients. The temptation is always present for one doctor or an entire center to arrange its statistics in such a way as to exaggerate the progress actually being made.

Research-oriented institutions, for example, may carefully select patients for clinical trials of new agents. In pilot research projects, doctors generally want to show high cure rates and long survival figures. Patients in such studies may be given the best possible backup care in order to increase their chances of survival.

"Clinical researchers don't like to treat dying patients," a scientist told Greenberg bluntly. "Poor risks can be sent elsewhere to die."

At the 1975 ACS Science Writers' Seminar, NCI director Frank Rauscher responded to Greenberg's charges: Greenberg's figures, while accurate, were out-of-date and did not reflect the progress of the war on cancer. ACS president Dr. George P. Rosemond even predicted that by 1978 "we will have reached the potential saving of one in two cancer victims" (*New York Times*, March 22, 1975). But when updated figures did appear, the new statistics did not support this argument.

The National Cancer Institute program issued "Cancer Patient Survival Report No. 5" in 1976. It is the most complete compilation of data on cancer survival ever made. By and large, the government report confirmed many of Greenberg's contentions and threw additional light on the frequent failure of orthodox therapy.

Although survival rates for six of the ten most common forms of cancer had improved since the early 1960s, the average improvement was minuscule. Large numbers of people were still dying of all types of cancer, despite adequate treatment with "proven" methods of therapy.

Figure 2
Five-Year Relative Survival Rates (Percent) For Ten Common Types of Cancer

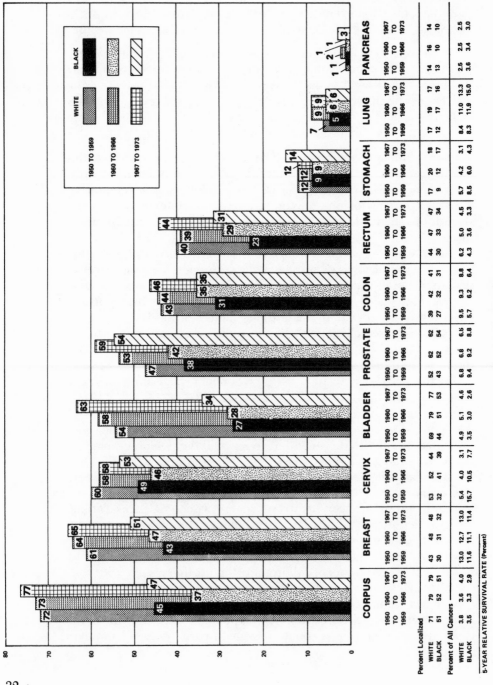

Source: *Cancer Patient Survival.* Report No. 5 NCI (1976)

In no common form of cancer had there been any real "break-throughs" between 1950 and 1973 (see Figure 2). For example, in that period the five-year survival rate (so-called cure rate) increased 4 percentage points for breast cancer (among whites), 9 for bladder, 3 for colon, 2 for lung, and 1 for pancreas. The so-called cure rate for stomach cancer remained static. It went down 2 percentage points for cancer of the cervix (NCI, 1976b).

In almost every case, the five-year survival rate for blacks was far less than for whites: 30 percentage points less for cancer of the corpus uteri; 29 points for cancer of the bladder, and so forth. NCI ascribed these differences to "socioeconomic factors not yet identified in detail."

The "cure" rate for pancreatic cancer was 1 percent—in other words, 99 out of 100 were dead five years after diagnosis. For lung cancer it was 9 percent, for colon—the most common cancer in males—it was 46 percent among whites, 35 percent among blacks.

Aside from these less than encouraging survival figures for most common cancers, the 315-page report also yielded many examples of a decline in survival for the less common tumors. For example, the one-, five-, and ten-year survival rates for lip cancer declined several percentage points in the latest figures. For pancreatic cancer, the one-year survival rate had been 17 percent for whites in 1950–54. This dropped to 10 percent in 1960–64 and climbed back to 14 percent in 1970–73, still several points below the 1950–54 figure, however. This decline coincided with the increased use of chemotherapy in the treatment of this malignancy: in 1950–53 only 2 percent of these patients had received chemotherapy, but in the 1970s over 20 percent received it (ibid.: 131).

There is even some doubt that these official figures, as unpromising as they are, really tell the whole truth. They may actually make the "proven" methods appear more successful than they actually are.

To begin with, these government statistics are based on results gathered from four "tumor registries" in Berkeley, New Orleans, Hartford, and Iowa City. Together they provide data on less than half a million patients out of the many millions who had cancer in the period 1950–73. The editors of the government study concede:

> It is difficult if not impossible to assess whether data contributed by these registries are a true reflection of cancer patient survival throughout the United States (*HEW News*, Bethesda, Md., September 19, 1977).

Dr. Hardin Jones, who died in 1978, was professor of medical physics at the University of California, Berkeley, assistant director of its Donner Laboratory, and an expert on statistics, aging, and the effects of drugs and radiation.

Jones spoke at the Eleventh Annual Science Writers' Seminar held by the American Cancer Society in New Orleans in March 1969. On this and numerous other occasions, Jones made sweeping and disturbing observations about the failure of orthodox therapy (Jones, 1969).

First, he said, the notion that patients treated by conventional therapies live longer than untreated victims "is biased by the methods of defining the groups." Thus, Jones claimed, if a person in the untreated category dies at any time while he is being studied, this is recorded as a death in the control group, and is registered as a failure of the "no treatment" approach. If, however, patients in the treated category die during the course of treatment (before the course is completed) their cases are rejected from the data since "these patients do not then meet the criteria established by definition of the term 'treated.' " The longer the period of treatment, the greater becomes the error.

"With this effect stripped out," Jones said to the 1969 gathering, "the common malignancies show a remarkably similar rate of demise, whether treated or untreated."

Second, said the Berkeley radiologist, beginning in 1940, various low-grade kinds of malignancies were redefined as "cancer." From that date, the proportion of "cancer" cases being cured increased rapidly "corresponding to the fraction of questionable diagnoses included."

Third, Jones's research showed no relationship between the intensity of treatment and survival rates. "Radical" surgery, for instance, did not seem to be more successful than more limited operations which removed only the tumor and small amounts of normal tissue.

Fourth, there is no proof that early detection affects survival. "Serious attempts to relate prompt treatment with chance of cure have been unsuccessful."

Jones concluded that

evidence for benefit from cancer therapy has depended on systematic biometric errors. . . . The possibility exists that treatment makes the average situation worse (ibid.).

To reporters, Jones once stated that, in his opinion, "radical surgery does more harm than good," and as for radiation treatment, "most of the time it makes not the slightest difference whether the machine is turned on or not" (Santa Ana [Calif.] Register, January 19, 1974).

While Jones's arguments certainly seem to contradict universally held beliefs on the value of therapy, little research refutes his arguments. In fact, since 1956 (when he first propounded his views) only three studies have tested the validity of his conclusions. All three upheld his theory (Houston and Null, 1978).°

It is also obvious that orthodox treatments have not been able to stop the rise in cancer mortality: there has been a steady increase in the cancer death rate in the United States in this century. Cancer accounted for one in 27 deaths in 1900, one in 16 in 1920, one in 12 in 1930, one in nine in 1940, one in seven in 1950, and one in six in 1960–70.

Since 1970 the percentage of people dying of cancer has increased at a slow but steady rate. In 1978 it passed the 20 percent mark—one in five of us will die of this disease (ibid.).

It might appear that the reason for this increase is simply that we are living longer and that cancer is a disease of old and middle age. This is not the only reason for the increase: these figures are *age-adjusted*, and have already taken into account the shift in seniority among the population.

In fact, people appear to be getting cancer earlier than ever before. Pediatrician Ronald Glasser notes that during the Christmas holidays of 1975, "of the twenty-three children admitted to the largest pediatric ward of the University of Minnesota Hospitals in a single day, eighteen had cancer." After noting that the cancer "death rate has been going up continuously," he adds:

As alarming as these figures are, they are still misleading. The cancers we are seeing today did not begin yesterday or the day before, but twenty, thirty and even forty years ago. Scientists now agree that most adult malignancies have their beginning in childhood . . . (Glasser, 1979).

Thus, the overall picture is not a bright one, despite the sugary optimism of the official pronouncements.

At best, only one-third of all cancer victims are surviving five years after diagnosis and treatment. Early detection, while seemingly beneficial in many cases, is no guarantee of success; the procedures used may themselves cause cancer later on. Even pin-sized tumors, such as Senator Humphrey's, can elude the surgeon's knife or the radiologist's beam.

Government statistics do not support the idea that great progress has been made in the treatment of cancer. In fact, progress appears to be slight in most cases, and in some cases "progress" has led to a declining cure rate.

° See articles by G. H. Green in *Australian and New Zealand Journal of Obstetrics and Gynecology* (vol. 10, 1970) and by B. Zumoff, H. Hart, and L. Hellman in *Annals of Internal Medicine* (vol. 64, 1966).

Meanwhile, as cancer strikes an increasingly youthful population, the cancer death rate and the cancer incidence rate relentlessly
edge upward.

The question inevitably arises then: if these current methods of
treating cancer are so inadequate, how and why are they considered
"proven cures"?

3

Surgery

The most common method of treating cancer is with the knife. Surgery has been practiced since the dawn of medical history to remove malignancies.

There is no doubt that in certain circumstances surgery is a highly effective and indispensable method of dealing with cancer. For example, five-year survival rate of patients with skin cancer, treated surgically, is 85 percent, for breast cancer 60 percent, for colon cancer 40 percent, and 70 percent for cancer of the uterus (Maugh and Marx, 1975:111).

Overall, most of the cancer patients who are cured today are cured because of surgery. Without denying this fact, however, it is important to take a serious look at cancer surgery. For the results of surgery are still so uncertain, and carry with them so many drawbacks, that new approaches are clearly necessary.

Cancer surgery, in general, was not in favor in the ancient world. Hippocrates (c. 460–c. 370 B.C.), who knew cancer well and even coined the term "carcinoma," urged doctors, "Above all, do no harm." Among his Aphorisms, number 38 states, "It is better not to apply any treatment in cases of occult cancer; for, if treated, the patients die quickly; but if not treated, they hold out for a long time" (cited in Shimkin, 1977:24).

To Hippocrates, cancer was caused by an excess of "black bile." Cancer was thus seen as a *systemic* ailment, caused by an imbalance of natural elements within the body, rather than a local problem.

The Roman medical encyclopedist Celsus (1st century A.D.) remarks that an advanced cancer is "irritated by treatment; and the more so the more vigorous it is." He goes on:

Some have used caustic medicaments, some the cautery, some excision with a scalpel; but no medicament has ever given relief; the parts cauterized are excited immediately to an increase until they cause death.

The best course, he suggests, is to use *mild* treatments:

After excision, even when a scar has formed, nonetheless the disease has returned, and caused death; while at the same time the majority of patients, though no violent measures are applied in the attempt to remove the tumor, but only mild applications in order to soothe it, attain to a ripe old age in spite of it (ibid.:26).

This principle remained in force for over a thousand years. For example, the Cordova physician Abul Qasim (1013–1106 A.D.) writes that surgery was acceptable in the earliest stages of the disease. "But when it is of long standing and large you should leave it alone. For I myself have never been able to cure any such, nor have I seen anyone else succeed before me" (ibid.:39).

There were two groups of healers who *did* attempt to treat cancer, however. The first were the folk healers and traveling medicine salesmen who provided some sort of medical service for the mass of impoverished serfs or city dwellers who could never afford a physician.

Then there were the surgeons. From the twelfth century on, the church-affiliated physicians abandoned surgery entirely to the lower-class barbers. These gentlemen would consent to remove cancerous growths, with much blood and very limited success (ibid.:32).

It is interesting to note that surgery entered the modern world as a very disreputable procedure, little better in the eyes of the medical orthodoxy than the herbalists and "quacks" with whom it competed for the same lower-class clientele. Surgeons could not write prescriptions, for example, without the countersignature of a physician nor could they perform operations except in the presence of a licensed physician.

From the start, there was tension between the surgeons and other healers, particularly the folk healers. According to a sixteenth-century document, the surgeons "mind only their own lucres [money]" and

sued, troubled and vexed divers honest men and women who without taking anything for their pains and skill had ministered to poor people for neighborhood, for God's sake and for charity. . . . [They] would undertake no case unless they knew they would be rewarded with a greater sum or reward than the case extended to . . . (Clark, 1964).

It is hard for us to realize just how ghastly surgery was until the mid-nineteenth century. According to one modern description:

The surgeon stropped his knife upon his boots. As he operated, he breathed and coughed into the incision, exposed also to the dust in the room and the particles falling from his beard and hair. The patient was strapped to the table and held down by attendants as the knife cut his quivering flesh or a saw hacked off his bones amid fearful shrieks of pain (Morris, 1977).

The predominant attitude toward what is now the standard treatment was generally disapproving and hostile.° Paracelsus (1493–1541), the extraordinary Renaissance physician, is quoted as having said:

It should be forbidden and severely punished to remove cancer by cutting, burning, cautery and other fiendish tortures. It is from nature that the disease arises and from nature comes the cure, not from the physicians (Issels, 1975).

How, then, did medicine arrive at the current situation, in which the same treatments are considered "orthodox"?

Surgery rose from quackery to respectability in the nineteenth century mainly because of two great discoveries: anesthesia and asepsis.

Ether anesthesia was originally a carnival sideshow sensation. With great difficulty a number of innovators attempted to promote its acceptance in surgery in the 1840s, but with little success. It was only after the Civil War that ether became a standard procedure in American hospitals (Collins, 1966). Once it did so, however, it made longer and more complicated operations possible and relatively painless.

Asepsis, the attempt to eliminate germs in the operating room, had an equally stormy history, including fierce opposition from the surgeons themselves (Shryock, 1962; Thompson, 1949). Nevertheless, once it was introduced, it made cancer operations and other surgery far less likely to end in death from infection, then a common occurrence.

These two developments in surgery coincided with several other trends which tended to increase the incidence of surgery. First, at least from 1900 on (and probably throughout the nineteenth century) cancer was increasing in frequency. This created a growing need for the services that surgeons provided. Second, there was the general tendency in the nineteenth century to use surgery freely as a kind of magic weapon to cure a variety of ills.

° Even less reputable was the use of chemicals to treat cancer. In the Renaissance, arsenic and metals were common ingredients in such "cures." Some metals apparently have an anti-cancer effect and recently a form of platinum has been used in the treatment of cancer at major cancer centers (MSKCC, 1976). Nevertheless, in their first appearance hundreds of years ago they "were abandoned because of their toxic effect, only to reappear in secret nostrums" (Issels, 1975).

This was particularly so in the treatment of women. In the nineteenth century, for example, hysterectomy (removal of the uterus, ovaries, and fallopian tubes) was even employed to treat women's "emotional problems," on the theory that the seat of a woman's emotions was her womb (Ehrenreich and English, 1973).

Once the technique of hysterectomy had been perfected, and anesthesia and asepsis were available, it was logical that surgeons would employ the knife to remove tumors. Hippocratic restraint was thrown out the window in the nineteenth century's enthusiasm for surgical progress.

This rapid rise of cancer surgery can best be illustrated by the early history of what is now Memorial Sloan-Kettering Cancer Center in New York.

The spiritual founder of Memorial Sloan-Kettering was a famous nineteenth-century "woman's doctor," J. Marion Sims. Sims received only a cursory medical training in the South before turning his hand to surgery. An enterprising young man, he resolved to extend the boundaries of surgery in the antebellum era. To do so, he gathered a group of slave women, upon whom he performed experimental operations in a kind of makeshift hospital behind his house.

These operations, says his biographer H. Seale Harris, M.D., were "little short of murderous." Some of these slave women received as many as thirty operations in a four-year period. This was the era before ether or antiseptics. Sims claims to have kept the women comfortable with opium (Seale Harris, 1950).

Sims perfected a new technique, for a once-common condition called "vesico-vaginal fistula," an abnormal passage between the urinary bladder and the vagina. The doctor then moved to New York City, where his innovation formed the basis of his professional and financial success. He helped to found the Women's Hospital, which is still in existence. One of the main functions of the hospital was to allow Sims and his colleagues to perform this operation on large numbers of women, many of them recent immigrants. In addition, Sims developed a select clientele of wealthy ladies.

The correction of vesico-vaginal fistulas thus became, for Sims and his colleagues, a thriving business. "Marion Sims tended to look upon the knife not as the last weapon, but as the first," says Dr. Harris.[*]

In the 1870s, Sims increasingly turned his attention to cancer. Apparently trying to duplicate the formula he had used successfully

---

[*] Ironically, it is now known that this condition is almost entirely iatrogenic—that is, it is *caused* by faulty procedures on the part of obstetricians and gynecologists. Thus, in a broad sense, Sims and his fellow doctors were unwittingly causing a disease and then curing it (Huffman, 1962; Green, 1971).

with vesico-vaginal fistulas, he began a series of unusually extensive operations on patients at Women's Hospital. Rumors began to spread that Sims was carrying out unnecessary and, in fact, barbaric operations (similar rumors had circulated in Montgomery, Alabama, years before concerning his slave experiments).

The Lady Managers (trustees) of the hospital became convinced that "the lives of all the patients in the institution were being threatened by . . . mysterious experiments," says Harris, and Sims was expelled from the hospital, a drastic step taken only in the most serious cases (Seale Harris, 1950; Considine, 1959). In addition, the aristocratic Sims and his followers were said to troop noisily through the wards and treat the women with contempt.

Although he was later reinstated to his position, Sims seems to have remained alienated from the women directors. When the wealthy Astor family, some of whose members were afflicted by cancer, offered $150,000 to Women's Hospital for a cancer wing, the Lady Managers hesitated. Cancer treatment and research was associated, in their minds, with Sims's experiments. Sims had no such hesitation, however, and opened private negotiations with the Astors' lawyer to obtain the money himself.

"A cancer hospital should be built on its own foundations," he wrote the lawyer, "wholly independent of all other hospitals." Consequently, the Astors' donation went to establish the New York Cancer Hospital in 1884, the first private cancer hospital in the United States. (The name was changed to Memorial Hospital in the 1890s, and to Memorial Sloan-Kettering Cancer Center in 1959.) Sims was to have been the first director of this center, but he died before he had a chance to fulfill this goal.

The existence of this and other cancer hospitals greatly increased the prestige of cancer therapy and of cancer surgery in particular. A stable base of patients provided "teaching material" for the development of new types of operations. Sims had written to the Astors: "Doubtful points of practice can be settled only in the wards of a great hospital."

Over a period of years, patients were persuaded to abandon home care and to entrust themselves to a hospital for treatment. After initial resistance, an increasing number of doctors were interested in making cancer a part of their practice.°

As medical techniques in general improved, so too did the scope of cancer surgery. "Talented assistants, blood banks to replace lost blood, a variety of anesthetics, antibiotics, strict antisepsis, tissue

° In the 1890s, the New York Cancer Hospital almost became a general hospital because of lack of cancer patients and of doctors interested in specializing in this disease (Considine, 1959).

replacements, information on the patient's physical and chemical status before, during, and following surgery and scores of other contributions by physicists, engineers, biologists, and biochemists" aided the aggressive surgeon (McGrady, Sr., 1964:304).

For the treatment of head and neck cancer, for example, ingenious surgeons devised an operation called the "commando." This involved removal of the patient's mandible, or jaw. Although the word meant literally "with the mandible," according to one surgeon, it "derived its wide acceptance and popularity from the fact that it brought to mind the slashing attack of the World War I commandos" (Crile, 1974).

For pancreatic cancer, Dr. Allen Oldfather Whipple, president of the American Surgical Association and clinical director at Memorial Hospital, designed the operation which bears his name. The "Whipple" involved removal of many organs adjacent to the affected gland, on the theory that they might be harboring nests of cancer cells. Yet, despite this "radical" procedure, the survival rate for pancreatic cancer remained persistently low: 5 percent five-year survival for localized pancreatic cancer and 0–3 percent when the disease had already spread (NCI, 1976).

Often unwilling to acknowledge the limitations of their methods, enamored of technology, and hostile to nonsurgical approaches, many surgeons conceived of progress in terms of greater and greater cutting. In 1948, for example, Dr. Alexander Brunschwig devised an operation which he called "total exenteration." This involved removal of the rectum, the stomach, the urinary bladder, part of the liver, and the ureter, all of the internal reproductive organs and the pelvic floor and wall, the pancreas, the spleen, the colon, and many of the blood vessels.

Patients were hollowed out in the desperate hope that, by doing so, all remaining cancer could be destroyed. Brunschwig himself called the operation "a brutal and cruel procedure" (New York Times, April 8, 1969).

But the ultimate operation was the hemicorporectomy—literally, the removal of half the body. Originated by Theodore Miller, like Brunschwig a Memorial Hospital surgeon, this operation involved the amputation of everything below the pelvis, in the treatment of advanced bladder or pelvic-region malignancy. Not surprisingly, many patients preferred to die rather than submit to Miller's invention (New York Times, November 30, 1969).

Surgery had clearly been taken about as far as it could go. Yet despite the fantastic ingenuity and skill of the surgeons, cancer was still not cured. In fact, as has been shown above, only one-third of cancer patients undergoing surgery and other "proven" methods live five years or longer.

Surgery works best on cancers that are detected before they metastasize to other parts of the body and create additional tumors. Once the cancer has spread, surgery is generally useless as a curative procedure although it may relieve symptoms caused by a large mass pressing against a nerve or organ.

Surgery has come under increasing criticism in recent years for a number of other reasons.

Some doctors and patients hold that much cancer surgery is either unnecessary or excessive in its scope. The fiercest argument has taken place over the question of breast cancer, but the issues raised in this debate appear applicable to other forms of cancer as well.

Breast cancer is routinely treated with an operation called the "radical mastectomy" or the "Halsted procedure," after its chief promoter. At the hearings of Senator Edward Kennedy's (D.-Mass.) Subcommittee on Health (of the Committee on Labor and Public Welfare) in May 1976, author and breast cancer victim Rose Kushner summarized the nature of the problem:

In the United States most of the 90,000 women who are expected to discover breast cancer in 1976 will be put to sleep without their knowing whether they will wake up with one breast or two. And most of the time, the amputation will be the Halsted radical mastectomy which leaves ugly scars extending into their armpits, and dips and hollows in their chests. Of course, the degree of disfigurement varies with the skill of the surgeon (U.S. Senate, 1976).

In addition, she noted, many women experience an "unattractive and sometimes painful swelling of the affected arm." She might have added the excruciating pain of the postoperative period, and the psychological and financial costs of the operation.

Incredibly, this operation is considered unnecessary by some of the leading experts in the field. A number of studies have suggested that about half of all breast cancer patients can receive much less radical, more sparing treatments without appreciably increasing their risk of a recurrence of the cancer.

The radical mastectomy is *not* routine in England, France, Canada, or the Scandinavian countries. Doctors in these countries regard it as ineffective and unnecessarily brutal. Questions have been raised about the wisdom of the procedure since it was first widely employed and popularized in the 1890s by Dr. William Halsted (1852–1922) of Johns Hopkins University, Baltimore.

The most determined criticism of the Halsted procedure has

come from George Crile, Jr., M.D., a retired breast surgeon and emeritus consultant in surgery at the Cleveland Clinic. Crile is orthodox in background and training. His father, George Crile, Sr., was in fact one of the most celebrated figures in American surgery. The younger Crile spent many decades treating and researching the causes of breast cancer.

Having started out an enthusiastic partisan of radical surgery he has become its most determined foe. Crile's comment on the radical is acerbic: "[It] seems to have been designed to inflict the maximal possible deformity, disfiguration and disability" on the women who receive it, he says, in his popular book, *What Women Should Know About the Breast Cancer Controversy* (Crile, 1974).

Crile generally favors the simple removal of the breast and some of the adjoining lymph nodes, but without the extensive mutilation of the Halsted procedure: "If the cancer is so advanced that it cannot be removed by an operation less than radical mastectomy, it has already spread through the system and is incurable by surgery." He also believes that in certain "properly selected cases, equivalent results can be obtained by even simpler operations in which only part of the breast is removed" (ibid.).

The new breast cancer detection procedures (mammography, thermography, etc.) are now detecting tumors so small that they cannot even be felt by manual examinations. Presumably, then, they have been located so early that they have not spread. Many of the women with these tumors understandably balk at having their entire breast, muscles, and armpit lymph glands removed. This has fueled the demand for the kind of limited operations practiced in much of Europe. Women also object to being pressured into signing release forms which allow the surgeon to remove their breast while they are still anesthetized, if their biopsy is positive. This procedure, common in American hospitals, takes the final decision out of the hands of the most interested party, the woman herself. According to Rose Kushner, in *Breast Cancer*, there is no appreciable increase in risk or cost in delaying surgery for a few weeks, during which time the patient can make an unpressured decision (Kushner, 1975).

Some recent scientific studies in this country support Dr. Crile's contention. In a survey conducted by Dr. Maurice S. Fox of the Massachusetts Institute of Technology, patients who have received the full-scale radical mastectomy were compared statistically to those who had only had the more limited procedures advocated by Crile and his supporters.

Fox found that the radical, disfiguring, and painful Halsted operation was "no more effective than more conservative, less mutilating treatment."

Dr. Bernard Fisher, a surgeon at the University of Pittsburgh, began a study in 1971 of 1,700 patients at thirty-four medical centers. In this study, patients whose tumors were believed to be confined to the breast were treated either with radical mastectomies or simple breast removal with or without postoperative irradiation. In 1979 he told reporters there was "no difference in survivals . . . between those who underwent radical surgery and those treated more conservatively." The study is continuing in order to pick up differences in long-term survival *(New York Times,* January 29, 1979).

The controversy over breast cancer surgery has been long and extremely bitter.

When Rose Kushner published *Breast Cancer* (now entitled *Why Me?*) in 1975, "the American College of Surgeons censured the book," she recalls, and "the American Cancer Society refused to recommend it. Remember, that was more than four years ago, and a lot has changed. But the medical establishment then thought I was a kook at worst and a pest and an agitator at best" *(New York Times,* October 22, 1979).

In fact, the minimalists appear to be winning this battle. Arthur C. Upton, director of the National Cancer Institute, has even nominated Kushner to serve on the National Cancer Advisory Board, and a Consensus Development Conference on the Treatment of Primary Breast Cancer in June 1979 decided that there should be a time lapse between the biopsy of suspicious breast tissue and any "definitive surgical procedure." They also decreed that the Halsted radical mastectomy should no longer be used as a treatment of choice for local breast cancer (ibid.).

Why, then, have American surgeons clung to the Halsted procedure for so long, making it, in Crile's words, the "central dogma" of all surgical practice in the United States? Crile's answers shed light not only on the breast cancer controversy but on other aspects of the cancer controversy, as well.

First, there are historical reasons. The radical mastectomy was an *American* innovation. (Although it was developed in England in 1867, it was not widely accepted until Halsted adopted it about twenty years later.) The use of the Halsted challenged for the first time the dominance of European physicians and surgeons over American medicine—a dominance which dated from before the American Revolution. The American surgeons were very proud of Johns Hopkins University with its famous "Big Four" of Halsted, Sir William Osler, William H. Welch, and Howard A. Kelly. Halsted was the chief of surgery and enjoyed an outstanding reputation. According to one history of Johns Hopkins:

Halsted was a perfectionist and his operations were works of art. His surgery was poetry—poetry of a sort few men understood. . . . When he dealt with cancer he struck for its roots without compromise. When he did a breast [sic] it was a finished piece of work. . . . (Bernheim, 1948).

Halsted's successors, however, were not perfectionists and sought ways to cut corners on his classic operation. "You can usually do with less," said Bertram Bernheim, M.D., a Johns Hopkins surgeon. It was another Hopkins surgeon, John M. T. Finney, first president of the American College of Surgeons (1913), who showed how to adapt the Halsted radical to "mass production" (Bernheim's phrase).

Where Halsted took four hours to do a cancer of the breast—and skin-grafted every case—Finney knew that that would never do for practical purposes and, using Halsted's main ideas, showed how much the same thing could be accomplished with no skin-grafting and in one-third the time (ibid.).

Yet Bernheim admits that the mass production surgeons' "percentage of cures never were quite so high as Halsted's."

The second reason for the veneration of the Halsted procedure, says Crile, is economic. Even when surgeons take shortcuts, the Halsted is a longer, more challenging, and difficult operation than the one it replaced. Surgeons, "almost by definition," prefer those procedures which require a maximum of skill over simpler operations because they are more challenging. "And, in a free-enterprise system," he adds, "the fee for a larger operation is also larger."

This factor is accentuated by the payment structure in the United States. Group payment plans pay surgeons two to three times as much for performing the Halsted than the simpler operation which leaves the patient's muscles and glands more or less intact. "The more appalling the mutilation," said George Bernard Shaw, "the more the mutilator is paid" (quoted in Crile, 1974).

When there are a lot of surgeons, who are paid "piecework," there will, ipso facto, be a lot of surgery, critics say. As the late Dr. John H. Knowles once put it, "We have surgical manpower creating its own demand. The more surgeons you have, the more surgery is going to be done, simply because the surgeons are there and they have to make a living" (quoted in ibid.).

Both Crile and Knowles believe that such pressure to perform more complicated and more expensive procedures "act through the subconscious." It is important to point out that surgeons do not sit around scheming how to mutilate patients for money. Rather, they evolve rationalizations and theories to justify a course of behavior which is in their collective economic interest.

A third reason for the persistence of the Halsted operation is the conservatism of the medical profession—especially the surgical division. It takes many years for a surgeon to perfect a procedure like the radical mastectomy. By this time, not only does part of his livelihood depend on it, but he is emotionally attached to it as well. He may have advised it for members of his own family, for friends, and, of course, for many patients. To admit that he was wrong may leave him open to criticism, attack, and possibly even malpractice suits.

Finally, most of the surgical faculty of most American medical schools, Crile says, is made up of practicing surgeons who teach only part-time. This has its good side, certainly, since it helps integrate teaching and practice. But the disadvantage is that the prejudices of today's generation of practitioners is passed on to the next generation almost without change. All of these factors have created an air of almost religious orthodoxy around the radical mastectomy.

But every orthodoxy must have its heretics. Crile is one of them. For many years he refused to publicize his views about the radical mastectomy, lest he be accused of propagating his beliefs in order to increase his surgical practice. He wrote his book on the subject after he had retired from practice and after numerous magazine articles had already appeared doubting the wisdom of the Halsted operation. Nevertheless, members of the surgical staffs of two Cleveland community hospitals saw fit to write to the Academy of Medicine and ask that Crile, a senior surgeon, be censured.

Some scientists, following the ancients, have questioned whether surgery itself does not accelerate the cancerous process. This question, too, is a highly emotional one for surgeons.

Since surgery inevitably disrupts the tumor, the danger of cutting into the tumor and spreading cancer cells throughout the body is always present. "A single cancer cell left alive," according to the *Science* report on cancer research, "can spell a patient's doom" (Maugh and Marx, 1975).

Some authorities believe that even rubbing a tumor may spread cancer cells throughout the system. According to one textbook, *Clinical Oncology for Medical Students and Physicians* (published jointly by the University of Rochester School of Medicine and the American Cancer Society):

> Massage of a tumor is followed by massively increased numbers of circulating tumor cells in the bloodstream in animals. A few clinical studies suggest the same phenomena (Rubin, 1971).

This textbook goes on to warn of two additional dangers of surgery and/or biopsy (the removal of a specimen for analysis):

Experimental data further suggest that surgical trauma decreases natural host resistance to the formation of metastases,

and

Needle biopsy is occasionally used, [but] . . . a needle track may harbor nests of cells which may form the basis for a later recurrent spread. . . . Incisional biopsy of certain highly malignant tumors through an open operative field may be contraindicated because of risk of spread of the tumor throughout the operative field (ibid.).

Thus surgical biopsy, a procedure used to detect cancer in its earliest stages and thus cure it, may contribute to the spread of cancer in some cases.

Other researchers have found, in experimental studies, that surgery per se has a deleterious effect on a patient's immune system and resistance to cancer. Drs. Gerald O. McDonald and Warren H. Cole, at the time of their studies with the University of Illinois, carried out an elaborate series of experiments to pinpoint the role of surgical stress in the spread of cancer. "Most surgeons," they told an American Medical Association meeting, "have encountered the patient whose cancer grows rapidly following operation, resulting in death within a few weeks" (McGrady, Sr., 1964:307).

In their animal experiments, the Illinois doctors subjected animals to various kinds of stress—operations, liver poisons, cold (of the type sometimes used as a "deep freeze" anesthetic), and chemical anesthetics. All of these, they found, decreased the animals' resistance to injected cancer cells. The chances of a tumor growing as a result of surgical operations increased anywhere from 50 to 450 percent. The liver poison, carbon tetrachloride, increased tumor take by 300 percent, ether 75 percent, and an anesthetic with "deep freeze" 60 percent.

The decreased resistance to cancer lasted two to three days after the stress—just the time when wayward cells in the human patient would be leaving the tumor site and attempting to establish themselves elsewhere in the body.

Cole, now an honorary life member of the American Cancer Society, presented additional evidence that many cancer cells were left behind during surgery and possibly even stimulated to invade the body by the stress of the operation.

In half of the patients he studied, Cole found cancer cells already circulating in the bloodstream, before, during, and after surgery. But in an additional 17 percent, these circulating cells could be found *only during* surgery. It is possible that these cells were liberated by the surgery itself.

Many other studies have shown that in 25 to 60 percent of patients, some cancer cells are left behind after an operation. Scientists have learned this by swabbing out the incised area after the operation and then examining the washings under a microscope. Such circulating cells *may* lead to further recurrences of cancer, although the subject is hotly debated among scientists (McGrady, Sr., 1964).

Such studies and statistics raise important questions about the extensive use of surgery in the treatment of cancer. But they leave out what may be the most important objection to the surgical treatment: the so-called human dimension.

Surgery hurts. Most of us are well aware of the excruciating pain that follows removal of a breast, a uterus, or a lung. Furthermore, the emotional pain may be worse than the physical. Much has been written about the psychological scars of mastectomy (Kushner, 1975). We might add the frightful prospect of laryngectomy, with the loss of one's natural voice; hysterectomy, with the premature onset of menopause; the loss of limbs in such childhood diseases as osteogenic sarcoma; or the castration of thousands of men in the treatment of prostatic cancer.

It is simply impossible to calculate the amount of human suffering caused by such surgery, as well-intentioned as it undoubtedly is in almost every case.

A team of psychiatrists, social workers, and psychologists studied the response of patients to their "cures" several years ago. They found that some "cured" patients had, quite simply, had their lives ruined by the successful therapy itself. For example, they cited the cases of:

—a previously dynamic corporation president confined to a wheelchair, with a nurse in attendance—ten years after successful cancer surgery.

—a fifty-year-old woman "a prisoner in my bathroom" compulsively (and unnecessarily) irrigating a colostomy [an artificial opening for fecal wastes in the abdomen] for twelve hours every other day—six years after successful cancer surgery.

—a thirty-five-year-old mother with three children . . . a virtual recluse—five years after the loss of a breast in a successful battle against cancer.

—a once-productive businessman, [who was prompted] to sell his business at a loss, become a non-functioning invalid, and settle down to await death—after successful cancer surgery eleven years earlier (Bard, 1973).

It must be emphasized that such patients figure among the *successes* of surgery and orthodox medicine—not its failures. Yet one of the psychologists who conducted this study was moved to remark:

Such stories of "death expectancy" reveal untold suffering for people whose lives have been saved, and for their families. They suggest a disturbing thought—more and more lives are being saved, but *for what?* (ibid.:166).

It is little wonder, then, that "a great many patients fear cancer treatment as much as or more than death itself," according to Dr. Robert Chernin Cantor, who has counseled cancer patients for seventeen years.

And the greatest source of anxiety is surgery:

Surgery is the most frightening of all treatment modalities. Consciously or unconsciously, everyone reacts to the recommendation of major surgery with great alarm. . . . Surgery and mutilation are fused, bound together in the image of a helpless victim subjected to violent assault (Cantor, 1978).

For this reason alone—if for none other—the search for safer, more effective, and less traumatic methods of treating cancer is one of the imperatives of modern medicine.

4

Radiation Therapy

The second so-called proven method of treating cancer is radiation therapy. A sharp controversy rages over the effectiveness and safety of this technique.

According to its defenders, radiotherapy is marvelously effective and safe. "Radiotherapists are among the few cancer clinicians who speak in terms of 'cures,'" says the *Science* cancer report. They claim to be able to cure 55 to 65 percent of patients with locally inoperable cancer of the prostate. In fact, according to Frederick W. George III of the National Cancer Institute (NCI), about 60 percent of *all* cancers are potentially curable with current techniques of irradiation (Maugh and Marx, 1975).

Since only about 33 percent of all patients are being "cured" (five-year survival) through the use of all methods, radiologists call for a stepped-up role for their techniques.

Radiation is already used on more than half of the cancer patients in the United States. "Radiation therapy, in use for seventy-five years, is more sophisticated, accurate and effective, with fewer side effects," says the American Cancer Society (ACS, 1978). "Enormous improvements have been made," says Jane Brody of *The New York Times* in *You Can Fight Cancer and Win*, a book she co-authored with an ACS vice-president. "Cancer specialists are now using radiation more and more. . . . Radiation therapy is often effectively used as a primary treatment. . . . [It can] cure cancers by totally eradicating them . . . extend life . . . [and] make remaining life more pleasant" (Brody and Holleb, 1977).

According to Brody's book, Senator Hubert Humphrey was a "famous beneficiary of modern radiation therapy." The reader will remember that the senator died of bladder cancer despite extensive surgery, radiation, and chemotherapy. The radiation treatment was the first line of defense, but failed to stop the relentless growth of his bladder tumor. Nevertheless, according to Brody and her American Cancer Society coauthor, he was a "beneficiary" because "he remained well for three years until the development of a new, more advanced cancer."

While many in the cancer field are calling for more radiotherapists, and the utilization of existing methods "to their maximum capacity" (Maugh and Marx, 1975:102), radiation's critics dispute both the value and the safety of the procedure.

The kinds of cancer that can actually be "cured" by means of radiation are few. Eighty percent of patients in the early stages of Hodgkin's disease (cancer of the lymphatic system) have five-year or more survival after radiation therapy. Radiation is also said to be very effective in cancer of the testicles, cancer of the cervix and of the prostate (Richards, 1972).

Many scientists dispute any further claims for radiation therapy. According to the prominent French oncologist Dr. Lucien Israël, in early cases of some kinds of cancer

radiotherapy sometimes gives brilliant results. Yet, apart from Hodgkin's disease and lymphosarcoma, there is much disagreement as to its effectiveness—indeed, there have been no conclusive trials. . . . Radiotherapists don't report their results . . . in such a way as to differentiate between the percentage of complete regressions and the percentage of objective partial regressions, and to indicate the distribution of length of those regressions (Israël, 1978).

In effect, Israël is saying that radiation therapy is an unproven—not a proven—method in many cases. Dr. Irwin D. J. Bross, director of biostatistics at the famed Roswell Park Memorial Institute, goes further:

For the situations for which most radiotherapy is given, the chances of curing the patient by radiotherapy are probably about as good as the chances of curing him by laetrile. This is because the chances of curing any patient in advanced stages of cancer are very poor, regardless of the method employed (Bross, 1979).

Israël embraces the use of radiation therapy, but as a palliative. It is "absolutely irreplaceable" in bringing about an "attenuation of symptoms," such as relief of pain, in advanced lung, esophageal, pancreatic, breast, and colon cancer.

"It is obvious that the limitations of this method are similar to that of surgical resection," says Michael B. Shimkin, M.D., a prominent specialist formerly with the U.S. Public Health Service. "The cancer is curable only if it is destroyed entirely by being within the field of radiation at levels lethal to the cancer" (Shimkin, 1973).

Radiation is frequently used as an adjuvant—i.e., along with surgery or chemotherapy. Such use is becoming more common, critics charge, as more and more women opt for limited breast surgery augmented by radiation. Dr. Bernard Fisher of the University of Pittsburgh has disputed the value of this procedure. In a 1968 study of 3,000 women at over forty institutions, he found that those receiving postoperative radiation did no better than those receiving only surgery in the treatment of breast cancer (Fisher, 1968).

Israël notes that with adjuvant radiation

we should observe a reduction in the rate of distant metastases. . . . [However], certain recent studies have thrown the medical community into confusion by showing that metastases may be more frequent in cases that have received radiation. . . . (Israël, 1978).

Why, then, is radiation used so extensively—if it is of such limited and questionable value in most cases? Basically, says Bross, because doctors regard it as *harmless.* "It is an added precaution and doesn't cost anything" is the surgeon's attitude when he sends a patient to the radiation therapy department. Many surgeons, adds the Roswell Park statistician, do not really believe in the value of the beam. "But if it's really harmless, it makes sense" (Bross, 1979).

Here we come to the nub of the controversy, for many critics charge that radiation is *not* harmless, but carries with it numerous dangers and drawbacks. In fact, they believe there is a massive, long-standing cover-up on the part of government officials and some scientists to hide the danger of radiation. An integral part of that cover-up has been to minimize the dangers of radiation therapy while extolling its supposed virtues.

Charges of radiation's dangers have often been voiced, but most often these charges have been ignored. Initially, this was because of the widespread enthusiasm for the new technique. In 1902, after one year of X-ray therapy at Memorial Hospital, the chairman of the board, John Parsons (the same Astor lawyer to whom Sims wrote his famous letter; see Chapter 3), exclaimed: ". . . the time is not far distant when a remedy for cancer may be found" (Considine, 1959).

Since radiation will often cause temporary remissions, some of the first reports were highly enthusiastic. William B. Coley, later to become famous for his Coley's toxins (see Chapter 7), wrote at the same time of ten cases of abdominal cancer with

. . . entire disappearance in one case of cancer of the cervix . . . marked improvement in three other uterine cases . . . more or less temporary improvement in most of the remainder. . . . In two cases of epithelioma of the head and face the tumors have entirely disappeared, one the size of a silver dollar on the forehead, one three-fourths of an inch in diameter on the face. . . . And one case of Hodgkin's disease, a practically hopeless condition, has shown the most remarkable improvement that has yet been reported. . . . The man has resumed his usual occupation" (Considine, 1959).

Coley soon noted that in many cases there was "a recurrence within a year." Disappointment with radiation apparently increased his interest in even more innovative approaches.

Slowly it became apparent that the "quiet, dreamlike process, in which nothing of significance seems to happen" (Glemser, 1969), was fraught with danger. Radiation enthusiasts ignored these signals, and some of them as a result succumbed to the toxic effects of radiation.

Within a year or two after the discovery of X rays (1895), it was found that the rays could cause skin disease and systemic problems. By 1902, 171 cases of accidental X-ray burns had been reported in the medical literature, including those of radiation pioneers Henri Becquerel and Pierre Curie.

In 1902 a German doctor recorded the first case of human cancer caused by radiation: the tumor had appeared on the site of a chronic ulceration caused by X-ray exposure. Experimental studies performed in 1906 suggested that leukemia (cancer of the blood) could be caused by exposure to the radioactive element radium. By 1911, 94 cases of radiation-induced cancer had been reported, more than half of them (54) in doctors or technicians. By 1922, over 100 radiologists had died from X-ray-induced cancer, and many other research workers, laboratory assistants, and technicians also succumbed (Hunter, 1978).

Many of these cases occurred because doctors refused to take warnings about radiation's dangers seriously. At Johns Hopkins, for instance, one of Halsted's students, Dr. F. H. Baetjer, became sick after administering X rays with few precautions.

"Even when it began to be noised about by word of mouth and in the medical journals that patients and X-ray operators especially ought to be protected against possible burns," writes a colleague, Dr. Bernheim, "Baetjer scoffed at it and then took only perfunctory precautions" (Bernheim, 1948).

Thus, although he "developed a huge private practice in X rays," Baetjer eventually developed cancer in his fingertips, which spread slowly and painfully to the rest of his body. After forty operations, he finally died of this X-ray-induced disease in 1933. This story was repeated dozens of times at most of the large medical centers in the country, and in many of the smaller clinics in which "X-ray fever" had taken hold. Both Marie Curie and her daughter Irène Joliot-Curie are believed to have died as a result of exposure to radioactive materials.

If the public needed convincing, proof of the danger of radiation came in the 1920s in a dramatic way. Soon after the discovery of X rays and radium, radioactivity was adapted for industrial use. One such use (employed until recently) was to luminize the dials of watches and instruments with a radium paint, which glowed in the dark.

There was tremendous demand for these instruments during World War I, and large factories were set up to process orders from the army. Working on a "piecework" basis, around the clock, the "luminizers"—mostly young women—developed a technique of expediting their work by sharpening the radium brush with their pursed lips.

Years later, veterans of this work began to succumb to one mysterious ailment after another. Out of approximately 800 women who had worked at a single New Jersey factory, 48 became seriously ill from radium poisoning, and 18 died of cancer of the jaw or related diseases.

Examples of industrial poisoning were not rare, of course, but what was unusual about this radium poisoning was the incredibly small amounts of the radioactive material needed to cause diseases, and the long latency period between exposure and clinical symptoms (Hunter, 1978).

Yet radiation continued to be used, especially at the larger medical centers. Why was this so, if it was common knowledge that radiation was a two-edged sword, capable of great harm?

A study of the record reveals an economic motive at work. One medical practitioner, for example, admitted to *The New York Times* in 1914 that radium therapy appeared to do more harm than good:

> Something is created which kills many patients. I cannot tell, nobody can tell, for four or five years just what the results will be. I simply feel that I've shoved those patients over a little bit quicker *(New York Times,* January 27, 1914).

But "I can double my money in a year," he said frankly, "while charging 4¢ per milligram per hour" (ibid.).

The search for radium became a big—and frantic—business. Marie Curie's daughter Eve Curie notes in the famous biography of her mother that "radium had acquired a commercial personality. It had its market value and its press" (Curie, 1943). American businessmen, inspired by radium's selling price of $150,000 a gram, attempted to corner a monopoly on radium-bearing lands.

In 1913, James Douglas, chairman of the Phelps-Dodge copper-mining empire, founded a "National Radium Institute" in collaboration with the U.S. Bureau of Mines. Simultaneously, Douglas made a

$100,000 gift to Memorial Hospital, then struggling with serious financial problems. But, as Bob Considine, Memorial's official historian, notes, "Douglas's enormous gifts came with strings attached."

First, Douglas insisted that his personal friend and physician, Dr. James Ewing, be made chief pathologist (later medical director) of the hospital;[*] second, that the hospital treat only cancer patients; and third, that it routinely use radium in that treatment. Once this was arranged, Memorial became in effect the distribution center for a new, and seemingly inexhaustible "product": radium emanations. Ewing proceeded, says the Memorial historian, to push "radium beyond the capacity of that mighty weapon to produce results" (Considine, 1959).

A similar process went on at other major centers. Dr. Howard A. Kelly, one of the famous "Big Four" at Johns Hopkins Hospital, was Douglas's partner in the "National Radium Institute." He constructed a private hospital adjoining his home in Baltimore. "One thing leading to another," wrote Dr. Bernheim, "he became owner of more radium than any other doctor in the nation." Under a convenient arrangement with Johns Hopkins, Kelly gave radium treatments to "all patients the Hopkins had—free as well as private" (Bernheim, 1948).

The press also had caught radium fever. "Radium Cure Free for All" cried *The New York Times* on page one in 1913, as it announced formation of the institute. "Not one cent's worth of radium will be for sale," proclaimed the head of the Bureau of Mines. "Every particle of the precious metal will be used in the cause of-humanity" (*New York Times*, October 24, 1913; January 27, 1914).

"Our special object," said Kelly, is "reaching and relieving the poor and large middle class to whom all unexpected expenses are a sore burden in any emergency."

Douglas confided, however, that "all this story about humanity and philanthropy is foolish. I want it understood that I shall do what I like with the radium that belongs to me. . . . I shall use it any way I like" (Langton, 1940).[**]

Contrary to the newspaper stories, radium and X-ray therapy were hardly free. In fact, radiation helped to save Memorial from

[*] Ewing's monumental work, *Neoplastic Diseases*, was dedicated to the memory of James Douglas.

[**] Douglas's motives for his involvement with radium were complicated. To many of his contemporaries, it appeared that he was out to corner a monopoly on radium-bearing lands for his own benefit. His "National Radium Institute" was eventually foiled by the opposition of other mineowners, including the Du Ponts. His belief in radium's value appears to have been genuine, however, since he used it on his daughter, dying of cancer, and even on his wife and himself, for trivial ailments. He died of aplastic anemia, probably caused by radium poisoning (*New York Times*, December 20, 1913; Considine, 1959; Langton, 1940).

bankruptcy during the 1920s and 1930s. In 1924 the rules and regulations of Memorial stipulated that "an extra charge will be made for Radium Emanations used in the treatment of patients" (Memorial, 1924). In that same year, the Radium Department was the greatest single source of income for the hospital. It administered over 18,000 treatments and brought in about $70,000—a large sum for those days.

Millions of dollars were now invested in radium and X-ray machinery. By 1934 more than 25,000 X-ray therapy treatments were administered annually at Memorial Hospital. In 1937, after initial opposition from the surgeons, radiation therapy was recognized as a "proven" method of treatment by the American College of Surgeons (Bailey, 1971).*

By 1977, this had increased to 73,037 radiation therapy treatments and implants annually, and 102,700 X-ray examinations and special procedures at Memorial (MSKCC, 1977a). In that same year, Memorial began a $4.5 million modernization program in the Department of Radiation Therapy, which aimed at replacing every piece of major equipment in the department by 1980. Eighty-nine professionals and technicians treat 160 patients a day with various forms of radioactivity (MSKCC Center News, July–August, 1977).

Radiation has always been lucrative—for hospitals, equipment and film manufacturers, and for the radiologists themselves. Once millions of dollars are invested in capital equipment there is a strong inducement to use that equipment, despite newer information suggesting its use should be curtailed.

In the late 1930s a more realistic attitude seemed to be forming toward the extensive use of radiation. In the 1934 Annual Report of Memorial Hospital, the doctors in the Breast Service wrote that because of excessive damage to the skin of their patients from "massive doses of high-voltage X rays" they had concluded that "this method of preoperative radiation was unsatisfactory" (Memorial, 1934).

Ewing continued to push the "continuous prolonged irradiation of the entire body" (ibid.) for practically every condition, but after his death even his most ardent supporters admitted that his view of radiation was excessively sanguine (Considine, 1959).

A realistic appraisal of radiation might have resulted if it hadn't

---

* Initial resistance to X-ray therapy was fierce, as it usually is to new methods of treatment. According to Dr. E. H. Grubbé of Chicago, the first man to treat cancer with X rays, the surgeons ridiculed and opposed his work. "They controlled medicine, and they regarded the X ray as a threat to surgery. At that time surgery was the only approved method of treating cancer. They meant to keep it the *only* approved method by ignoring or rejecting any new methods or ideas. This is why I was called a 'quack' and nearly ejected from hospitals where I had practiced for years" (Bailey, 1971).

been for the events of August 1945—the bombing of Hiroshima and Nagasaki, which ushered in the "atomic age." Suddenly radiation, which had been merely a medical subspecialty and an arcane branch of physics, moved to center stage in world history.

The question of radiation therapy's effectiveness and *especially its safety* became a burning political question. There were now powerful reasons, beyond the profitability of the procedures themselves, both to exaggerate the benefits and to obscure the dangers of radiotherapy.

As the government pressed forward with its open-air testing program and its creation of a nuclear weapons arsenal, it ran into ever-increasing opposition in the United States and around the world (see, for example, Pauling, 1958).

Atomic *medicine* provided excellent public-relations copy for the purveyors of atomic bombs. Atomic energy "can be used for man's destruction or as a tool by which he can make himself a better world," said the chairman of the Atomic Energy Commission, Lewis Strauss. Strauss wore many hats: Wall Street investment banker, admiral of the U.S. Navy, trustee of Memorial Sloan-Kettering, the Rockefellers' personal financial adviser, and a "hawk" on matters atomic. The implication clearly was that radiation per se was neutral, but could be used for good or for ill. A "good" use of radiation was "the focusing of the powerful beams of deadly radiation on cancerous growths" *(New York Times, April 8, 1954).*

Key scientists, such as Cornelius P. "Dusty" Rhoads, director of Memorial Hospital, made public statements on the harmlessness of open-air atomic bomb testing during the 1956 Eisenhower–Stevenson campaign *(New York Times, October 21, 1956).*

During this time evidence was accumulating that radiation could have many deleterious effects on the body. High doses of radiation could cause acute radiation sickness. For example, an accident victim at the Los Alamos Scientific Laboratory (May 21, 1946) was accidentally exposed to about 2,000 roentgens of radiation.° According to Linus Pauling:

> During the first few hours he vomited several times. Then for several days his condition was good. On the fifth day the number of white cells in his blood fell rapidly, and on the sixth day his temperature and pulse rate rose. On the seventh day he had periods of mental confusion, then he gradually sank into a coma and died on the ninth day (Pauling, 1958:79).

This was a very large dose, but even seemingly minute doses, it was soon found, could cause various kinds of cancer and leukemia. It

° A roentgen (named after the discoverer of X rays) is the unit used to measure the X rays or gamma rays to which a body is exposed.

could also increase the probability of death and shorten a person's life span, cause chromosomal damage, affecting future generations, destroy the bone marrow and the vital immune system produced therein, and—in cancer patients—create burns, cell and tissue death (necrosis), and fibrosis of the internal organs (Israël, 1978:73; Pauling, 1958).

The Atomic Energy Commission was quite successful in hiding these troubling facts, not only from the general public but from the medical community which actually administered the therapeutic beam. The AEC provided much of the information for the medical textbooks on radiation and its hazards. Thus, physicians have generally received a biased education concerning the appropriate uses of radiotherapy (Bross, 1979).

The AEC's attitude toward low-level radiation was aptly summarized by Dr. Edward Teller, the "Father of the H-Bomb," and Dr. Albert Latter in *Life* magazine (February 10, 1958): "The only thing these statistics prove is that radiation in small doses need not necessarily be harmful—indeed may conceivably be helpful" (quoted in Pauling, 1958:119).

Even in 1979, *Science* magazine was forced to conclude:

> The radiation research community has lived almost entirely off the energy and defense establishments. . . . For anyone seeking objective scientific advice it is practically impossible to find someone knowledgeable who was not trained with AEC money *(Science, April 13, 1979)*.

This may appear at first sight to be yet another "honest debate" over a scientific question—the danger of radiation versus the value of radiotherapy. But recently released documents apparently show that the pro-nuclear side of the argument consciously covered up what they knew to be real dangers of radiation and atomic fallout.

In the 1950s, President Eisenhower instructed the Atomic Energy Commission to "keep them [the public] confused" on questions of radiation. The commissioners sought to protect their bomb-testing programs from irate citizens. "People have got to learn to live with the facts of life," said one AEC commissioner, "and part of the facts of life is fallout." "It is certainly all right," said Strauss, "if you don't live next door to it." "Or *under* it," added another commissioner *(New York Times, April 20, 1979)*.

Since that time the "nuclear establishment" has continued to promote industries and procedures which expose Americans to low levels of ionizing radiation. The rapid development of nuclear energy has added new pressure to declare low-level radiation safe. If it is *not* safe, then not only the nuclear arsenal but also the nuclear power plants are called into question, since such plants can emit radiation.

Scientists who have tried to expose the dangers and ineffectualness of diagnostic and therapeutic radiation have often suffered for their sins. Dr. Bross, who holds important positions at both Roswell Park and at Johns Hopkins and has published over 300 articles and communications, failed to get a renewal of his government grants when he spoke out on this topic. There was a congressional hearing on February 14, 1978, on this matter, and at that time he was asked to resubmit his proposal.

In 1979 Dr. Bross's grant application was approved by the National Cancer Institute, but only for $50,000 a year, far less than the $350,000 which he claims is needed to answer the question, "What are the long-term hazards of radiation therapy?"

Bross pinpoints a thirty-year cover-up of radiation's hazards and in particular the role of doctors in promoting that danger:

It is almost impossible to get "peer review" that will accept a study of iatrogenic [doctor-caused] disease. You just can't get people associated with the medical profession to accept a study that is frankly dealing with doctor-caused cancer. Everybody said I was crazy to do that, and they were right. But on the other hand if I called it something else and they turned me down anyway, then the public would not know why they turned me down. I figured it's better the public should know that the National Cancer Institute won't support this kind of research.

For 30 years radiologists in this country have been engaged in massive malpractice—which is something that a doctor will not say about another doctor (Bross, 1979).

In conclusion, radiation therapy appears to be of limited value in the treatment of cancer. There is little controversy over the number of patients who are currently being cured by radiotherapy—it is small.

Most doctors believe that radiation is a relatively harmless procedure. They therefore recommend it to patients (especially advanced cases) as a palliative. It is also being used with increasing frequency in earlier cases, such as in conjunction with limited mastectomy.

Some researchers believe that this use of radiation is not only ineffective, but positively harmful for its recipients, and part of a disastrous national policy that serves as a smoke screen for the hazards of radiation.

5

Chemotherapy

Third among the so-called "proven" methods of treating cancer is chemotherapy: the use of drugs to kill cancer cells. Few topics in medicine today are as controversial as the use of these drugs.

In theory, a drug cure for cancer is highly appealing. Just as specific drugs cure many bacterial and parasitic infections, so should cancer chemotherapy ideally kill cancer cells without harming excessive quantities of normal tissue. In reality, however, orthodox chemotherapy has not yet developed an agent specific and safe enough to restrict its attack to cancer cells. Most chemotherapeutic agents work by blocking an essential metabolic step in the process of cellular division. Since cancer cells often divide more rapidly than normal cells, this lethal "antimetabolite" action should be directed preferentially against cancer cells. However, most normal tissues engage in cell division at varying rates. Thus chemotherapy poisons many normal tissues as well—especially the rapidly dividing cells of the bone marrow, intestinal wall, and the hair follicles.

The bone marrow is the foundation of the immune system. The use of chemotherapy is often accompanied by destruction of this immune system, which serves the dual function of preventing infections and combating the spread of cancer. Chemotherapy often brings in its train a host of blood-deficiency diseases (such as leukopenia, thrombocytopenia, and aplastic anemia). These in turn, can give rise to massive, uncontrollable infections. Cancer patients on chemotherapy have been known to die of something as innocuous as the common cold.

Because of its effects on the immune system, chemotherapy stands in contradiction to another form of therapy: immunotherapy. This form of treatment is still considered experimental at most cancer centers. "Immunotherapy holds hope of harnessing the body's own disease-fighting systems to combat cancer with essentially no overt toxicity," says the American Cancer Society's 1979 edition of *Cancer Facts and Figures.* "In laboratory animals, substances such as

BCG (Bacillus Calmette-Guérin) can stimulate immune mechanisms. These substances now are being used in humans alone or with other forms of treatment" (ACS, 1979).

Since immunotherapy is generally used as a treatment of last resort, almost all patients receiving it have first received chemotherapy, or are given drugs in combination with the immune-stimulating agents. The clinical results with BCG and other immune stimulants have generally been disappointing, and some doctors believe this is because the prior or concurrent use of immunity-destroying anticancer drugs wipes out whatever beneficial effects these newer agents may have.

Chemotherapy's effect on the gut can be equally disastrous. Cancer patients often have difficulty in eating or absorbing their food. Cancer drugs may cause nausea, bleeding sores around the mouth, soreness of the gums and throat, and ulceration and bleeding of the gastrointestinal tract. Because some forms of chemotherapy particularly affect rapidly dividing cells, and the mucous cells are quick dividers, this form of therapy has resulted in the sloughing of the entire internal mucosa of the gut. Death may result.

Some people withstand chemotherapy with few side effects. Many others become nauseated, vomit, lose their hair, or develop infections. Some have a wide range of toxic reactions.

There are about thirty drugs in use against cancer (see Table 1). Some of them are what are called "alkylating agents," which react with the genetic material of the cells (DNA). These drugs produce a cross-linking of the bases of the DNA chain, which blocks replication of nuclear DNA during mitosis. Some of these drugs are nitrogen mustard, Thio TEPA, Leukeran, Myleran, and Cytoxan.

Another major category of drugs are the antimetabolites. These chemicals prevent cells from making nucleic acids and proteins essential to their survival. The drugs' molecules mimic necessary constituents in the cell. One of them, methotrexate, competes with folic acid, a B vitamin, and prevents the vitamin from being utilized. This leads to the death of the cell. It is thus literally an antivitamin. Other drugs in this category are 6-mercaptopurine (6-MP) and 5-fluorouracil (5-FU).

In addition, chemotherapists use antibiotics, which have anti-tumor activity; plant alkaloids—poisons derived from the periwinkle plant; and even a close cousin of DDT, called o,p-DDD.

All of these drugs have one characteristic in common: they are all poisonous. They work because they're poisons. Methotrexate, for example, carries with it the following warning:

METHOTREXATE MUST BE USED ONLY BY PHYSICIANS EXPERIENCED IN ANTI-METABOLITE CHEMOTHERAPY.

TABLE 1

NATIONAL CANCER INSTITUTE

INVESTIGATIONAL DRUGS USED AGAINST CANCER

September 1977

Drug categories and agents (column headers, Common name / Other names):

ALKYLATING AGENTS:
- Busulfan — Myleran
- Chlorambucil — Leukeran
- Cyclophosphamide — Endoxan, Cytoxan
- Dibromomannitol — DBM, Mylobromol
- Nitrogen mustard — HN2, Mustargen, Mechlorethamine
- Phenylalanine mustard — L-Sarcolysin, Melphalan, Alkeran
- Thio TEPA — TSPA
- Triethylene melamine — TEM

ANTIMETABOLITES:
- Azacytidine
- Cytosine arabinoside — Ara-C, Cytarabine, Cytosar
- 5-fluorouracil — 5-FU
- 6-mercaptopurine — 6-MP, Purinethol
- Methotrexate — Amethopterin
- Thioguanine — TTG

MITOTIC INHIBITORS:
- Vinblastine sulfate — Velban
- Vincristine sulfate — Oncovin

ANTIBIOTICS:
- Actinomycin D — Dactinomycin, Cosmegen, Mereidnomycin
- Adriamycin
- Bleomycin
- Daunomycin — Rubidomycin, Daunorubicin
- Mithramycin — Mithracin
- Mitomycin C

RANDOM SYNTHETICS:
- VP-16
- BCNU — 1,3-Bis(2-chloroethyl)1-nitrosourea
- CCNU
- CIS-Platinum (II) — CIS-dichlorodiamine
- DTIC — Hydrea
- Methyl CCNU — Dacarbazine
- o,p'-DDD — Mitotane, MIH, Ibenzmethyzin
- Procarbazine
- Streptozotocin

HORMONAL AGENTS:
Adrenal cortical compounds:
- Prednisone
- Prednisolone
- Dexamethasone
Androgens:
- Fluoxymesterone
- Testosterone propionate
Estrogens:
- Ethinyl estradiol
- Diethylstilbestrol
Other:
- Progesterone

ENZYMES:
- L-asparaginase — EC-2

(Hormonal agents and trade names are known by a variety of trade names.)

Disease	Drugs marked
Leukemia — Acute — Granulocytic	Adriamycin, Actinomycin D, 6-mercaptopurine, Methotrexate, Cytosine arabinoside
Leukemia — Acute — Lymphocytic	L-asparaginase, Prednisone/Prednisolone, Adriamycin, Actinomycin D, Vincristine, 6-mercaptopurine, Methotrexate, Cytosine arabinoside
Leukemia — Chronic — Granulocytic	Methyl CCNU, Busulfan
Leukemia — Chronic — Lymphocytic	Prednisone, Chlorambucil
Adrenal cancer	o,p'-DDD
Bladder cancer	Adriamycin, Methotrexate, 5-fluorouracil
Brain tumors	BCNU, CCNU, Procarbazine, Vincristine
Breast cancer	Fluoxymesterone, Testosterone propionate, Ethinyl estradiol, Diethylstilbestrol, Prednisone, Adriamycin, Methotrexate, 5-fluorouracil, Cyclophosphamide, Vincristine, Thio TEPA
Burkitt's lymphoma	Methotrexate, Cyclophosphamide
Choriocarcinoma	Adriamycin, Methotrexate, Vinblastine
Colon cancer	CCNU, Mitomycin C, Mithramycin, 5-fluorouracil
Endometrial cancer	Progesterone
Ewing's sarcoma	Adriamycin, Actinomycin D, Cyclophosphamide
Head & neck cancer	Bleomycin, Methotrexate
Hodgkin's disease	Prednisone, BCNU, CCNU, Procarbazine, Bleomycin, Adriamycin, Vinblastine, Vincristine, Nitrogen mustard, Cyclophosphamide, Thio TEPA
Lung cancer	CCNU, Adriamycin, Bleomycin, DTIC, Methotrexate, Cyclophosphamide
Lymphosarcoma	Prednisone, BCNU, Adriamycin, Bleomycin, Methotrexate, Nitrogen mustard, Cyclophosphamide
Melanoma	Methyl CCNU, DTIC, CCNU, BCNU, Adriamycin
Multiple myeloma	Prednisone, Adriamycin, Cyclophosphamide, Phenylalanine mustard
Mycosis fungoides	Bleomycin
Neuroblastoma	Adriamycin, Vincristine, Cyclophosphamide
Osteogenic sarcoma	CIS-Platinum (II), Adriamycin, Methotrexate, Cyclophosphamide
Ovarian cancer	Adriamycin, Methotrexate, Cyclophosphamide, Nitrogen mustard, Thio TEPA
Pancreatic islet cell tumors	Streptozotocin
Polycythemia vera	Busulfan
Prostatic cancer	Ethinyl estradiol, Diethylstilbestrol
Reticulum cell sarcoma	Prednisone, BCNU, Adriamycin, Bleomycin, Methotrexate, Cyclophosphamide, Nitrogen mustard
Retinoblastoma	Cyclophosphamide, Nitrogen mustard
Rhabdomyosarcoma	Adriamycin, Vincristine, Cyclophosphamide
Sarcomas (general)	Adriamycin
Stomach cancer	DTIC, Mitomycin C, Methotrexate
Testicular cancer	CIS-Platinum (II), Bleomycin, Mithramycin, Adriamycin, Methotrexate, Cyclophosphamide
Wilms' tumor	Adriamycin, Actinomycin D, Vincristine

Source: *Drugs vs. Cancer*, DHEW Publication No. (NIH) 78-786

BECAUSE OF THE POSSIBILITY OF FATAL OR SEVERE TOXIC REACTIONS, THE PATIENT SHOULD BE FULLY INFORMED BY THE PHYSICIAN OF THE RISKS IN-VOLVED AND SHOULD BE UNDER HIS CONSTANT SUPERVISION (*Physician's Desk Reference*, 1978).

The package insert then goes on to describe the "high potential toxicity" of the product. This includes the abovementioned symptoms, as well as malaise, undue fatigue, chills and fever, dizziness, and various problems of the skin, blood, alimentary system, urogenital system, and central nervous system. Finally, the doctor is warned that

Other reactions related or attributed to the use of methotrexate such as pneumonitis; metabolic changes, precipitating diabetes; osteoporotic effects, abnormal tissue, cell changes, and even sudden death have been reported (ibid.).

How successful are these drugs in combating cancer? This question is important; if they were highly effective, one might tolerate their admittedly harsh side effects to get the benefit of a cure.

It is generally agreed that in certain uncommon forms of cancer, chemotherapy is highly effective. Choriocarcinoma, a rare tumor which afflicts pregnant women, can be cured in about 70 percent of cases with methotrexate, Dactinomycin, and Vinblastine.

Another type of tumor which has yielded quite well to chemotherapy is Burkitt's lymphoma. Through the use of Cyclophosphamide, methotrexate, and other drugs, doctors have been able to achieve about a 50 percent cure rate. However, this type of cancer is exceedingly rare in the United States. It is found primarily in certain parts of Africa, where it is believed to be caused by a virus (Maugh and Marx, 1975:26).

Acute lymphoblastic leukemia, which most often attacks children, is in some ways the "showpiece" of the chemotherapists. Through the use of such drugs as Daunorubicin, Prednisone, Vincristine, 6-MP, methotrexate, and BCNU, often in complex combinations, doctors at certain specialized cancer centers have been able to achieve 90 percent remission, and 70 percent survival beyond five years. This is remarkably better than the grim prognosis for this disease only a decade or so ago.

Other forms of cancer which have responded to chemotherapy include testicular tumors (30–40 percent respond, 2–3 percent cured); Wilms' tumor (treated in combination with surgery and/or radiation: 30–40 percent cured), and neuroblastoma (5 percent cured), and Hodgkin's disease, stage IIIB and IV (70 percent respond, 40 percent survive beyond five years) (ibid.).

In other forms of cancer, chemotherapy can offer palliation (partial or temporary remission of the disease) and occasionally prolongation of life.

Unfortunately, the types of cancer which respond to chemotherapy are generally among the least common forms of the disease. The most common forms of cancer—the big killers such as breast, colon, and lung malignancies—generally do not respond to treatment with drugs. Furthermore, according to Maugh and Marx, chemotherapy is not very effective against tumors that have grown large or spread. Its greatest successes are against small tumors that have only recently developed.

Chemotherapy has other drawbacks. There is an increased incidence of second, apparently unrelated malignancies in patients who have been "cured" by means of anticancer drugs. This is probably because the drugs themselves are carcinogenic. When radiation and chemotherapy were given together, the incidence of these second tumors was approximately twenty-five times the expected rate (ibid.:123):

Since both radiation and chemotherapy suppress the immune system, it is possible that new tumors are allowed to grow because the patient has been rendered unable to resist them. In either case, a person who is "cured" of cancer by these drastic means may find himself struggling with a new, drug-induced tumor a few years later.

Interest in cancer chemotherapy developed in part out of frustration with the limitations of surgery and radiation therapy. Even scientists sympathetic to these two methods admit that they "have been near the limits of their utility for many years" (Maugh and Marx, 1975).

The inspiration for cancer chemotherapy was the antibiotic revolution of the 1930s. Coupled to this was the "crash program" concept popularized during World War II.

"I am convinced that in the next decade, or maybe more, we will have a chemical as effective against cancer as sulfanilomides and penicillin are against bacterial infection," said Sloan-Kettering director C. P. "Dusty" Rhoads in 1953 (*Denver Post*, October 3, 1953).

"There is, for the first time, a scent of ultimate victory in the air," read an article on anticancer drugs in *Reader's Digest* in February 1957.°

"We can look forward confidently to the control and ultimately the eradication of cancer," said the director of the National Cancer

° *Reader's Digest* is often a barometer of orthodox thinking on the cancer problem. Laurance S. Rockefeller, chairman of the board of Memorial Sloan-Kettering, is a director of the magazine's parent company, and the *Digest's* publisher, DeWitt Wallace is, in turn, a major contributor to the New York cancer center.

Institute in the 1950s. He promised Congress major new gains "in the next few years" (*Denver Post,* October 3, 1953).

In fact, announcing the imminent demise of cancer has become something of a subspecialty within the medical profession, especially around the month of April, when the American Cancer Society conducts its annual appeal drive.

"Nothing short of spectacular . . . a work of monumental importance" was how one New York chemotherapist described a new drug treatment for breast cancer (*New York Daily News,* February 17, 1976).

The public has become cynical and disgruntled about these claims, which usually only succeed in raising false hope in the minds of cancer victims and their families. "Cancer chemotherapists have a lingering poor reputation among large segments of the lay public," say the authors of the *Science* report, who are generally well-disposed toward the field. They attribute this in part to the "bitter disappointment" of chemotherapy's painfully slow progress (Maugh and Marx, 1975).

Many scientists have begun to question the basic premise of cancer chemotherapy, which is the use of toxic agents to kill every last cancer cell in the body. Dr. Victor Richards, for example, calls chemotherapy "at best an uncertain method of therapy" because it cannot harm or kill cancer cells "without producing comparable effects on normal cells." Chemotherapy succeeds because it is a systemic poison, and it fails for the same reason. Richards compares the use of such poisons to the difficulty of controlling

an expanding colony of mice by shooting them with a smaller number of bullets than the number of mice. No matter how we calculate the firing system, one could see that inevitably, if even two mice capable of mating remained, doubling of the population would resume (Richards, 1972).

"With chemotherapy," he adds, "we have no sure shot. . . . It is clear that we can never eliminate the last cancer cell by using antimetabolites" (ibid.).

Given the generally poor performance of chemotherapy, its often horrendous side effects, and the limitations built into its very nature, why do orthodox doctors continue to promote this form of treatment as the wave of the future, and a "proven" method of treatment?

Among other factors, there are economic forces which help shape the direction of cancer therapy, diagnosis, prevention, and management. Drugs are central to the American economy, and it is perfectly logical from a business point of view to seek a cure for cancer in the form of a patentable and marketable drug.

The long-standing interest in such a cure, dating from before

World War II, has led to the creation of a "chemotherapy establishment" at all the major medical centers. These individuals are tied to
the pharmaceutical industry not only philosophically but often ma-
terially as well. Some of them are consultants to drug companies,
while others are directors or executives. No law requires companies
or consultants to reveal their relationships. Thus it is possible that
drug company influence at cancer centers is greater than appears
from the public record. In addition, a number of drug company
officials serve on NCI advisory committees (Table 2).°

Grant money and gifts are available to those centers which work
on drugs in which the companies have a proprietary interest. Money
is not generally available for substances or approaches in which drug
companies have no such interest. Thus the "invisible hand" of the
marketplace has chosen toxic chemotherapy for development and
ignored other approaches which might be as promising from a medical, but not an economic, point of view (see Chapter 17).

Chemotherapists are latecomers to the cancer scene. ". . . lack of
regard for chemotherapists . . . has historically been exhibited by
many surgeons and radiologists," according to the *Science* report on
cancer (Maugh and Marx, 1975). Understandably, the chemotherapists have spoken in glowing terms about the effects of their agents,
while underplaying the drawbacks. A steady stream of positive reports has made chemotherapy fully acceptable to medical practitioners.

Finally, if cancer specialists were to admit publicly that chemotherapy is of limited usefulness and often dangerous, the public
might demand a radical change in direction—possibly toward unorthodox and nontoxic methods, and toward cancer prevention.

By constantly touting the promise of anticancer drugs, orthodox
practitioners ward off this challenge to their expertise and researchers parry the threat radically new concepts represent to their
long years of research. The use of chemotherapy is even advocated
by those members of the establishment who realize how ineffective
and dangerous it can be.

Richards, for example, admits that in the major forms of cancer
(lung, bowel, stomach, pancreas, cervix, etc.) even *palliation* occurs

° Patricia E. Byfield, associate research scientist, Upjohn, serves on NCI's Breast Cancer
Task Force Committee; Hans J. Hansen, director, department of immunology, Hoffmann–La
Roche, serves on NCI's Developmental Therapeutics Committee; Bruce Johnson, analytical
research department, Pfizer, serves on the Large Bowel and Pancreatic Cancer Review Committee; Irving Johnson, vice-president for research, Lilly, serves on the Developmental Therapeutics Committee; Gary L. Neil, head of cancer research, Upjohn, also serves on the
Developmental Therapeutics Committee; and Arthur Weissbach, head, department of cell
biology, Roche Institute, serves on NCI's Cause and Prevention Scientific Review Committee
(NIH, 1979).

TABLE 2
Commonly Used Anticancer Agents in the United States

Common Name	Trade Name	Marketing Company	Associates in Cancer Establishment*
1. Busulfan	Myleran	Burroughs-Wellcome	none known
2. Chlorambucil	Leukeran	Burroughs-Wellcome	none known
3. Cyclophosphamide	Endoxan, Cytoxan	Mead-Johnson	none known
4. Nitrogen mustard	HN_2, Mustargen	Merck	Good, MSKCC
5. Pipobroman	Vercyte	Abbott	Shubik, NCAB
6. Thio TEPA	TSPA, Thiotepa	Lederle (Am. Cyanamid)	Fisk, MSKCC
7. Triethylene melamine	TEM	Lederle (Am. Cyanamid)	Fisk, MSKCC
8. Cytosine arabinoside	Ara-C, Cytosar	Upjohn	Byfield, Neil, NCI
9. 5-fluorouracil	5-FU	Hoffmann–La Roche	Bobst, ACS; Weissbach, NCI
10. Methotrexate	Amethopterin	Lederle (Am. Cyanamid)	Fisk, MSKCC
11. Vinblastine sulfate	Velban	Lilly	Dixon, NCAB; I. Johnson, NCI
12. Vincristine sulfate	Oncovin	Lilly	Dixon, NCAB
13. Adriamycin	Adriamycin	Adria Labs (Farmitalia, Hercules)	none known
14. Mithramycin	Mithracin	Pfizer	B. Johnson, NCI
15. Mitomycin C	Mitomycin C	Abbott	Shubik, NCAB
16. Hydroxyurea	Hydrea	Squibb	Thomas, Furlaud, MSKCC
17. Procarbazine	Matulane	Hoffmann–La Roche	Bobst, ACS
18. Delta-1-testalolactone	Teslac	Squibb	Thomas, Furlaud, MSKCC
19. Cluoxymesterone	Halotestin	Squibb	Thomas, Furlaud, MSKCC
	Ultandren	Ciba-Geigy	none known
20. Progesterone	Delalutin	Squibb	Thomas, Furlaud, MSKCC Byfield, Neil, NCI
	Depoprovera	Upjohn	
21. Nandrolone phen-proprionate, N.F.	Durabolin	Organon	Seitz, MSKCC
22. Nandrolone decanoate, N.F.	Deca-durabolin	Organon	Seitz, MSKCC

* Individuals who hold leading positions in the cancer field, as well as a formal association (president, director, or consultant) with a drug company.

only "for brief duration in about 5 to 10 percent of the cases." Yet he urges the use of drugs for such patients as well. His reason is revealing:

> Nevertheless, chemotherapy serves an extremely valuable role in keeping patients oriented toward proper medical therapy, and prevents the feeling of being abandoned by the physician in patients with late and hopeless cancers. Judicious employment and screening of potentially useful drugs may also prevent the spread of cancer quackery. . . . Properly based chemotherapy can serve a useful purpose in preventing improper orientation of the patient (Richards, 1972:215).

In Richards's view (and he is not alone) it is worthwhile to risk putting patients through the harrowing experience of nausea, vomiting, dizziness, hair loss, mouth sores, and possibly even premature death, simply in order to keep them "oriented toward proper medical therapy" and away from "cancer quackery."

The drug industry is not indifferent to developments in cancer research and therapy.

"A cancer cure will be worth a fortune," a drug-company executive said in the 1950s (Applezweig, 1978). Although no infallible "cure" has been discovered for any form of cancer, chemotherapy has become a $200-million-a-year industry. Stock analysts project a $1-billion-a-year business before long (ibid.).

For many years the drug industry showed only lukewarm interest in investing its own money in the search for anticancer drugs. According to Alan Klass, a Canadian surgeon and former chairman of the Manitoba Cancer Institute,

> more effort is devoted in the [drug] industry towards research in the area of fast sellers, for the potentially unlimited market of coughs, colds, pain relief, depressions, tensions, than to grim cancer. Prospects of financial success are immeasurably greater in the less grim group (Klass, 1975).

"These [anticancer] drugs are costly to develop and sales are still limited," an industry analyst wrote several years ago (de Haen, 1975).

Other pharmaceutical spokesmen have worried that an effective cancer cure would upset the medical marketplace. "Nobody will be able to hold onto a cancer cure," a drug company executive predicted. "It would be too hot to handle" (Applezweig, 1978).

The president of Merck Sharpe & Dohme told *Fortune:*

> I've always had a horror of Merck having an exclusive position in a cancer drug. It's just so emotional. I have a feeling that if we gave it away free, people would say we were charging too much (Robertson, 1976).

Despite these fears and reservations, since the 1950s all the major drug companies have maintained a presence in the cancer field. "All companies regard this work as a public service," Dr. C. Chester Stock of Sloan-Kettering Institute claimed in 1956. "For drug companies there won't be much money in anticancer drugs, but there will be a lot of prestige" (Wall Street Journal, February 8, 1956).

If only prestige were involved, however, as Stock claimed, the companies were working at it with unusual zeal. Between 1946 and 1953 Parke-Davis alone sent 1,500 different chemical compounds to Sloan-Kettering for testing, according to the president of that drug firm (Wakefield [Mass.] Item, September 17, 1953).

Many of the hundreds of thousands of compounds tested at Sloan-Kettering or the National Cancer Institute were submitted by industry, usually the largest pharmaceutical houses. A standardized legal agreement, drawn up by Frank Howard, a Standard Oil executive, was used to bring about a formal partnership between the company and Sloan-Kettering. The compounds were tested free of charge to the company. The agreement guaranteed a patent or a "perpetual non-exclusive, royalty-free license" for the company involved (Howard, 1962, contains a copy of the agreement). Howard was a firm advocate of patenting medical discoveries, such as cancer drugs. Speaking at George Washington University in 1956, he said:

To undertake a costly industrial research or development project without inquiring into the patent situation is like drilling an exploratory oil well without finding out who owns the property on which you drill (Howard, 1956).

"Dusty" Rhoads, who shared with Howard the original idea for a cancer drug testing institute, told a group of patent attorneys in 1940:

In the near future patents may well control its [medicine's] entire development. . . . The patent lawyers can and do control the support of industrial science. I wish to establish clearly the need for, as well as the profits to be obtained from, intelligent study of the factors which influence the course of illness (Memorial, 1940).

In fact, almost every anti-cancer drug marketed since World War II has been patented by its manufacturer, although most of the research was done at government-supported institutions. The agreement between industry and Sloan-Kettering paid off in one case, that of methotrexate (amethopterin), which was patented by Lederle Laboratories, a division of American Cyanamid, Inc. in 1951.° Under

---

° MSKCC overseer and former Sloan-Kettering chairman James Fisk, Ph.D., is a director of American Cyanamid, Inc. (see Appendix A).

the "standard form" agreement, first used with Lederle, the company was given a patent, was allowed to keep drug research secret, and merely had to provide the substance for testing.

The agreement was so favorable to industry not only because of the business orientation of Memorial Sloan-Kettering's leaders, but because of the difficulty of getting profit-oriented drug companies to invest in the seemingly "grim" field of cancer.

Sales figures for methotrexate were recently estimated at about $5 million a year. With the adoption of a "high-dose methotrexate" regimen for a number of different cancers, however, these sales figures have probably increased considerably. Methotrexate costs around $9 for 500 milligrams (International Workshop, 1975). The high-dose regimen requires the use of hundreds of grams of this substance per patient.

Today, the attitude of the drug companies toward cancer has changed considerably. This is due in part to the progress that has been made in the past twenty-five years in understanding cancer, progress which makes effective drug treatment more possible. Drug companies have also been enticed into the field by government grants disbursed by NCI.

In 1955, the center of drug testing shifted from Sloan-Kettering Institute to NCI's Cancer Chemotherapy National Service Center in Bethesda, Maryland. Congress allocated $25 million to test 20,000 chemicals a year at "The Wall Street of Cancer Research," in the words of the center's director, Dr. Kenneth M. Endicott (*Newsweek*, January 20, 1958).

Under this plan the government directly subsidized drug companies to do research which, if successful, would create new products for them. For example, Chas. Pfizer & Co. received $1.2 million in 1958, Upjohn & Co. $150,000, and Abbott Laboratories $208,000 (ibid.).

Most important in changing industry attitudes, however, have been market factors. The drug industry traditionally has been one of the most profitable businesses in the world. "For many years," says Dr. Klass, "the profits of the drug industry have been twice the average for all other American industries" (Klass, 1975:76). Most of these profits came from antibiotics, painkillers, or mood-altering drugs such as Valium.

As patents have run out, and as the industry has faced increasingly costly government regulations and other problems, profitability has also fallen. From a pretax profit of 21 percent in 1973, the entire industry experienced a slump in the latter 1970s. "Drug profitability is not what it used to be," *Chemical & Engineering News* complained in 1976. "Profit margins have dropped to a 10-year low" (*Chemical & Engineering News*, March 1, 1976). These worries have been compounded in recent years. "Evidence of the slow-down in ethical pharmaceutical volume abounds," writes Standard and Poor's *Industry Survey* (Standard and Poor's, 1979).

One of the main reasons for this drop has been a lack of new markets to exploit. Patents have run out on many of the most profitable drugs of the 1950s and 1960s.

"What the drug industry needs is a major new product line," a Wall Street analyst told *Business Week*. Not surprisingly, one of the areas he pinpointed as a potentially lucrative area was cancer chemotherapy *(Business Week*, January 17, 1977).

Although new cancer drug research is usually shrouded in secrecy, it is known that such giant firms as Eli Lilly, Merck, and Hoffmann–La Roche are now spending an increasing proportion of their research budgets on cancer° *(Dun's Review*, December 1974; Robertson, 1976).

General disappointment with cancer chemotherapy has made the drug companies look in other directions for an effective (and patentable) cancer medicine. One candidate is interferon—or more accurately, the interferons. These are naturally occurring substances which appear to have anticancer and antiviral effects.

Interferon was discovered in the 1950s and little interest was shown in developing its potential in the United States, mainly because of the difficulty of producing commercial amounts. Interferon is a natural substance which is formed by cells when they are attacked by viruses.

European studies showing anticancer results, plus an increased possibility of synthesizing an active anticancer drug, have whetted the appetites of the drug companies. The American Cancer Society has now allocated $2 million to buy European interferon and test it in a "crash program" (ACS, 1978).

Should interferon turn out to be an effective agent, and should a way be found to market it (or a substance which could stimulate its production in the human body), it could turn out to be a profitable breakthrough for the pharmaceutical industry.

The potential profits to be derived from interferon production are huge, and the competition is fierce.

Interferon, like radium seventy-five years ago, is fabulously expensive. One ounce of interferon is worth $1.8 billion *(Omni*, July 1979). In 1975 it was estimated that interferon treatment for cancer costs $500–5,000 per patient per day, depending on the dosage given (International Workshop, 1975:12). It was hoped at the time that

---

° The drug industry is said to be "notorious for secrecy" *(Dun's Review*, December 1974:55). Nevertheless, the chairman of Merck has acknowledged that his company is working on a cancer vaccine (ibid.).

new techniques would bring this cost down five to tenfold within a
few years. But one industry spokesman has said the price is likely to
be *multiplied* by three (ibid.:85).

The cost has come down, but not that much. At the present time
150 cancer patients are being treated with interferon at ten U.S.
cancer centers at an average cost of $50,000 per patient (*New York
Post,* June 28, 1979).

Even should the price drop, the cost will certainly remain considerable. In the clinical trials conducted in Sweden at the Ka-
rolinska Institute, interferon was given three times a week for one
and a half years. At 1975 prices, this equals between $117,000 and
$1,170,000 per patient.

This represents a considerable potential market for the drug
companies. Several patents already have been taken out on interferon purification processes. Not surprisingly, then, there is intense
competition for techniques, contacts, and markets.

The 1975 International Workshop on Interferon, chaired by Dr.
Mathilde Krim of Sloan-Kettering, noted:

A separate "workshop" session . . . dealt with the cost of production of
human interferon. This session was attended by a number of representatives
from the [drug] industry, obviously interested in the development of production facilities. However, there was considerable reluctance on the part
of industry representatives to quote cost estimates in a public forum. (Interestingly enough, the same individuals were quite eager to discuss the problem in their competitors' absence.) (International Workshop, 1975:66).

When the American Cancer Society, Memorial Sloan-Kettering,
National Cancer Institute, and the National Institute for Allergy and
Infectious Diseases sponsored the Second International Workshop on
Interferons at Rockefeller University, April 22–24, 1979, the list of
contributors to the meeting read like a Who's Who of the drug field.
It included Baxter-Travenol Laboratories, Bristol-Myers Co., Bur-
roughs Wellcome Co., Cutter Laboratories, Hoffmann–La Roche,
Inc., Johnson & Johnson, Merck Sharpe & Dohme, Miles Labora-
tories, Monsanto Co., Pfizer Inc., Schering-Plough Corp., Searle Lab-
oratories, Smith Kline and French, U.S.V. Pharmaceuticals, and
Warner-Lambert (Second International Workshop, 1979).°

Nor have the big companies been neglecting the chemical approach to cancer, although it has been plagued with disappoint-

---

° Industry speakers were well represented in most of the scientific sessions, which testifies
to the seriousness with which it regards this research. An Upjohn scientist spoke at the morning
session (April 22) on "interferon inducers," a Burroughs Wellcome researcher spoke that afternoon on "antiviral activities of interferons *in vivo*," etc. In all, fifty-seven drug company
representatives attended.

ments. Thus, in recent years, Bristol-Myers has won approval for the commercial marketing of Platinol (cis-platinum), a drug used in the treatment of bladder cancer (MSKCC, 1976). Bristol-Myers also won approval in March 1977 to market BiCNU. And I.C.I. Americas received approval from the U.S. government to sell Nolvadex, a drug used in the treatment of advanced breast cancer *(New York Times,* July 23, 1978).

Cancer drugs represent a tantalizing possibility to the drug companies. In a few special instances it has paid off well. In the United States, the best seller has been Adriamycin, an anticancer antibiotic noted for its extreme toxicity. It is owned outright by Adria Laboratories, a joint venture of Hercules, Inc., and the Montedison Group of Italy. The drug is said to produce regressions in such conditions as lymphoblastic leukemia, acute myeloblastic leukemia, Wilms' tumor, and various other kinds of carcinoma, including Hodgkin's disease (de Haen, 1975).

During its first year on the market (1974) Adriamycin sold an impressive $10 million. And although the U.S. government routinely hides sales figures on drugs—"to avoid disclosing figures for individual companies"—it is believed that sales have increased considerably since then.°

Adriamycin illustrates how the public pays for these drugs to be developed and then pays again—this time at monopoly prices—to purchase these drugs from private companies. Montedison, the Italian conglomerate, attempted to find a U.S. licensee for its product in 1969. At that time, however, the U.S. drug industry still had little interest in investing in cancer drugs. The Italian firm finally made an arrangement with the National Cancer Institute under which the U.S. government and Sloan-Kettering Institute would test the drug in animals and humans. U.S. researchers did much of the work to develop the drug in this country and even obtained permission from the Food and Drug Administration to market it. Of course, U.S. taxpayer money paid for this expensive work. But the patent remained in the hands of its original owners, who have profited handsomely by this arrangement (Applezweig, 1978).

Even more profitable has been the Soviet drug Ftorafur. This compound has been patented by the Soviet Institute of Organic Synthesis, which has licensed the Japanese Taiho company to market the drug in Japan.

Analysts are not sure of the exact composition of Ftorafur. It

---

° Quote from a government report on pharmaceutical preparations (U.S. Department of Commerce, Bureau of the Census, 1977). "Data on new prescriptions are compiled privately for drug manufacturers by a company that copyrights its figures. Thus, they rarely work their way directly into public hands . . ." *(Wall Street Journal,* July 8, 1976).

appears to be an oral, relatively nontoxic form of the American drug 5-fluorouracil.*

Ftorafur is doing better than any American drug for cancer. Sales in 1976 were $100 million, or roughly ten times the best-selling drug in the United States.

The main reason for Ftorafur's success, however, was the unusual—some would say reckless—way in which the drug has been marketed. "Some Japanese physicians," it is said, "now tend to identify 'precancerous' states, 'risk of cancer' or 'susceptibility to cancer' and treat the patient prophylactically [i.e., preventively] with anticancer drugs" (Applezweig, 1978).

This situation arises because Japanese physicians routinely sell drugs to their patients. Ftorafur reputedly comes with a high retail markup, which naturally encourages the physician to sell more drugs. If "risk of cancer" now makes one a candidate for an anticancer drug, then every Japanese (and American) could now be considered a candidate for Ftorafur. Because of the radically different way in which drugs are marketed in the United States, however, it is unlikely that American companies could repeat the success of their Japanese counterparts (ibid.).

The drug industry is a kind of "silent partner" in the cancer research enterprise. It has managed to invest relatively little in the cancer problem, yet stands to reap tremendous benefits when and if a "breakthrough" is found.

Through its many interlocks with the research centers and the American Cancer Society, and through selective funding of specific research projects such as interferon, it maintains its presence in the field. The domination of investment bankers and industrialists over the cancer field guarantees that the ultimate "cure for cancer" will come marked "Patent. Pending" and, most probably, "Made in U.S.A."

---

* The patent on 5-FU, as it is called, was held for seventeen years by Hoffmann–La Roche and the American Cancer Society (25 percent). Perhaps by coincidence, one of the founders of the ACS, Elmer Bobst, is a former president of Hoffmann–La Roche.

PART TWO

Unproven Methods

6

Unorthodox Therapies

The "proven" methods of treating cancer are in a state of crisis. At best, only one-third of today's cancer victims are living five years or more after discovering they have cancer. Even if everyone followed the American Cancer Society's advice, received regular checkups and so forth, this would not substantially increase the cure rate. Given the current methods, at most one-half of all cancer victims could be "saved" for an average of five years.

The remainder of cancer's victims will continue to waste away and die, despite the best efforts of their physicians and families.

Clearly, the cancer problem cannot be solved in any ultimate sense by sticking to today's "safe and sound" methods. Something radically new is needed—approaches that are fresh and daring.

Where will these radical new ideas come from? Many people believe they will come from the well-funded, orthodox research centers. It is only logical, they think, that those with the best credentials, finest equipment, and amplest research funds will make the big breakthroughs in cancer. No one can say with certainty that this will not happen.

Another possibility, however, is that the most fundamental breakthroughs will come from innovative clinicians or small research laboratories, which have the advantage of independence, so vital to a creative scientist. Many such laboratories exist around the world, and a number of them have put forward alternate views of the cancer problem, and alternate solutions. To the establishment, in general, such independent researchers are not innovators. They are not really scientists. They are advocates of unproven methods or, more bluntly, "quacks."

"Quack" is one of the ugliest words in the English language. The idea of exploiting a desperate, dying person's hope of a cure is so repulsive that most people are instantly deterred from looking any further once this label is applied.*

If we are to find a cure for cancer, however, it is necessary to examine all alternatives. In the case of "quack" cures, it is necessary to ask, first of all, on what basis these methods are condemned.

Since the American Cancer Society has taken the lead in condemning such unorthodox procedures, its book *Unproven Methods of Cancer Management* can serve as a guide to orthodox thinking on quackery.

Unproven Methods (as well as the larger index and files that complement it) is part of a plan to investigate new methods in the treatment, diagnosis, and prevention of cancer. The American Cancer Society asserts that the book is only meant to be informative, and not to stigmatize any scientist. In fact, it resembles the list of "subversive" organizations once maintained by the House Un-American Activities Committee. Merely including a scientist's work on the list has the effect of damning a researcher's work, and of putting the tag of "quackery" on him and his efforts.

One scientist, recently added to the list, noted that from 1973 to 1976 he received a basic research grant from the National Cancer Institute. But, he notes, once his method was placed on the ACS's "unproven" list "we could not get a renewal, by hook or crook—no matter how good the application itself was" (Gold, 1979).

The orthodox characterization of "unproven" methods is based on several serious charges. Each of these will be examined in some depth.

First, it is said that unorthodox practitioners and researchers are basically without the requisite knowledge of cancer to make any intelligent statements about the disease.

The proponents of new or unproven methods of cancer management range from ignorant, uneducated, misguided persons, to highly educated scientists with advanced degrees who are out of their area of competence in supporting a particular form of treatment. A few hold Ph.D. or M.D. degrees. . . .

They may have multiple unusual degrees such as N.D. (Doctor of Naturopathy), Ph.N. (Philosopher of Naturopathy), M.T. (Medical Technologist), DABB-A (Diplomate of American Board of Bio-Analysts), or

---

* The American Cancer Society changed the name of its Committee on Quackery to the Committee on Unproven Methods of Cancer Management in the 1950s (Young, 1967:398). But Richards (1972), himself affiliated with the Society, still uses the designation "cancer quackery" and an ACS official in Rockland County, New York, called Michael Schachter, M.D., a "quack" for his use of laetrile and other unconventional therapies (*The Journal-News,* Rockland, New York, December 28, 1977). "Unproven method," for the American Cancer Society, appears to be simply a euphemism for "quackery."

Ms.D. (Doctor of Metaphysics); these degrees may have been received from correspondence schools (ACS, 1971b).

Table 3 lists sixty advocates of unorthodox therapies whose credentials are given in the ACS book on unproven methods. It is immediately apparent that there is a discrepancy between what the ACS says about the advocates of these methods and the facts, as revealed in the Society's own chapters on the individuals involved.

According to information provided by the ACS itself, of these sixty, thirty-nine, or almost two-thirds, hold bona fide medical degrees from such universities as Harvard, Illinois, Northwestern, Yale, Dublin, Oxford, or Toronto. Only one holds a medical degree from what the ACS describes as a "class C institution which went out of existence." Two are osteopaths who became medical doctors (M.D.s) when the two healing professions merged in California in 1962.

Three of these medical doctors also hold doctorates (Ph.D.s) in scientific disciplines from reputable institutions.

In addition, eight other proponents of new methods received Ph.D.s in such fields as chemistry, physiology, bacteriology, parasitology, or medical physics from universities such as Yale, Johns Hopkins, University of California-Berkeley, Columbia, and New York University.

Thus, over 75 percent of these "snake oil salesmen," as they are sometimes called, are medical doctors or doctors of philosophy in scientific areas. In most cases, if they hold medical degrees, they have spent their working lives treating and/or researching cancer; the doctors of science have usually attempted to apply their knowledge of a particular area of research to the cancer problem.

Recall, however, that the ACS primer on unproven methods states that "a few" hold M.D. or Ph.D. degrees; a few in this case is 75 percent.

Of the other 25 percent, three individuals hold honorary doctorates of science (D.Sc.)* There are also a dentist, nurse, chiropractor, bachelor of arts, and registered nurse. There are also two "naturopaths" and three laymen, without any known degrees.

There are no M.T.s, DABB-As, or "Doctors of Metaphysics" on the list. In fact, in general it is difficult to distinguish most of these "quacks" from orthodox cancer doctors in the matter of education, training, or scientific background.

A second common charge concerns the nature of the methods proposed by unorthodox practitioners. These are supposed to be highly bizarre and exotic, and therefore patently worthless and absurd.

---

* Ernst T. Krebs, Jr., codiscoverer of Laetrile, received this honorary degree after the ACS article was written. This fact is noted in other ACS publications.

TABLE 3

Advocates of Unorthodox Cancer Therapies

(Information from American Cancer Society, *Unproven Methods of Cancer Management*)

Name	Sci. Degree(s)	From **	Professional Status
1. William P. Aiken	M.D.	Northwestern University	General practitioner; pulmonary specialist.
2. Eleanor Alexander-Jackson	Ph.D.	New York University	Bacteriologist, New York University; University Hospital, Michigan; New York State Dept. of Health; Cornell Medical College; College of Physicians and Surgeons, Columbia University.
3. Manfred von Ardenne	Ph.D.	[not given]	"Connected with development of cathode ray and oscilloscope tubes and worked on the electron miscroscope." Work supported by E. German government.
4. H. H. Beard	Ph.D.	Yale University	Professor of chemistry and physical science, Tulane University.
5. Joseph Blaszczak	D.V.M.	University of Bologna	Veterinarian; vitamin therapy (B group).
6. Johanna Brandt	N.D., Ph.N.	First National University of Naturopathy	Advocated the "Grape Cure" for cancer.
7. Dean Burk	Ph.D.	University of California, Berkeley	Founder and head, Cell Chemistry, National Cancer Institute (ret.).
8. Mildred Cates	R.N.	[not given]	Harry Hoxsey's nurse.
9. Robert R. Citron	M.D.	University of Illinois	General practitioner; member, American Medical Association.
10. William B. Coley †	M.D.	Harvard University	Chief of Bone Service, Memorial Hospital.
11. Ernesto Contreras	M.D.	Army Medical School, Mexico City	House Officer-Pathology, Children's Hospital, Boston; pathologist, Army Hospital.
12. William M. Crofton	M.D.	Dublin University	Fellow, Royal Society of Medicine; lecturer, University Hospital, Dublin.
13. Sergio M. DeCarvalho	M.D.	Lisbon University	Licensed to practice in California; laboratory medicine.
14. Philip L. Drosnes	[not given]	[not given]	"Convicted of practicing medicine without a license"; acquitted on appeal.
15. Isaac Newton Frost	M.D.	Memphis Hospital Medical College	General practitioner.
16. Max B. Gerson	M.D.	Freiberg, Baden Universities	Internal medicine, neurology, Gotham Hospital, N.Y.C.
17. Donald F. Gibson	M.D.	Yale University	General surgery and urology.
18. Thomas J. Glover	M.B. (M.D.)	University of Toronto	"Licensed to practice medicine in Ontario in 1913."
19. Joseph Gold	M.D.	State University of New York–Upstate Medical College	Director, Syracuse Cancer Research Institute.

Name	Sci. Degree(s)	From **	Professional Status
20. Oskar C. Gruner	M.D.	Royal College of Physicians, London	Licensed to practice in Canada, 1936.
21. Henry G. Hadley	M.D.	Washington University, St. Louis	Certified by American Board of Internal Medicine; chest specialist.
22. Bruce Halstead	M.D.	College of Medical Evangelists	Marine biologist, Loma Linda University.
23. Wendell G. Hendricks	M.D. (D.O.) *	College of Osteopathic Physicians and Surgeons	"Accused of administering the Lincoln, Koch, and other agents. . . ."
24. John E. Hett	M.D.	University of Toronto	Developer of "Hett serum."
25. Harry M. Hoxsey	[none]		Developer of Hoxsey Method (herbs).
26. Andrew C. Ivy	Ph.D., M.D.	[University of Chicago, Rush Medical College]	Executive director, National Advisory Cancer Council; director, American Cancer Society.
27. Barbara J. Johnston	M.D.	New York University	Board-certified internist; head of oncology, St. Vincent's Hospital, N.Y.C.
28. Herman H. Kahlenberg	Ph.D.	University of Wisconsin	Assistant, Rockefeller Institute; laboratory owner.
29. William Donald Kelley	D.D.S.	Baylor University	Orthodontist.
30. William F. Koch	Ph.D., M.D.	[University of Michigan, Detroit College of Medicine]	Developer of Glyoxylide.
31. Byron Krebs	M.D. (D.O.) *	College of Osteopathic Physicians and Surgeons, Los Angeles	Full-time general practitioner.
32. Ernst T. Krebs, Sr.	M.D.	College of Physicians and Surgeons, San Francisco	Co-developer of laetrile.
33. Ernst T. Krebs, Jr.	A.B.	University of Illinois, Urbana	"Biochemist"; co-developer of Laetrile.
	[D.Sc.(Hon.)]	[American Christian College, Tulsa]	
34. Lillian Lazenby	[not given]	[not given]	"Convicted of practicing medicine without a license"; acquitted on appeal.
35. Andrew J. Lewis	B.A.	John Carroll University	Owner, Lewis Laboratory for Cancer Research.
36. Robert E. Lincoln †	M.D.	Boston University	General practitioner.
37. Virginia Livingston	M.D.	New York University	General practitioner.
38. Jack G. Makari	M.D.	American University, Beirut	Research positions at Royal College of Physicians and Surgeons, England; WHO fellow, Harvard; fellow, Johns Hopkins; associate professor, University of Texas; immunologist, M. D. Anderson Hospital; director of research, Muhlenberg Hospital, New Jersey.
39. A. Ernest Mills †	M.D.	Tufts University	Internist.
40. Norman Molomut	Ph.D.	Columbia University	Bacteriologist, Pasteur Institute, Michigan; College of Physicians and Surgeons, Columbia University; director of research, Waldemar Medical Research Foundation.

Name	Sci. Degree(s)	From **	Professional Status
41. Paul A. Murray	M.D.	University of Pittsburgh	General practitioner.
42. Gaston Naessens	[not given]	[not given]	"Claims to have studied biology at University of Lille."
43. Perry L. Nichols	M.D.	University of the South	"A class C institution which went out of existence."
44. Paul Niehans	M.D.	University of Bern	Surgery; endocrinology.
45. James W. Ollerenshaw	B.Ch., B.M. (M.D.)	Oxford University	Fellow of Royal Society of Medicine; Associate of Industrial Medical Officers.
46. Robert C. Olney	M.D.	Eclectic Medical College, Cincinnati	Medical director, Providence Hospital, Lincoln, Nebr.
47. Morton Padnos	Ph.D.	New York University	Parasitologist, U.S. Army, New York Aquarium, Waldemar Medical Research Foundation.
48. James H. Rand, III	D.Sc. (Hon.)	University of Berlin	Development engineer, chemist, inventor; son of founder of Remington-Rand, Inc.
49. Wilhelm Reich	M.D.	University of Vienna	Associate of Sigmund Freud.
50. Emanuel Revici	M.D.	University of Bucharest	Director, Institute of Applied Biology, and Trafalgar Hospital, N.Y.C.
51. Jules Samuels	M.D.	University of Gent	ACS turned down offer to bring Samuels to U.S. to explain his "endocrinotherapy."
52. Michael J. Scott	M.D.	Creighton University	"Member of the College of Surgeons."
53. Franklin L. Shivley	M.D.	Northwestern University	Licensed to practice in Ohio.
54. Leo L. Spears	D.C.	Palmer School of Chiropractic	Founder, 600-bed Spears Chiropractic Clinic.
55. Charles F. Swingle	Ph.D.	Johns Hopkins University	Plant physiologist in "government service."
56. Eli J. Tucker	M.D.	Tulane University	General practitioner; orthopedic surgery.
57. Henry K. Wachtel	M.D.	University of Vienna	Associate Professor of physiology, head of Cancer Research Dept., Fordham University.
58. Morvyth McQueen Williams	M.D., Ph.D.	Yale University	Certified in diagnostic roentgenology by American Board of Radiology.
59. Joseph W. Wilson	M.D.	University of Pittsburgh	General practitioner; general surgery.
60. George S. Zuccala	B.S., D.Sc. (Hon.)	Physicians and Surgeons College of Microbiology, Chicago	Serologist, City of New York, 1926–1944; laboratory owner.

† Name eventually removed from unproven methods list.
* California osteopaths became medical doctors (M.D.s) in 1962.
** Information in brackets from sources other than ACS.

In the 19th and 20th centuries, literally thousands of unproven cancer remedies were promoted or sold in this country. These "remedies" cover a wide range of materials, methodology and rationale.

Among the simpler ones are escharotic fluids used to treat external cancer; natural products, such as cobwebs saturated with arsenic powder liquid applied as a poultice, or clover blossom tea; and raw food diets, such as the "grape cure" . . . (ACS, 1971b).

Richards's book on cancer offers an alternative list of bizarre remedies:

Tear extract? Ox bile? Llama placenta? Lemon juice enemas? Clam extract? Diamond carbon compound? These substances and many others have been or are currently being offered for the treatment of cancer (Richards, 1972:271).

This sort of "criticism" can have profound implications. In Justice Thurgood Marshall's 1979 decision concerning the legal status of laetrile, he cites the following in support of the government's argument:

Since the turn of the century, resourceful entrepreneurs have advertised a wide variety of purportedly simple and painless cures for cancer, including liniments of turpentine, mustard oil, eggs, and ammonia; peat moss; arrangements of colored flood lamps; pastes made from glycerin and Limburger cheese; mineral tablets; and "Fountain of Youth" mixtures of spices, oil and suet *(New York Times,* June 19, 1979).

The fact is that none of these methods has been widely marketed for the treatment of cancer within living memory. Neither cobwebs, nor clover blossom tea, nor tear extract, ox bile, llama placenta, lemon juice enemas, nor *any* of the purported methods named in Marshall's decision are even mentioned in the ACS list.

The methods which Marshall mentions, if they once existed, did so at or before the turn of the century—not in the present period. They sound characteristic of an earlier age of medicine, when patent medicines of dubious value dominated medical practice, not just the treatment of cancer.

But another point must be made. Many of the most effective orthodox medicines are derived from substances which, at first sight, do seem absurd, and possibly even dangerous.

The well-known drug Premarin, used by millions of women to relieve the signs of menopause, is derived from *pregnant mares' urine* (Epstein, 1978). Penicillin is derived from mold. The orthodox anticancer agent Mustargen is a form of poisonous mustard gas; another anticancer agent comes from the periwinkle plant. Digitalis, for the heart, comes from the common foxglove. The list goes on.

Imagine how it would be possible to attack these present-day conventional therapies, which are derived from mare's urine, mold, weeds, and poison gases. This is no more nor less absurd than the lists given above. *Any* substance may offer a therapeutic effect: the only way to tell is to test the substance in the laboratory or with patients.

As the late Sloan-Kettering chemotherapist David Karnofsky once stated:

The relevant matter in examining any form of treatment is not the reputation of its proponent, the persuasiveness of his theory, the eminence of its lay supporters, the testimony of patients, or the existence of public controversy, but simply—does the treatment work? (Karnofsky, 1959).

The public, and much of the medical profession, is under the impression that unorthodox methods of cancer management are routinely subjected to fair and impartial analysis, before the "quack" label is pinned upon them.

This idea is embellished for the general reader in the chapter "Cancer Quackery" in Dr. Richards's book (the chapter was written by Denise Scott):

Many agencies throughout the U.S. and indeed in many other countries carry on such investigations [of quackery] and report on their findings in a wide variety of scientific journals and other publications.

These investigating agencies include the National Cancer Institute, the American Medical Association, the Federal Food and Drug Administration, the U.S. Public Health Service, and certain independent agencies. They have strict standards of investigation. These include examination of clinical evidence presented by the treatment proponent (as the examination of biopsy slides and of X-ray pictures); analysis of the new drug; experiments in animals; tests for consistency (through treatment of a large number of patients); and reviews of the results of the autopsies of patients who have died after having received the new remedy or treatment (Richards, 1972:271).

This sort of investigation is so reasonable that, as the author states, "no honest and serious researcher can have any objection to scientific investigation of his method" along these lines. Unfortunately, such an investigation almost never takes place before a method is condemned as quackery.

Table 4 lists fifty-eight "unproven" methods included in the ACS book in the 1970s. In twenty-four out of fifty-eight cases (or 41.4 percent) *no investigation at all* was carried out by the American Cancer Society or any other agency before the method was condemned.

In seven cases, or 12.1 percent, it appears that the results of the investigation were not negative at all, but actually *positive*. This does not mean, of course, that these seven methods are "cures for cancer." Rather, the scanty data points in a positive, rather than a negative, direction.

For example, one of the methods included on the ACS list is chaparral tea. This, it is said, is "an old Indian remedy made by steeping the leaves and stems of a desert shrub." Yet many bona fide drugs originated as old Indian remedies (cf. Vogel, 1970).

The American Cancer Society states:

After careful study of the literature and other information available to it, the American Cancer Society does not have evidence that treatment with chaparral tea results in objective benefit in the treatment of cancer in human beings (ACS, 1971b:55).

The story of chaparral tea began, it says, when an eighty-five-year-old man was brought to the University of Utah with a proven malignant melanoma (deadly form of skin cancer) of the right cheek. He refused surgery and treated himself, instead, with chaparral tea. "He returned eight months later," the ACS report continues, "with marked regression of the cancer."

Such regressions do occur spontaneously on occasion—but less than one in several thousand cases (Everson and Cole, 1966). University of Utah scientists then used the tea on other patients. "Four patients have responded to some extent to treatment with the tea, including two with melanomas, one with choriocarcinoma metastatic [spread] to the lungs and one with widespread lymphosarcoma." One of the other melanoma patients "experienced a 95 percent regression" whereupon the remaining growth was removed by surgical excision (ibid.).

Research then performed at the National Cancer Institute by Dean Burk, Ph.D., showed that in laboratory cultures "this is a very active agent against cancer," in the words of Dr. Charles R. Smart, associate professor of surgery at the University of Utah Medical Center.

The tea was also being used by scientists at other medical centers, including the chairman of the biochemistry department at the University of Nevada. An Arizona scientist received an $81,000 contract "to investigate treatments which might be developed from desert plants," and doctors in Reno had begun to use chaparral tea on their cancer patients.

Dr. Smart does warn that in some cases the tea may have accelerated the growth of some tumors; otherwise, there is nothing negative about this treatment in the ACS summary. Yet based on the above information the Society placed chaparral tea on its unproven methods list.

TABLE 4
ACS Unproven Methods—Results of Testing

Method	Nature of Investigation	Results*
1. Anticancergen Z-50	National Research Council	(−)
2. Antineol	4 investigators, 15 patients	(−)
3. Bamfolin	no objective regression, but "subjective amelioration" — a French magazine	(+/−)
4. H. H. Beard Methods	test canceled midway by California Dept. of Public Health	(?)
5. Biomedical Detoxification	no investigation	(0)
6. Bonifacio Anticancer Serum	worthless—Commission of the National Institute for the Study and the Cure of Tumors, Milan	(−)
7. Cancer Lipid Concentrate	no investigation	(0)
8. Carcin or Neo-carcin	ineffectual—French Ministry of Public Health (undocumented by ACS)	(−)
9. Carzodelan	no investigation	(0)
10. CH-23	ineffective—Medical Association of Bavaria, quoted in *Journal of AMA,* Aug. 5, 1968	(−)
11. Chaparral Tea	some positive clinical data; effective in animal studies	(+)
12. Chase Dietary Method	no investigation	(0)
13. C.N.T.	no investigation	(0)
14. Coley's Mixed Toxins	positive in double-blind study at NYU (withdrawn from ACS list, 1975)	(+)
15. Collodaurum, etc.	no investigation	(0)
16. Contreras Methods	no investigation	(0)
17. Crofton Immunization Method	no investigation	(0)
18. Ferguson Plant Products	positive effects in animals and possibly man	(+)
19. Fresh Cell Therapy	no investigation	(0)
20. Frost Method	no investigation	(0)
21. Gerson Method	data reviewed by AMA, NCI, and NY Medical Soc.	(−)
22. Gibson Methods	no investigation	(0)
23. Glover Serum	12 patients reviewed. Physician dissent.	(−)
24. Grape Diet	no investigation	(0)
25. H-11	mostly negative, but in some cases rate of growth appeared slow or inhibited	(+/−)
26. Hadley Vaccine	no investigation	(0)
27. Haematoxylon Dissolved in DMSO	hospital research committee, Harris County, Texas	(−)
28. Heat Therapy or Hyperthermia	no genuine investigation; now in use at most major cancer centers	(0)
29. Hemacytology Index (HCI)	conflicting reports: "must await further investigation"	(?)
30. Hendricks Natural Immunity Therapy	no investigation (license removed for violating Cancer Anti-quackery law by using banned methods, such as Koch, Lincoln, etc.)	(0)
31. Hett "Cancer Serum" and Gruner Blood Smear Test	no "independent clinical investigation"	(?)

Method	Nature of Investigation	Results *
32. Hoxsey Method	visiting committee of six doctors from British Columbia, for three days	(−)
33. Hydrazine Sulfate	negative results at Sloan-Kettering [positive results by Gold, Gershanovich, et al. not cited]	(−)
34. Iscador (Mistletoe)	no investigation	(0)
35. Issels Combination Therapy	five-day visit by English doctors	(−)
36. Kanfer Neuromuscular or Handwriting Test	"a means of separating high-risk groups from low-risk groups," worth "further investigation"	(+)
37. KC-555	positive in animals; tests terminated	(+)
38. Kelley Malignancy Index	no investigation	(0)
39. Koch Antitoxins	four medical commission reports	(−)
40. Krebiozen or Carcalon	NCI committee retrospective of 504 cases	(−)
41. Laetrile	retrospective on 44 patients	(−)
42. Lewis Methods	inconclusive—Cleveland Society of Pathologists	(?)
43. Livingston Vaccine	no investigation	(0)
44. Makari Intradermal Cancer Test	VA Hospital use, etc.	(+)
45. M.P. Virus	three patients tested: "does seem to affect malignant tissue" but dangerous	(+)
46. Mucorhicin	improvement in 2 out of 15 cases reviewed	(+/−)
47. Multiple Enzyme Therapy	no investigation	(0)
48. Naessens Serum, or Anablast	French Ministry of Public Health	(−)
49. Nichols Escharotic Method	Bureau of Investigation of AMA (1933); also 1943 study of 19 cases	(−)
50. Orgone Energy Devices	no investigation	(0)
51. Polonine	no investigation	(0)
52. Rand Coupled Fortified Antigen	"further investigative and research data" needed—Cleveland Academy of Medicine	(?)
53. Revici Cancer Control	33 cases evaluated in clinical trial	(−)
54. Samuels Causal Therapy	condemned after investigation by chairman of Amsterdam Health Council	(−)
55. Spears Hygienic System	no investigation	(0)
56. Staphylococcus Phage Lysates (Lincoln Method)	no objective evidence, but "marked symptomatic improvement" (since removed from list)	(+/−)
57. Ultraviolet Blood Irradiation	no investigation; resolution of Nebraska doctors against Koch methods	(0)
58. Zen Macrobiotic Diet	no investigation	(0)

* Key:
    (−)   Ineffective according to data given in ACS book
    (0)   Never investigated
    (+)   Effective according to data given in ACS book
    (+/−)   Contradictory results found in investigation
    (?)   Inconclusive results

A similar case is that of Ferguson Plant Products, otherwise known as the Jivaro Head Shrinking Compound. This was given to an American explorer, Wilburn Ferguson, by an Indian chief in Ecuador.

In the early 1950s, the compound was analyzed by scientists at the Los Angeles County Hospital, who successfully isolated an active agent from the compound. It turned out to be a "highly potent antibiotic" (ACS, 1971b), which is significant, since antibiotics form one whole class of known anticancer agents.

The compound was then tried against known animal tumors and leukemias "with some degree of success" according to the hospital staff (ibid.:116). In 1952 a representative of the National Cancer Institute visited Ferguson in Ecuador and reviewed the scientific data which had been gathered there. He reported:

Ferguson did not claim to me that he had a cure for cancer in humans, but did claim to have a cure for cancer in animals. He did say that he believed that his drug caused regression of human cancer and showed me evidence of this that was rather convincing. All of his treated patients still have cancer, some have died, but the ones which I saw, providing the previous observations were truthfully presented, had regressed considerably (ibid.).

The ACS report then adds that in the spring of 1953, the Merck Institute for Therapeutic Research, an offshoot of the Merck Sharpe & Dohme pharmaceutical company, "initiated studies with Ferguson anticancer material. A report on these studies has not been published."

Again, there is nothing negative in this account, which comes from the ACS article. Yet, on the basis of the above facts, the ACS added the Ferguson compound to its list, claiming that there was no evidence it "results in objective benefit in the treatment of cancer in human beings."

In some cases, the ACS and its confreres have condemned a method only to silently remove it from the list years later.

Coley's toxins is such a instance (see Chapter 7). Another was the case of Robert E. Lincoln, M.D. Lincoln's name was added to the ACS list in 1964, when the controversy over his work was still alive.

Lincoln was a graduate of Boston University School of Medicine, who had done postdoctoral work at Harvard, and then gone into general practice in the small town of Medford, outside Boston. For many years he was an unremarkable small-town doctor, a member in good standing with the American Medical Association and its state affiliate, the Massachusetts Medical Society.

In the 1940s, in the midst of an influenza epidemic, Lincoln made what he felt were some important discoveries concerning the bacterial origin of various diseases—discoveries which he later extended to cancer. He also believed that he had discovered a possible cure for some forms of these diseases in bacteriophage—viruses which parasitically attack and destroy specific bacteria.

Lincoln began to treat patients with injections of these viruses and claimed to see some remarkable results, including remissions of cancer. In 1946, therefore, he submitted these clinical results to the *Journal of the American Medical Association.* His paper was rejected.

He then submitted the same paper to the *New England Journal of Medicine,* published in Boston. This time it was rejected for "lack of space" (Morris, 1977).

Undaunted, Lincoln wrote three letters in succession to an editor of the New England journal, asking for his assistance in preparing the article for publication. He received no reply to any of these letters. In March 1948 Lincoln asked the director of a large Boston hospital to visit him and study the clinical results he had assembled and the methods by which he had achieved them. The director wrote back that he "couldn't find the time."

The general practitioner next wrote to the Massachusetts Medical Society, asking for a chance to present his work to his colleagues at a meeting. The Society stalled, but in the meantime began sending out a form letter to inquirers stating that Lincoln's method was ineffective.

Lincoln was perturbed and wrote to the president of the AMA itself, asking him to send someone to Medford to investigate the situation. This medical leader, however, referred Lincoln back to the Massachusetts Medical Society.

This stalemate was dramatically broken when Lincoln happened to treat the son of Charles Tobey, a United States senator. Tobey, claiming that Lincoln had cured his son of cancer, excoriated the Massachusetts medical establishment from the floor of the Senate.

Stung by this criticism, the Massachusetts Medical Society finally dispatched a team of surgeons and radiologists to Medford, where they interviewed some patients on the back porch of Lincoln's house. They claimed to be unable to see any signs of actual, objective benefit, however, but did concede that there were some "cases of marked symptomatic improvement," which they attributed to "the tremendous force of faith and hope" (ACS, 1971b:197).

When Lincoln read this, he complained publicly of the "high degree of stupidity" shown by this report. The leaders of the Massachusetts Medical Society then demanded his resignation; when he refused to resign, he was expelled on April 8, 1952. One year later, Lincoln sued the Society for $250,000 for libel, but he died in the following year and the case never came to trial (Morris, 1977; ACS, 1971b).*

In 1975 the ACS quietly took Lincoln's name off the unproven methods list, a tacit admission of an error on its part. However, it is virtually impossible for cancer patients to receive his treatment.

But Lincoln is hardly alone in the treatment he received. Table 5 shows that 53.5 percent of the methods on the ACS list were either not investigated at all before being condemned, or were actually found positive in the tests conducted. In another 6.9 percent the data was contradictory, while in 8.6 percent the investigators could not reach a definitive conclusion. Thus, over 70 percent of the methods on the unproven methods list have never been shown to be ineffective by any sort of rational scientific procedure.

In the remaining 30 percent, some sort of investigation was carried out, and the method in question was judged negative by the investigators (if not by the proponent). But did these investigations conform to the fair and scientific standards outlined in the Richards book, and most other orthodox writings on "quackery"? Only very rarely, it turns out.

For many of these methods, it is impossible to say whether the investigation was adequate, since the ACS critics rely on secondhand or thirdhand reports. Five investigations were carried out by foreign medical organizations, and for some the only source of information appears to be magazine articles. These may be valid investigations of fraudulent or worthless remedies, but it is hard to tell merely from the information the ACS provides.

For only about a dozen methods does the ACS offer documented evidence of failure. This in itself is significant, since it represents only about 20 percent of the total.

But were these methods subjected to adequate investigation before they were condemned? Again, the answer would have to be no.

Included in this negative category are such therapies as laetrile, hydrazine sulfate, Krebiozen, the Gerson method, the Hoxsey method, Glover's serum, Koch antitoxins, and Revici Cancer Control.

As the reader will see in the following pages, many of these methods have been tested and condemned in a one-sided manner. In *no* case, for example, has a clinical double-blind study been carried out on any of these procedures. (A double-blind test is one in which neither the patient nor the physician knows the nature of the medication being given. It is generally considered the most objective form of testing.)

---

* Much of the information on Lincoln comes from sources favorable to his approach, particularly Morris. The ACS account does not contradict these, but is scanty.

The National Cancer Institute long resisted performing such tests on Krebiozen, despite the fact that fifty-six U.S. Congressmen co-sponsored a resolution calling for one (ACS, 1971b:2). For many years, of course, the establishment has similarly refused to conduct a clinical trial of laetrile, on the grounds that this would be "a criminal abuse of hopes" (Dr. Daniel Martin in *Medical World News,* October 26, 1975).

Sometimes, the investigation has been highly informal. Hoxsey's treatment, which on the surface appears closer to true "quackery" than any in the ACS book, was never subjected to either animal studies or clinical trials of any sort. The only negative investigation cited in the book, in fact, was a three-day visit to his clinic by several Canadian physicians, who came away unimpressed.

Glover's serum, which is a predecessor of the Livingston technique (see Chapter 13), was subjected to some cursory animal studies and a review (but no clinical trial) of twelve patients, before it was condemned.

It would be extremely surprising and unlikely if this list did *not* contain instances of mad delusion and outright fraud. After all, it *is* a list of purportedly quack remedies, and one would expect to find at least some such treatments there.

However, what is at issue here is whether these methods have been fairly and adequately tested before being condemned. Richards proposed excellent criteria for the testing of such methods: examination of clinical evidence, including biopsy slides and X-ray pictures; analysis of the drug or agent proposed for therapy; experiments in animals; testing in a large number of patients; and reviews of autopsies.

In addition, one should add the trial of putative methods by means of double-blind studies, of the kind currently proposed by the director of the National Cancer Institute for laetrile.

A careful examination of the ACS manual shows that these criteria are almost never met in the study of unorthodox therapies. Rather, the Society appears to have made an a priori judgment on the worthlessness of uncommon cancer therapies, and then stretched the facts to fit its preconceptions.

Not all of these methods are valid, of course, and some are probably fraudulent. But taken as a whole the unproven methods are a repository of new ideas from which cancer scientists should be able to draw freely. The stigma of "quackery" attached to these methods by the American Cancer Society and others may prevent them from doing so.

This opposition on the part of orthodoxy is antiscientific and ultimately self-serving. As Pat McGrady, Sr., a former American Cancer Society official, has said:

The Establishment has turned the terror of this ugly disease to its own ends in seeking more and more contributions from a frightened public and appropriations from a concerned Congress. Still, undismayed by the futility of funds dumped into the bottomless barrel of its "proven" methods, it remains adamant in refusing to investigate "unproven" methods. . . .

Forgetful of the fact that of the few really useful treatments, all, or almost all, were initiated under the kind of abuse now heaped upon "unproven" remedies, the Establishment may be denying help for tomorrow's cancer patients as well as today's (McGrady, Sr., 1975).

TABLE 5
Statistical Analysis of Investigations of ACS Unproven Methods

Kind of Investigation		Method Number (total = 58) *	Percentage
I.	No investigation made	5, 7, 9, 12, 13, 15, 16, 17, 19, 20, 22, 24, 26, 28, 30, 34, 38, 43, 47, 50, 51, 55, 57, 58 [total = 24]	41.4%
II.	Investigation made: method found to be positive (+)	11, 14, 18, 36, 37, 44, 45 [7]	12.1%
III.	Investigation made: contradictory data (+/−)	3, 25, 46, 56 [4]	6.9%
IV.	Investigation made: inconclusive results (?)	4, 29, 31, 42, 52 [5]	8.6%
V.	Investigation made: method found to be negative (−)	1, 2, 6, 8, 10, 21, 23, 27, 32, 33, 35, 39, 40, 41, 48, 49, 53, 54 [18]	31.0%
			100.0%

* See Table 4.

7

Coley's Toxins

In the late nineteenth century a young Memorial Hospital surgeon, fresh out of Harvard Medical School, stumbled across one of the most intriguing findings ever made in cancer research. His discovery was first tolerated, then ridiculed, and finally suppressed. Today, although given lip service by some doctors, its potential is still largely unexplored.

The doctor's name was William B. Coley, and his discovery is known as Coley's toxins, or "mixed bacterial vaccine."

Coley's first patient at Memorial was a young woman of nineteen with a cancer of the bone. Coley amputated her arm, and the prognosis seemed good. Yet a short while later the girl died. The young doctor was horrified at his complete failure to effect a cure, despite the seemingly early detection of the growth (Nauts, 1976b).

Coley could not accept the supremacy of surgery, a technique which was often dangerous, mutilating, and futile in the treatment of cancer. Nor could he accept the commonly held belief that cancer was incurable and unconquerable. This determined young man began a long and tedious search for a cure for cancer (ibid.).

Coley began methodically searching the patient records at New York Hospital. Researching in the dusty archives, he went back fifteen years and examined the case records of all bone cancer patients treated at that hospital. Most of these cases ended in failure and death. To his amazement, however, Coley discovered one patient who had been given up for lost by his doctors and yet had walked out of the hospital in apparently perfect health (Cancer Research Institute, 1976).

What had happened? On his deathbed, the patient had suffered two attacks of erysipelas, a severe and sometimes life-threatening infection of the skin caused by the bacteria *Streptococcus pyogenes.*

Today erysipelas is controlled by antibiotics, but at the turn of the century it was a fairly common infectious disease, whose side effects included severe fever and chills similar to those accompanying typhoid fever.

This one patient recovered from the erysipelas and miraculously his tumors also began to shrink and disappear. In a short while this man, on whom the doctors had operated four times to no avail, was discharged from the hospital. His doctors shook their heads as he left and called his case a "spontaneous remission"—a cure with no apparent cause (Everson and Cole, 1966).

The man's records had lain in New York Hospital's dusty record room until that day in 1888 when Coley dug them out and stared at them in amazement. Coley copied down the man's address and went to his house, but the man had moved. He found a neighbor who knew his forwarding address, and from there he went to yet another address. Up and down the stairs of New York's tenements Coley trekked in search of this "miracle man." And, finally, he found him. It had been seven years since his discharge from New York Hospital, yet despite that length of time, as Coley discovered, the man was still in complete remission of his cancer (Burdick, 1937).

Coley's next step was to try to create the same curative conditions that had occurred accidentally years before: he would deliberately infect a terminally ill cancer patient with erysipelas. One can imagine the consternation of Coley's surgical colleagues at this suggestion—after all, what was the sense in giving a patient with one fatal disease *another* nearly fatal disease to contend with?

Coley found a supporter at Memorial, however, in Dr. W. J. Bull, chief of the Bone Service, Coley's own department. After due preparations, a volunteer was found and was injected with a culture of strep in 1891.

There was no reaction. Again and again, using different cultures, Coley injected his patient. Again nothing happened. What disappointment—another dead-end lead. And there it might have ended, had not a friend brought Coley a particularly active, virulent culture of strep germs from the famous German "microbe hunter," Robert Koch.

When Coley administered this culture, the patient's temperature shot skyward and he contracted a severe case of erysipelas. Doctors and nurses feared for the patient's life. But within a few days another "miracle" had occurred: the tumors on his tonsils and neck completely disappeared, and only a scar remained. This man was in total remission of cancer (ibid.).

Unbelievable? Remember that this happened right at Memorial Hospital, in full view not only of Coley, but of his chief, Dr. Bull, and other distinguished Memorial surgeons and pathologists. In 1893 Coley published his first paper on the new method, "A Preliminary Note on the Treatment of Inoperable Sarcoma by the Toxic Product of Erysipelas" (Coley, 1893).

Over the years, Coley was to publish dozens of such papers, recording what he said was the success—and sometimes the failure—of his new treatment method.

Coley began a creative experiment with the microbial treatment of cancer which lasted over forty years. Between 1891 and 1893 he treated ten cases of inoperable cancer with live erysipelas germs at the old Memorial Hospital on 104th Street and Central Park West in Manhattan.

Coley also studied a number of other cases of "spontaneous remission" in cancer which followed erysipelas infections. In 1893 he tabulated these initial results: of the seventeen cases of advanced carcinoma studied, four were permanently cured, ten showed improvement, which did not lead to a cure but added years to their lives (palliation), and three showed no improvement at all (ibid.).

In sarcoma, cancer of the bone and connective tissue, Coley's claims were even more impressive: 41 percent complete cures. If these statistics were true, these were probably the best results ever achieved in cancer until that time. The results would even compare favorably with any mode of therapy used today. Nevertheless, there were drawbacks to the erysipelas treatment.

For one thing, it was an ordeal for the patient: high fever, malaise, and the danger of death from the infection itself. For another, live strep, an infectious agent, posed a potential health threat to the workers and other patients in the hospital. Nearly 6 percent of the first group of patients died of the infection itself.

Another serious drawback was the uncertainty of erysipelas therapy. Often it was impossible even to induce the disease, even when the patient was placed in a so-called erysipelas bed—the unchanged bed of a recently deceased victim of the disease. It was a temperamental microbe.

Coley therefore attempted to improve his invention. Instead of using bacteria, live or dead, he mixed the toxins of the strep (normally formed during the metabolism of the microbe) with those of another germ, *Bacillus prodigiosus*. "Prodigiosus" in Latin means "wonderful," and the wonder of this germ was that it had the power of intensifying the activity of other microbes, such as strep. (Today it is called *Serratia marcescens*.)

The first patient treated with the mixture was a sixteen-year-old German immigrant boy, who had a huge inoperable growth on his abdomen. The doctors at Memorial despaired of even treating him. As a last resort, he was referred to Coley for treatment with the mixed bacterial vaccine. Coley began the treatment on January 24, 1893, injecting directly into the tumor, and continued injections for four months. Memorial Hospital records tell the story:

These injections produced within eight hours a rise in temperature from 0.5 to 6 degrees, a pulse running from 100 to 106. The chill and tremblings were extreme. . . . [There were also] severe headaches. . . . The tumor gradually diminished in size, at times for a few days after injection it would be enlarged, but the final diminution was indisputable (cited in Nauts et al., 1953).

On May 13 the boy was discharged from Memorial—his tumor reputedly one-fifth the size it had been upon admission. Two weeks later, the growth was no longer visible. Coley presented this patient a number of times to doctors at the New York Academy of Medicine and the New York Surgical Society. This patient lived on for another twenty-six years and died suddenly of a heart attack in 1919. At autopsy, the coroner is said to have found no evidence of cancer (Cancer Research Institute, 1976).

For those hearing of Coley's results for the first time, this will undoubtedly seem hard to believe. Yet, as Dr. Lloyd J. Old, a Sloan-Kettering vice-president, and Dr. Edward Boyse, FRS, member of Sloan-Kettering Institute, wrote a few years ago; "Those who have scrutinized Dr. Coley's records have little doubt that the bacterial products that came to be known as Coley's toxins were in some instances highly effective" (Old and Boyse, 1973).

Coley's voluminous results have been tabulated by his daughter, Mrs. Helen Coley Nauts, executive director of the Cancer Research Institute, Inc., New York, N.Y. In seventeen monographs and numerous papers, she and her medical colleagues have documented 894 cases treated with her father's vaccine.

Patients with inoperable tumors of various kinds had 45 percent five-year survival, while those with operable tumors had 50 percent. The best results were in giant cell bone tumors where 15 out of 19 (or 79 percent) of the inoperable patients and 33 out of 38 (or 87 percent) of the operable patients had five-year survival.

In breast cancer the results were equally impressive. Thirteen out of 20 of the inoperable (65 percent) and 13 out of 13 of the operable had five-year survival. Comparable results were seen in other types of cancer (for example, 67 percent in Hodgkin's disease, 67 percent in inoperable ovarian cancer, 60 percent in inoperable malignant melanoma) (Nauts, 1976a).

In addition, the toxin therapy brought other beneficial effects, including a marked decrease or cessation of pain, improved appetite and weight gain (up to 50 pounds), and a "remarkable regeneration of bone" in a number of cases (ibid.).

Since these results are generally much better than those achieved with any conventional therapy today, how is it that most non-professionals as well as many cancer scientists have never heard of this method?

From the start, many doctors were skeptical of Coley's unorthodox treatment, even when they saw what appeared to be proof before their very eyes. Today a "cure for cancer" is still a dream. Eighty years ago it must have seemed like an impossibility, for most doctors believed that cancer was basically an incurable disease (Considine, 1959).

The fact that an unknown but ambitious young man was somehow curing cases they themselves were unable to cure may have irked some established cancer therapists. The fact that he, a surgeon, may have done so by nonsurgical means may have seemed disloyal.

Coley obtained the support of the powerful Huntington railroad family in his efforts. Not long afterward, however, Dr. James Ewing became medical director of Memorial Hospital, with the support of the even more powerful Douglas–Phelps-Dodge interests. While Coley was not hostile to radiation, and in fact supervised the first tests of X-ray therapy at Memorial, Ewing was almost fanatical about the use of radium (see Chapter 4).

The contrast between the two competing, alternate methods could not have been greater. Radium was costly—a fabulous $150,000 a gram. Coley's toxins were remarkably inexpensive. The major cost was in paying the salary of a skilled technician to grow the germs properly. Since radium interests had invested millions of dollars in that metal, and since radium could be given in easily measurable and predictable doses, it had great appeal.

Coley's toxins were more difficult to administer, and less certain in their results. There were four basic reasons the toxins varied in their effects.

The preparations were made from living organisms which varied unpredictably in their strength (virulence). When they were made with care, under Coley's supervision, they appeared to be highly successful.

But when Coley or a colleague did not supervise their production, the results tended to be rather less impressive. Parke-Davis, the pharmaceutical company, produced the toxins commercially for many years. Unlike Coley's collaborators, however, the company heated the formula for two and a half hours, thereby allegedly destroying much of its effectiveness. Yet despite its relative weakness, Parke-Davis formula #IX showed a 37 percent cure rate for inoperable patients.

Second, the toxins produced fevers, and not all physicians knew how to deal with temperatures ranging as high as 104° F. Many doctors felt that such fevers and discomforts should be combatted with analgesics. Other doctors attempted to *use the fever* itself as a therapeutic tool—an idea said to date back to Hippocrates. These doctors appear to have achieved far better results.

Third, clinical results depended on the stage of cancer being treated—and this appears true of all treatment modalities. Those who received the toxins early in the course of their illness appeared to do much better than those who received the treatment when the disease had already spread. A high percentage of the patients in the operable group who received adequate toxin therapy remained free from recurrence five years or more (Nauts, 1976b).

Finally, the toxins worked best when they were given *before* other methods of therapy. These other methods, particularly radiation, suppressed and damaged the immune system. Coley's toxins appeared to work by jolting the immune system of the cancer patient into greater activity. One could therefore predict that attempts to give Coley's toxins to patients in a terminal condition who had already received surgery, radiation, and/or chemotherapy were unlikely to produce highly beneficial results.

Such unpredictability, although based on controllable factors, was highly damaging to the reputation of Coley's toxins. Many doctors wrote to the New York surgeon and complained that they had received ineffective batches, especially those which had been prepared commercially.

Coley remained a member in good standing of the medical fraternity, and was in fact heaped with honors. At the age of thirty-six, he became the youngest Fellow of the American Surgical Association. In 1935, he was made an Honorary Fellow of the Royal College of Surgeons of England, a plaudit rarely given to Americans (Burdick, 1937). At his retirement, Coley was given a banquet at the Waldorf-Astoria. Even Ewing spoke in his honor. Coley was honored mostly for his work as a surgeon, however. His work with the toxins was rarely mentioned; it was treated as a kind of eccentricity.

After Coley's death on April 16, 1936, there was a real possibility that his innovative methods of treating cancer would be forgotten. This danger was not lessened when Coley's son, Bradley, succeeded him as head of Memorial Hospital's Bone Service. The younger Coley discontinued use of the toxins in the bone therapy department, and therefore in the hospital as a whole.

In the 1936–39 hospital report, the younger Coley spoke of his father's "voluminous contributions" but omitted all mention of the toxins. With Coley gone, and his method no longer in use at Memorial, Ewing inserted a brief mention of the treatment in the last edition of his encyclopedic *Neoplastic Diseases:*

Coley's toxins have been used with other methods in certain cases of osteogenic sarcoma which recovered. I have been unable to form any definite estimate of the part played by this agent in the disease. But in some recoveries from endothelioma of bone, there is substantial evidence that the toxins played an essential part (Ewing, 1940:314).

Though the toxins appeared to have value, their use gradually slipped into disuse, since no one in a prominent position was interested in promoting Coley's discovery. Unfortunately, Coley's death coincided with the beginning of enthusiasm for chemotherapy and the introduction of new, high-voltage X-ray machines.

In fact, Coley would most likely have been doomed to obscurity had it not been for one member of his family: not his son, who officially followed in his footsteps, but his young daughter. Helen Coley Nauts, without a scientific background, believed that her father's work would vanish unless something was done quickly to rescue it. Without help from her brother, she finally undertook the arduous task of publicizing Coley's work on her own.

In 1945 she presented a paper at an American Association for the Advancement of Science (AAAS) meeting. She was encouraged to do so, despite the fact that she was a layperson, by Dr. Kanematsu Sugiura, Memorial's long-time chemist and a friend of her father (Nauts, 1976b).

Mrs. Nauts's approach was to gather "ironclad" cases of cures or remissions definitely attributable to the toxins. She had hoped to gather 100, but after several years she had almost 1,000. These she published in her monographs and papers, which have been distributed to libraries and interested individuals around the world.

The response from the leadership of Memorial Sloan-Kettering was not encouraging. Until this time, Sloan-Kettering had continued to produce a small amount of the toxins for research purposes. Parke-Davis also continued to produce a small amount of the toxins.

By 1953, however, all production of the toxins in the United States stopped. Through persistent pressure, however, Mrs. Nauts was able to get a clinical test performed at New York University–Bellevue Hospital, a double-blind study in which neither the patients nor the principal investigator knew who received the toxins and who a fever-inducing placebo.

This study was conducted by Barbara Johnston, M.D. and was supported by Mrs. Nauts's group. Dr. Johnston, now head of medical oncology at St. Vincent's Hospital, New York, attempted to conduct

a study which would eliminate the criticisms leveled at earlier studies. How she did this is part of the scientific record (Johnston, 1962).
In addition to the double-blind test, a larger number of other patients were treated with Coley's toxins in relatively uncontrolled
situations.

The results of both series of patients appear quite clear-cut. In
the double-blind test, the group treated with a placebo, only one
patient out of 37 showed any sign of improvement: a questionable
decrease in the size of the bladder tumor for a few weeks.

"Of the 34 patients treated with Coley's toxins," she wrote, "18
showed no improvement. Of the remaining 16, 7 noted decreased
pain," while 9 showed such benefits as tumor necrosis, apparent
inhibition of metastases, shrinkage of lymph nodes and disappearance of tumors. The New York internist wrote:

It is the impression of the authors that Coley's toxins has definite onco-
lytic [tumor-destroying] properties and is useful in the treatment of certain
types of malignant disease.

When the study was completed, however, the chairman of
the Department of Medicine at NYU School of Medicine, Lewis
Thomas, M.D., invited Dr. Johnston to leave the hospital. Thomas is
now the president of Memorial Sloan-Kettering Cancer Center
(Johnston, 1976). "They let us finish [the test] so as to prove that it
was wrong," Dr. Johnston has said. "But it didn't turn out that way"
(ibid.).

To illustrate the doublethink which has surrounded the double-
blind test—one of the few ever performed on an "unproven
method"—one need only consider the manner in which the American Cancer Society interpreted this experiment when it included
Coley's toxins in Unproven Methods in 1965.

"There was little objective basis offered for believing that bacterial toxin therapy had significantly altered the course of disease in
any of the treated cancer patients," the ACS wrote (ACS, 1971b).

The Johnston articles contained striking confirmation of Coley's
claims, in both series of experiments. Perhaps most impressive are
the photographs that accompany the article, which appear to show
dramatic, objective remissions of tumors of the neck in a short period
of time under treatment with bacterial toxins. But somehow this
evidence was not enough to dissuade the American Cancer Society
from issuing a negative judgment.

More recently, Coley's toxins have been enjoying a kind of vogue
in some research circles. Scientists promoting their own interests in
cancer immunotherapy have tried to make Coley out to be a wise

godfather of the movement. Yet the use of Coley's methods is practically nonexistent.

A recent issue of the Cancer Research Institute's *Annual Report* revealed no clinical use in the United States, but did mention some tests being conducted in the Federal Republic of Cameroon, in western Africa.

Mrs. Nauts has preferred to join the establishment rather than fight it. A member of the powerful Grace chemical empire has become chairman of the board of her organization and a Sloan-Kettering vice-president is its medical director. Mary Lasker, honorary chairperson of the American Cancer Society, was appointed to the board of trustees.

In October 1975 the Cancer Research Institute, Mrs. Nauts's once-controversial organization, was welcomed back into the fold at a Hotel Pierre banquet. Laurance S. Rockefeller gave the keynote address at the exclusive black-tie affair, and fifteen establishment scientists, including Drs. Old, Good, and Boyse of SKI, received bronze medals and cash awards from the CRI (MSKCC, *Center News*, December 1975). Quite inevitably, the Cancer Research Institute has become a respectable member of the cancer establishment.

Quietly in 1975 the American Cancer Society removed Coley's name from its unproven methods list. But the desperate cancer patient, for whom Coley's method might offer hope, still finds it very difficult to get an injection of Coley's toxins in the United States.

8

The Laetrile Controversy

Few controversies in cancer therapy have been as fierce or prolonged as that over the proposed anticancer agent laetrile.

According to the Food and Drug Administration, "Laetrile has been sold for treating cancer for around 25 years, yet there is still no sound, scientific evidence that it is either effective or safe. It is therefore classified as a 'new drug'" (FDA, 1975). In the words of an American Cancer Society official, Helene Brown, laetrile is "goddamned quackery" (Schultz and Lindeman, 1973).

According to its proponents, laetrile is neither "new" nor really a "drug." And far from being quackery, when used correctly as part of an overall nutritional program, it is one of the most promising and effective treatments for cancer.

The widespread fear of cancer and the growing bitterness over orthodox medicine's failure to find a cure, despite billions of dollars spent, has fueled the laetrile controversy. According to Charles Moertel, M.D., of the Mayo Clinic, laetrile is "a dominant unresolved problem for American medicine today" (Moertel, 1978).

To understand why this is so, it is necessary to look more closely at the substance itself and the long history of its use.

Although the term "laetrile" is of relatively recent coinage,* the chemical most often sold as laetrile has been used as a folk remedy

---

* The definition of laetrile and its relationship to amygdalin can be confusing. Crystalline amygdalin was first isolated in 1830 from bitter almonds by two French chemists. The chemical formula of amygdalin is given in the Merck Index.

Laetrile, on the other hand, is a coined word, registered by Ernst T. Krebs, Sr. and Ernst T. Krebs, Jr. in 1953. It is a contraction of *"laevo-rotatory mandelonitrile* beta-diglucoside." This is a purified form of amygdalin, which turns polarized light in a left-handed (hence "laevo-") direction. For various reasons, the Krebses believed that only the "laevo-" form of this subfor cancer or related diseases for many centuries. The laetrile sold to cancer patients today is another name for amygdalin, a glycoside, or type of carbohydrate, which occurs frequently in living organisms, especially in plants and their derivatives. All glycosides have one thing in common: in reactions with water they can be split into a sugar (or sugars) and a noncarbohydrate substance(s). Usually, an enzyme must be present to facilitate this cleavage.

There are different kinds of glycosides in nature. The kind we are concerned with releases cyanide (HCN) when broken down. It is therefore called a cyanogenic (or cyanogenetic) glycoside. Included in this category are plant chemicals such as prunasin, found most commonly in wild cherry bark; dhurrin, found in sorghum; lotusin, from the *Lotus arabicus* plant; and, of course, amygdalin.

Laetrile is found all over the globe, occurring naturally in about 1,200 different plants. One could compare it, in its ubiquity, to glucose. Like sugar, laetrile does not normally occur in a purified form, but it can be extracted quite readily from its sources.

We have all ingested amygdalin, or "taken laetrile," at one time or another and some of us take it every day, without knowing that we are engaging in medical controversy. Chickpeas and lentils, lima beans and Chinese sprouts, cashews and alfalfa, barley, brown rice, and millet—all these foods, and many more, contain laetrile. For commercial purposes, laetrile is derived from the kernels of the apricot, the peach, and the bitter almond, after which amygdalin is named (Gr. *amygdale* = almond).

According to some experts, laetrile-rich foods, including fruit kernels, were eaten by our ancestors, including Peking man (Brothwell and Brothwell, 1969:130). Laetrile's use in medicine dates from the time of the great herbal of China, credited to the legendary culture hero Emperor Shen Nung (28th century B.C.), which is said to list kernel preparations useful against tumors. Ancient Egyptian, Greek, Roman, and Arabic physicians were all familiar with the biologic properties of "bitter almond water" (*aqua amygdalarum amarum*). Celsus, Scribonius Largus, Galen, Pliny the Elder, Marcellus Empiricus, and Avicenna all used preparations containing laetrile to treat tumors. The same is true of the medieval pharmacopoeia (Halstead, 1977; Summa, 1972).

---

stance would be useful in cancer. Laetrile (with a capital L) usually refers to the Krebses' original product, whose purification process was patented by them.

In this book, laetrile (with a small l) refers to the commercial forms of amygdalin which are currently in use and around which the debate rages. Most of these are probably racemic (i.e., mixed left-turning and right-turning forms). Krebs, Jr., believes that these commercial products are less than one-third as effective as his original Laetrile (Krebs, Jr., 1979).

Such ancient use does not, of course, constitute proof that laetrile is effective. For those familiar with the course of medical history, however, it does remove it from the realm of simple quackery and make it a prime candidate for serious scientific testing. Other natural products have already demonstrated their usefulness in the treatment of cancer. Antibiotics such as bleomycin, dactinomycin, doxorubicin, mithramycin, and mitomycin C; plant alkaloids such as vincristine and vinblastine, and biologicals such as BCG and C. Parvum have all been accepted as orthodox treatments—but often after fierce resistance by the establishment. Ancient prescriptions are being rewritten in modern terms by cancer researchers. Remedies that were long thought of as pure "quackery" are now being found to have a rational basis.

Folk remedies from around the world have shown promise in cancer therapy. For example, the Penobscot Indians long used the mayapple (Podophyllum peltatum) as a folk remedy for cancer. This was even recorded in a medical book in 1849, but for over one hundred years this was scorned or ignored.

Most cancer researchers "shied away from such weird-sounding therapies, lest their scientific reputations suffer," according to Margaret B. Kreig in Green Medicine, a study of the search for plants that heal. A few researchers, like NCI's Jonathan Hartwell, decided to investigate mayapple and found that this "quack cure" actually retarded the growth of cancer. Now called VM-26, it has been found to be effective in the treatment of brain cancer in some cases, and is routinely used for certain warts, which are, after all, benign growths (Kreig, 1964; also, ACS, 1975).

The autumn crocus, which was advocated as a cancer cure by Dioscorides, the famous Greco-Roman physician and botanist, has been found to contain a chemical useful in the treatment of chronic granulocytic leukemia (Kreig, 1964).

Mistletoe (Viscum album), which was recommended by Pliny the Elder 2,000 years ago, was found to cause more than 50 percent tumor inhibition in mice in experiments at Roswell Park Memorial Institute, Buffalo, New York (ibid.).

Garlic, ginseng, and other herbs have given some indication of anticancer activity (ibid; Brown University, 1976).

Most recently, the NCI announced that it is conducting tests on maytansine, a drug derived from an East African shrub. It, too, was used by natives to treat cancer (ACS, 1975).

Because of its natural origin, and the great antiquity of its use, laetrile would be a likely candidate for scientific investigation, even if the current controversy had not developed.

Holistic Medicine

Howard Goldstein, M.D., an anti-laetrilist, has said: "There is no proven case of a person with bona fide cancer who has received no other treatment than laetrile being cured of his disease" *(Nyack* [N.Y.] *Journal-News,* December 21, 1977).

Even if this statement were true—and there are qualified physicians who would dispute it—it misses the point of the entire debate. Laetrile involves much more than the use of a single drug for the treatment of cancer. Laetrile and the movement that has grown up around it pose a major challenge to the current methods of treating cancer as they are practiced at most medical centers. This challenge has not only medical but also philosophic and socioeconomic implications.

Laetrilists are not just advocating a single substance, but, like the advocates of other unorthodox therapies, are proposing the marketing of a new kind of treatment for the patient's body and mind.

There is apparently an irreconcilable difference between laetrilists and orthodox doctors in how they understand cancer.

Since the time of John Hunter (1728–1793), orthodox oncologists have tended to see cancer as a localized disease that, as Hunter said, "only produces local effects" (Shimkin, 1977). Such a disease should therefore be curable through localized means; e.g., removing the growth through surgery or other techniques.

Hunter's view led to an enormous increase in surgery and spurred the development of new operative techniques. Nevertheless, experiments in this century, and particularly in the past twenty years, have shown that the body has natural immune mechanisms against cancer analogous to those that function in microbial infections. The logical corollary of this view is that cancer can be controlled by enhancing the body's normal immune functions, which orthodox methods tend to destroy.

Laetrilists are not alone in adopting this view, but they propose some novel methods of influencing the body's natural curative powers. First of these is with the cyanogenic glycosides, consumed either through the ingestion of laetrile-rich foods or introduced as medicine in a concentrated form. Laetrile per se is not an immune stimulant, but neither does it apparently harm the natural defense mechanisms. Since laetrilists regard this class of substances not as drugs but as "vitamin B-17," they advocate its daily ingestion for the maintenance of a cancer-free state, as well as its use in concentrated form when cancer has already developed.

In addition, they utilize megadoses of recognized vitamins such as (emulsified) vitamin A and vitamin C, as well as other vitamins and minerals (e.g., selenium) believed to have anticancer properties.

Enzymes are usually added to this regimen, following the theory of Krebs, Jr. (1970) and Beard (1911) that the pancreatic enzymes—trypsin and chymotrypsin—are intrinsic anticancer factors. To free these enzymes to kill cancer cells, laetrilists advise their patients to eat only small amounts of animal protein. They advise their patients to eat large amounts of fresh fruits and vegetables, in part to make up for the loss of animal protein and in part for the other enzymes and nutrients that these foods contain. Supplements are often given in the form of Wobe Mugos, which contain enzymes from pancreas, calf thymus, peas, lentils, and papaya (Wolf and Ransberger, 1972).

The laetrile diet of Ernesto Contreras also forbids such items as alcohol, coffee, soft drinks, white bread, ice cream, butter, canned and prepared foods, and it encourages the use of "health foods" such as whole grains, herb teas, and honey [see Table 6, page 120].

In addition, laetrilists sometimes employ other relatively non-toxic and unorthodox therapies, such as those mentioned in the following chapters of this book or included in the ACS handbook on unproven methods.

Finally, laetrile-using physicians generally attempt to treat the *whole person*—body, mind, and spirit—hence the designation *holistic medicine*. Although there is no single method of psychotherapy employed, there has been a great deal of interest in the work of Dr. O. Carl Simonton, who attempts to use biofeedback techniques to concentrate a patient's conscious and subconscious mind on the destruction of his tumor and the restitution of his health (Simonton and Matthews-Simonton, 1978).

All of this adds up to a new and radically different approach to cancer, one that many patients report to be a positive, healing experience, both mentally and physically. This is in sharp contrast to those methods currently employed in orthodox medicine that, whatever their medical value, are extremely trying on the patient's mind, body, and bank account. Opponents of the laetrile movement sometimes make the mistake of regarding the concept of holistic medicine as a clever ruse being used to fool a gullible public that simply doesn't want to take some very bitter medicine. Such an attitude is contradicted by the observations of two sociologists, neither of whom is connected to this movement, who view holistic medicine as a radical challenge to orthodoxy:

In these revolutionary periods, nothing less than the very definition of the discipline is at stake. After a new paradigm emerges, all previous research in an area may be defined as irrelevant, if not false.

Laetrile research is clearly an attempt at paradigm creation or revolutionary science (Markle and Petersen, 1977).

The fact that laetrile therapy threatens to change current methods of treating a major disease accounts in part for the vehemence with which it has been opposed by the medical establishment.

Is Laetrile a Vitamin?

Laetrilists contend that purified amygdalin is not a drug, new or old, but a food factor—specifically, that it is vitamin B-17 (Burk, 1975). This concept has been attacked by Dr. David M. Greenberg in an article entitled "The Vitamin Fraud in Cancer Quackery" in which he proposes several properties that distinguish a bona fide vitamin:

(1) It is a nutritional component of organic composition required in small amounts for the complete health and well-being of the organism.
(2) Vitamins are not utilized primarily to supply energy or as a source of structural tissue components of the body.
(3) A vitamin functions to promote a physiologic process or processes vital to the continued existence of the organism.
(4) A vitamin cannot be synthesized by the cells or the organism and must be supplied *de novo*.
(5) In man and in other mammals, deficiency of a specific vitamin is the cause of certain rather well-defined diseases (David Greenberg, 1975).

Vitamin B-17 certainly conforms to requirements (2) and (4). Whether it conforms to the others hinges on a single, central issue: does it help prevent cancer? If it does, it would certainly seem to be a vitamin—even by Greenberg's criteria.

Greenberg states that "no evidence has ever been adduced that laetriles are essential nutritional components"; "laetriles have never been shown to promote any physiological process"; and "no specific disease has been associated with a lack of laetrile in any animal." Yet no studies of the effect of laetrile on cancer are cited by this author, although such studies do exist.

There are three main arguments in favor of laetrile's vitamin status. None of these is ironclad, but each suggests that this theory deserves a serious reception.

First, cancer is a chronic, metabolic disease. As the well-known British chemist J. D. Bernal remarked:

After the successes early in the century of the understanding and cure of such external deficiency diseases as scurvy (vitamin C) and beriberi (vitamin

B), and internal deficiency diseases such as goitre (thyroxin) and diabetes (insulin), it began to be apparent that a very large number of chronic diseases were deficiency diseases, though in some cases the deficiency might be the effect of an earlier infection (Bernal, 1971:928).

Why should we rule out the possibility that cancer, or at least some forms of it, could be prevented or controlled by naturally occurring substances?

Second, there is epidemiological data suggesting that populations which have relatively large amounts of isolated laetrile in their diets are also relatively free of cancer. The Hunzakuts, who live in a kingdom near Pakistan, have often been reported to be virtually free of cancer. It is well established that apricots and apricot kernels form a staple in their diet to a degree unparalleled in the rest of the world (Leaf and Launois, 1975; Renée Taylor, 1960).°

Third, experiments performed to test laetrile's *preventive* value at Sloan-Kettering did show a prophylactic effect, according to Dr. Kanematsu Sugiura (see Chapter 9).

The idea of laetrile as vitamin B-17 is therefore not simply a ruse or cancer quackery, but a scientific hypothesis which deserves serious attention.

The Biochemistry of Laetrile

In the late 1940s, biochemist Ernst T. Krebs, Jr., purified a crude apricot-kernel preparation and proposed a biochemical rationale for its use in the treatment of cancer. On the basis of extensive work reported in the scientific literature, Krebs proposed a "cyanide theory" to explain laetrile's effect on cancer. Bruce W. Halstead, M.D., a toxicologist, has recently summarized the long debate over laetrile's mode of action (Halstead, 1977).

Two separate pathways have been suggested for laetrile's activity in the body. The first pathway is not controversial. The second—the one proposed by Krebs—has been sharply questioned by a number of critics (David Greenberg, 1975; J. P. Ross, 1975).

According to this second pathway, the glucuronide form of amygdalin is synthesized in the liver of people who ingest natural amygdalin. This glucuronide is then broken down at the tumor site to release cyanide, which selectively attacks the cancer cells, but

° A great deal of nonsense has been written about this "paradise" principality, much of which seems intended to show that life is better under semi-feudalism.

spares normal cells. Some scientists have in fact found glucuronide formation in the liver and, to a lesser extent, in the intestine and kidneys (Halstead, 1977).

In order for this glucuronide to be broken down, the enzyme beta-glucuronidase must be present. In some studies this enzyme has been found in cancerous tissues of the breast, uterus, stomach, mesentery, abdominal wall, and esophagus, in amounts about 100 to 3,600 times more than is present in noncancerous tissues. More recently, Sloan-Kettering Institute researchers have found that "in many cases beta-glycosidase and glucuronidase activities were higher in cancerous than homologous normal tissues. . . ." (Sloan-Kettering, 1974:60).

The breakdown of laetrile by beta-glucuronidase at the site of the tumor would cause general cyanide poisoning in normal cells were it not for the presence of another enzyme, rhodanese, which is capable of detoxifying cyanide.

Rhodanese was discovered by K. Lang in 1933, and a number of scientific reports have shown that normal cells contain a relatively high concentration of rhodanese and low levels of beta-glucuronidase (Halstead, 1977). Sloan-Kettering researchers found variable levels of rhodanese.

If the glucuronide is in fact formed in the liver, as Krebs postulated, and if this glucuronide then reaches the tumor site, where it is broken down by the high level of beta-glucuronidase, the resulting cyanide could conceivably poison cancer cells deficient in rhodanese, while sparing those normal cells that have high levels of this enzyme.

At the same time, benzaldehyde, a known painkiller, would also be released, accounting perhaps for the analgesic properties often associated with laetrile.

Some scientists believe that benzaldehyde itself may be an active anticancer chemical in laetrile. According to Andrew A. Benson of the Scripps Institution of Oceanography in La Jolla, California, the Japanese scientist Kenji Sakaguchi of the Kasei Institute of Biological Sciences in Michida, Japan, has found that benzaldehyde "is effective against human lung cancer" (*Science News*, February 3, 1979).

A number of other possible mechanisms of laetrile activity have also been proposed (Passwater, 1977; McCarty, 1975; Halstead, 1977). Krebs's original explanation is still widely respected among laetrilists and in some ways is the most appealing since it comes close to the long-sought "magic bullet" for cancer, which could kill cancer cells while leaving normal cells unharmed. Ironically, the basic principle behind laetrile's use resembles chemotherapy's rationale. In fact, when laetrile was originally proposed in the early 1950s, it was called "chemotherapy." Halstead has summarized the current status of the controversy over laetrile's mode of action:

Despite Krebs' critics and a number of unanswered questions about the "cyanide theory," it continues to remain the most biochemically rational explanation of some very complex chemical events revolving around the use of amygdalin (laetrile) in cancer metabolic therapy. This theory is now under critical review by a number of investigators and only time and further research will determine its ultimate reality (Halstead, 1977).

The Question of Toxicity

A great deal has been made of the alleged toxicity of laetrile. In 1977–78 the FDA took the extraordinary step of posting large "Laetrile Warning" posters in 10,000 post offices and sending an FDA *Drug Bulletin* on the subject (November–December 1977) to hundreds of thousands of health workers. As a result, laetrile, once known as a remarkably nontoxic form of therapy, is today widely considered to be a dangerous and toxic drug.

The FDA *Bulletin* contained numerous misstatements about laetrile. For example, it stated that "this glycoside [amygdalin] contains cyanide." Of course, amygdalin does not contain cyanide, but can be hydrolyzed into benzaldehyde, hydrogen cyanide, and two sugars, given the presence of beta-D-glucosidase and beta-oxynitrilase (David Greenberg, 1975). This is more than a semantic difference. Unless the proper conditions are met, cyanide is as firmly bound in the amygdalin molecule as a brick in a solid brick wall. One might as well state that table salt is poisonous because it contains chlorine!

According to the poster, thirty-seven poisonings and seventeen deaths have been caused by "ingestion of laetrile ingredients (apricot and similar fruit pits)." Apricot pits are not ingredients of laetrile. If anything, laetrile is an ingredient of apricot pits (kernels), which also contain other substances, such as enzymes, not found in purified amygdalin. (The whole kernel contains only 2 to 4 percent laetrile.) The thirty-seven poisonings, culled from the entire world over many years, refer to circumstances quite different from those encountered by cancer patients ingesting laetrile as medicine.

In the United States, three deaths have been attributed by the government to laetrile ingestion. Two women died of apparent cyanide poisoning after swallowing vials of laetrile meant for injection purposes only (*Journal of the American Medical Association,* April 14, 1978).

The third case was that of Elizabeth Hankin, an eleven-month-old daughter of a laetrile-using cancer patient. According to the FDA, the child "accidentally ingested up to five tablets (500 mg./tab) of laetrile" and died. Laetrilists (including the parents) contend that the child may never have taken laetrile, and was off the critical list when doctors decided to administer a powerful anticyanide antidote. The child subsequently slipped into a coma and died (*The Choice*, December, 1977).

The FDA *Bulletin* contains other "warnings" that appear to be primarily designed to frighten cancer patients away from an alternative form of cancer therapy. For example: "Indeed, some deaths ascribed to cancer, particularly in debilitated patients, may have been either due to or accelerated by cyanide from the drug." A frightening prospect—but what is the evidence for this? The FDA hedges by saying, "Further studies should be undertaken to determine whether this is true or not."

At the present time it is estimated that 50,000–100,000 cancer patients are taking over 1 million grams of laetrile a month (Moertel, 1978). So far, two or possibly three deaths have been reported from an accidental overdose of this substance. Several cases of minimal toxicity have also been reported. Based on these facts, laetrile does not seem to be a "dangerous" or "toxic" substance when it is taken correctly.

In 1978 anti-laetrile reseachers killed dogs by infusing large amounts of cyanide into their stomachs through feeding tubes. The cyanide had been derived from laetrile prior to the "feeding." The amount necessary to kill the animals was figured out scientifically, and then the animals were given drugs to prevent them from regurgitating the mixture (Schmidt, 1978). This finding—that laetrile, when first broken down by enzymatic action or heat, can poison those who ingest it—made headlines around the world. But it is not really news. The potentially poisonous nature of a slurry of bitter almond kernels has been known since the time of the pharaohs, when it was used to execute prisoners (Summa, 1972).

Since 1837 it has been known that under the proper chemical conditions amygdalin can be hydrolyzed to release hydrogen cyanide. This does not normally happen to a dangerous extent in the human gut, and certainly not when purified amygdalin (without enzymes) is administered by injections, which avoid the digestive tract. When administered properly by a physician, laetrile does not appear to be a significantly toxic substance. The record reveals no deaths or serious injuries of persons injected with laetrile.

This observation is borne out by Sloan-Kettering's five-year study of laetrile. In one case, laetrile was injected into mice in doses as high as 8 grams per kilogram per day, with no sign of acute or chronic toxicity. This is the equivalent of giving a human being a pound a day of this "toxic" substance! In another test, mice were given 2 grams per kilogram per day for thirty months. Sugiura reported that the treated mice in his experiments exhibited better health and well-being than the controls, which did not receive laetrile (Stock et al., 1978).

When advocates of orthodox chemotherapy accuse laetrile of being toxic it is a case of the pot calling the kettle black. As was shown above, most standard chemotherapeutic agents are truly toxic in the extreme. Methotrexate alone can produce such blood diseases as anemia, leukopenia, and thrombocytopenia, as well as liver atrophy, necrosis, cirrhosis, fatty changes, fetal death, congenital abnormalities, diarrhea, ulcerative stomatitis and, occasionally, death from intestinal perforation (*Physicians' Desk Reference*, 1978).

In comparison to such agents, laetrile is indeed nontoxic, although one could certainly imagine situations in which it could be toxic or even fatal (the same is true of water or air). Paracelsus (1493–1541), sometimes called the "Father of Chemotherapy," could very well have been commenting on this controversy when he wrote, "All substances are poisons; there is none which is not a poison. The right dose differentiates a poison from a remedy."

The Testing of Laetrile in Animals

Although spokesmen for orthodox medicine continue to deny that there have been any animal study data in favor of laetrile, this is contradicted by a number of studies, including—but not limited to—those at Sloan-Kettering.

For example, the SCIND Laboratories in California conducted several experiments in preparation for an Investigative New Drug (IND) application filed by the McNaughton Foundation in 1970. (The application was approved and then suddenly revoked.)

In the second study on carcinoma of rats (Walker 256), with amygdalin in dosages of 500 milligrams per kilogram injected intraperitoneally on days one, three, and six after tumor take, the following results were found:

DAYS' SURVIVAL TIME

Controls: 19, 19, 19, 19, 20, 20, 22, 22, 22, 22, 24, 24, 24, 25, 25, 26, 26, 26, 26

Treated: 27, 28, 28, 28, 29, 29, 29, 30, 30, 30, 30, 30, 31, 32, 32, 32, 60, 60, 60, 60 (U.S. Senate, 1977:419).

The mean survival time of the controls was thus 23 days, while of the amygdalin-treated group it was 38 days, or a 70 percent increase over the controls. Notice that the survival time of *every* amygdalin-treated animal was greater than that of *every* control animal.

As Dr. Carl Baker, then director of the National Cancer Institute, wrote in a letter to Congressman Edward Edwards, "The data provided by the McNaughton Foundation certainly indicates some activity in animal tumor system" (McCarty, 1975). In Europe as well, a number of experiments were performed that appear to show anticancer activity in animal systems. For example, in a test by Dr. Paul Reitnauer, chief biochemist of the Manfred von Ardenne Institute, Dresden (East Germany), 20 of 40 H strain mice were given bitter almonds, in addition to their standard diet. Bitter almonds contain relatively high levels of laetrile.

Fifteen days after initiation of this regimen, all 40 mice were inoculated with 1 million Ehrlich ascites cells. The 20 control mice lived an average of 21.9 days following this injection. The 20 mice receiving the bitter almond supplement lived an average of 25.8 days, which was statistically significant (Reitnauer, 1973).

Dr. T. Metianu, director of research in pharmacology-toxicology of the Pasteur Institute, Paris, using an adenocarcinoma adapted for mice, showed that 10 mice treated subcutaneously with amygdalin two to three times per week for 20 to 25 days with 500 milligrams per kilogram lived an average of 58 days past the time of tumor take. A group of 10 control mice averaged 21 days' survival time. A repetition of this experiment showed 47 days' survival for the laetrile-treated mice and 27 for the controls. Less striking results were observed at higher dosages, and no effect was seen at 100 milligrams per kilogram in this system (cited in Burk, 1975).

Combination Therapy

Laetrile is rarely used alone in the treatment of cancer. Thus, laetrilists have always argued that research institutes such as Sloan-Kettering or NCI should use this "vitamin" in combination with other vitamins, minerals, and enzymes to achieve optimal results.

The first scientist to attempt such an experiment on a large scale in animals was Harold Manner, Ph.D. Dr. Manner, chairman of the biology department at Loyola University, Chicago, used a combination of emulsified vitamin A (A-mulsin, produced by the Mugos Company), the company's Wobe Mugos enzymes, and laetrile.

The results were dramatic. As stated in Manner's recent book, *The Death of Cancer:*

After 6–8 days an ulceration appeared at the tumor site. Within the ulceration was a puslike fluid. An examination of this fluid revealed dead malignant cells. . . . The tumors gradually underwent complete regression in 75 of the experimental animals. This represented 89.3% of the total group. The remaining 9 animals showed partial regression. No attempts were made to determine increase in life span or changes in metastases (Manner et al. 1978a).

These startling results took place in mice which develop spontaneous mammary tumors, the female C3H/HeJ strain acquired from the Jackson Laboratories, Bar Harbor, Maine.

Manner's results were greeted with skepticism by most cancer researchers. Manner was criticized for first presenting his findings to a laymen's group—the National Health Federation—rather than to his scientific colleagues. Manner replied that it would take years before these results could be accepted and published, and that hundreds of thousands of people would die needlessly in that time.

In addition, Manner was criticized for not testing laetrile, enzymes, and vitamins separately. Specifically, his study did not determine if laetrile in and of itself had any effectiveness against cancer.

In a follow-up experiment, involving a total of 550 C3H/HeJ mice, Manner attempted to clarify some of these problems. Enzymes alone, combinations of enzymes and laetrile, or of vitamin A and enzymes, produced between 52 and 54 percent total regressions of cancer. Laetrile alone hd no appreciable effect but a combination of enzymes, vitamin A, and laetrile were significantly more effective than just enzymes and/or vitamin A. The triple combination produced total regressions in 38 out of 50 cases, or 76 percent. Manner has subsequently published these results (Manner, 1978b).

The establishment had much to say against Manner but, as the Chicago scientist has often pointed out, the orthodox cancer research doctors have never availed themselves of the opportunity to refute his claims *by reproducing his tests*.

Clinical Studies

In modern times, laetrile was one of the first purified chemicals to be tried for cancer treatment in a hospital setting. The substance was used by the Russian physician Fedor J. Inosemtzeff in 1844; after several months "the patient was declared cured, and he left the hospital. He had received about one and a half ounces of pure amygdalin without showing any signs of toxicity" (Inosemtzeff, 1845).

Laetrile was employed in the treatment of cancer in the early 1950s by Ernst T. Krebs, Sr., a San Francisco physician, and a Los

Angeles doctor, Arthur Harris. In a 1962 paper, Harris claimed that of the 82 cancer patients treated with laetrile between 1951 and 1953, 3 were alive and free of disease almost ten years later, 24 were alive with their cancers under control, and 55 had received only temporary, palliative results (H. H. Beard, 1962).

These and other early clinical reports were challenged in a retrospective study of 44 cancer patients treated with laetrile, reported in an article by the California Cancer Commission (CCC). The Commission claimed that laetrile was "completely ineffective" in man, in laboratory animals, or *in vitro* (California Cancer Commission, 1953).

For many years this report stood as the definitive anti-laetrile study, but it has recently come under sharp attack. For example, all the doctors questioned by the CCC reported important subjective benefit from laetrile. In addition, the discussion of "toxic cellular changes" in cancer cells was omitted from the official 1953 report, even though the original laboratory studies had mentioned this occurrence. In addition, the patients had all received either very few injections or dosages considered to be minute by today's standards (Culbert, 1976:110).

Since that time, laetrile has been used by an extraordinary number of cancer victims. Although the aura of illegality that has surrounded laetrile in this country has undoubtedly discouraged scientific publication, there are a number of clinical papers that report positive results with regard to both safety and efficacy.

In 1962, for example, John A. Morrone, an attending surgeon at the Jersey City Medical Center, reported "a dramatic relief of pain" in ten cancer patients treated with laetrile, as well as other effects that "suggest regression of the malignant lesion" (Morrone, 1962).

At both the sixth and the ninth International Cancer Congresses, sponsored by the International Union Against Cancer, Ettore Guidetti of the University of Turin and his colleagues reported positive effects of laetrile on cancer patients (Rossi et al., 1966).

One of the most prolific authors in the field has been a Philippine physician, Manuel D. Navarro. He has published almost twenty articles on his experiences with laetrile therapy since 1954 (bibliography in McNaughton, 1967). Navarro has called laetrile "the ideal drug for the treatment of cancer."

Hans A. Nieper, M.D., is a well-known West German oncologist who uses laetrile and synthetic analogs of laetrile in his medical practice. He is the author of several papers on laetrile, including one on the results of sixty cases treated with laetrile (Nieper, 1970).

In 1977, John A. Richardson, M.D., published detailed case histories of cancer patients treated by him selected from about 4,000 patients whom he claims to have treated with some success at his Albany, California, clinic. "Almost all of them have shown a positive response to their initial course of therapy before returning home" (Richardson and Griffin, 1977).

In addition, there have been numerous journalistic accounts of the Clinica del Mar of Ernesto Contreras, M.D., in Tijuana, Mexico, where cancer patients have been treated with laetrile since the early 1960s. According to these accounts, Contreras claims that 35 percent of his patients (most of whom were terminally ill at the inception of treatment) experienced no response at all. 65 percent received some benefit from laetrile, but almost half of these had recurrences of the disease after its temporary arrest; in the remaining cases, there were "more definite responses," ranging from slight improvement to the dramatic disappearance of all symptoms. Contreras estimates that perhaps 5 percent of the terminal patients he has seen have been actually "saved." These are modest claims, which belie the picture often painted of his Tijuana clinic as the haunt of crackpots and thieves. Nevertheless, Contreras has never published his results in a scientific form, despite numerous promises to do so (Schultz and Lindeman, 1973).

There have been a number of clinical studies attesting to laetrile's effectiveness, especially as a palliative. What has been lacking has been the randomized, double-blind study which has become a standard part of new-drug testing in the United States. Responsibility for the lack of such double-blind tests rests mainly with the federal government and especially the FDA, which has opposed such a test, even when it has been proposed by established cancer scientists.

Instead, in 1978 the National Cancer Institute undertook a retrospective study of cancer victims treated with laetrile. This study came under criticism from the laetrile movement because it placed its main emphasis on tumor shrinkage as an index of anticancer effect, and omitted reduction in pain or other palliative aspects of laetrile's action. One pro-laetrile organization, the National Health Federation, therefore refused to cooperate in the government's study. The NCI sought patients who had received laetrile, and only laetrile, in the treatment of cancer. Twenty-two cases were finally found who met all of the NCI panel's criteria for judging drugs. These cases were then "blinded," i.e., reviewed in such a way that any pro- or anti-laetrile bias on the part of the reviewers was theoretically removed.

Of the 22 cases deemed evaluable by NCI, 2 showed complete responses, i.e., total elimination of their tumors; 4 showed partial responses, i.e., greater than 50 percent reduction in tumor size; 9

cases had "stabilized disease"; and "3 additional patients showed increased disease-free intervals." Thus 18 out of 22, or 82 percent, appear to have had a beneficial response to laetrile therapy (Ellison, 1978).

There is no way of knowing how typical these responses might be of laetrile patients in general, but such a response rate, if it were consistent for all patients, would compare quite favorably with orthodox methods of therapy.

Although NCI officials adduced other possible reasons for these results, Dr. Arthur Upton, the director of the National Cancer Institute, shortly afterward asked permission from the Food and Drug Administration to conduct clinical trials on patients at either NCI itself or the major cancer centers around the country (ibid.). More than a year later the FDA had still failed to grant approval for this test.

At the same time, according to one source, Hans Nieper, the German physician who uses unorthodox therapies, met at Sloan-Kettering with its vice-presidents Lloyd J. Old, M.D., and C. Chester Stock, Ph.D., and with the honorary chairperson of the American Cancer Society, Mary Lasker. The meeting was held to arrange tests on new synthetic variants of laetrile, or mandelonitrile, which Nieper claims are far more effective than laetrile itself (Chowka, 1979).

Conclusions

In part because of the federal government's intransigence on the question of testing, laetrilists have taken to the courts and the legislatures. Laetrile has been legalized in twenty states and action is pending in a number of others. In New York, pro-laetrile bills have been passed by wide margins in the state legislature, only to be vetoed by an anti-laetrile governor.

Before the Supreme Court decision of June 1979, cancer patients were able to receive laetrile legally from their physicians under an affidavit system set up by federal circuit judge Luther Bohanon. The 1979 Supreme Court decision was widely interpreted in the press as a rebuff to Bohanon's opinions (*New York Times*, June 19, 1979). Yet according to Judge Bohanon's law clerk, Tim Kline, the main practical effect was to remand the case to the Circuit Court of Appeals for review (Kline, 1979). The affidavit system still remains in effect.

Bohanon's original twenty-page opinion still contains valuable insights for everyone concerned with this controversy. Bohanon's ruling was not, as sometimes depicted, a call for unlimited "freedom

TABLE 6
Laetrile Diet

	Laetrile Diet	Forbidden Food
Beverages	Chamomile tea, clear tea, mint tea, papaya tea, Sanka.	Alcohol, cocoa, coffee, milk, soft drinks.
Bread	Rye bread, soya bread, whole wheat or bran muffins, whole wheat bread.	All other. White bread.
Cereals	Buckwheat, cornmeal, cracked wheat, millet, oatmeal, sesame, fine ground grits.	All other. Refined and bleached flour.
Cheese	Cottage cheese only in limited quantities.	All other.
Dessert	Fresh fruits, stewed fruits, Jell-O.	All pastries, puddings, custards, junket, sauces, ice cream.
Eggs	Poached or boiled eggs, not fried, one a day.	Any other form.
Fat	Cold-pressed oils, preferably safflower or soya oil, soya lecithin spread.	Butter, shortening, margarine, saturated oils and fats.
Fish	White flesh fish only (very fresh).	All other fish and seafood.
Fruits	Fresh fruits only: apples, pears, apricots, bananas, cherries, currants, grapes, guava, mangos, melon, nectarines, papaya, peaches, plums, ripe oranges, quince, tangerines, avocados, ripe pineapple. Following dried fruits (unsulfured) can be stewed: apples, apricots, dates, figs, prunes, peaches, pears, plums, raisins.	Canned fruits.
Juices	Only fresh juices. May be selected from lists of fruits and vegetables permitted, including the following green leaves: chicory, endives, escarole, lettuce, swiss chard, and watercress.	All canned juices, and juices with artificial coloring and sweetening.

	Laetrile Diet	Forbidden Food
Meat	Lean, grilled, broiled, roasted, or baked beef, chicken, lamb, turkey, and veal. Internal organs: only heart and extra-fresh calf liver permitted.	No pork, fat, fried or smoked meat sausages.
Milk	Yogurt, buttermilk, and nonfat milk allowed in limited quantities.	Other dairy products.
Nuts	All types of fresh raw nuts (except peanuts), almonds, 6 to 10 a day.	Roasted and salted nuts and peanuts.
Potatoes	Baked boiled and mashed. Potato salad seasoned with salad dressing substitute, brown rice, or corn.	French fried, chips, white rice.
Salads	The following raw vegetables, shredded or finely chopped, separately or mixed: carrots, cauliflower, celery, chicory, green pepper, lettuce, radishes, swiss chard, watercress, onions, ripe tomatoes, turnips, brussels sprouts, broccoli.	Any other.
Seasoning	Chives, garlic, onion, parsley, herbs, laurel, marjoram, sage, thyme, savory, cumin, oregano, salt substitutes or other potassium salt, and sea salt in small amounts.	Spices, pepper, paprika.
Soups	Vegetable soup, barley, brown rice, and millet can be added.	Canned and creamed soup, fat stock, consommé.
Sweets	Unpasteurized honey, unsulphured molasses, raw sugar, or dark-brown sugar. Carob.	Candy, chocolate, white sugar.
Vegetables	Raw or freshly cooked: artichokes, asparagus, carrots, cauliflower, celery, chives, corn, endives, green onions, spinach, green peas, green pepper, leeks, lentils, lima beans, potatoes, radishes, tomatoes, wax beans, yams, eggplant, squash. Any vegetables listed under salads.	All canned ones.

Any Variations in This Diet Should Be Done Only With Doctor's Permission.

(Information from Ernesto Contreras, M.D.)

of choice" without consumer protection. In the jurist's view the argument over laetrile was an unresolved scientific dispute and needed to be treated as such:

Unquestionably, the administrative record in this case reveals a substantial and well-developed controversy among medical professionals and other scientists as to the efficacy of laetrile.

Advocates of laetrile's use in cancer treatment include many highly educated and prominent doctors and scientists whose familiarity and practical experience with the substance vastly exceeds that of their detractors. To deem such advocacy "quackery" distorts the serious issues posed by laetrile's prominence and requires disregarding considerable expertise mustered on the drug's behalf.

While the record reveals an impressive consensus among the nation's large medical and cancer-fighting institutions as to laetrile's ineffectualness, a disconcerting dearth of actual experience with the substance by such detractors is revealed. . . .

The current debate is fierce. The issue appears largely unresolved as to laetrile's true effectiveness, in large part because FDA has prevented adequate testing on humans. . . .

It is only when the substance is openly used, and its results carefully observed and fully reported that this controversy will be resolved (Bohanon, 1977).

9

Laetrile at Sloan-Kettering: A Case Study

June 15, 1977, was a bright, balmy day on Manhattan's Upper East Side. Within Memorial Sloan-Kettering Cancer Center (MSKCC) that morning, almost one hundred reporters and observers and half a dozen film crews from the leading television stations had assembled to hear the long-awaited official verdict on laetrile from the world's most prestigious cancer research center.

On the dais of the new conference room sat men whose credentials in the scientific world, and even among the public, appeared impeccable: Robert Good, Ph.D., M.D., director and president of Sloan-Kettering Institute, whose face was familiar to many from the cover of *Time*. Lewis Thomas, M.D., president of the overall Center and author of popular books and articles on science. Dr. Daniel Martin, a leading cancer researcher at the Catholic Medical Center, Queens, as well as eight other Memorial Sloan-Kettering scientists. °°

All of them agreed, apparently, in the words of the official press release prepared for the occasion, that "laetrile was found to possess neither preventive, nor tumor-regressant, nor anti-metastatic, nor curative anticancer activity," after almost five years of testing at the private research center (Zimmermann, 1977:127).

The officials of the center cleared their throats, reporters put down their danishes and coffee and picked up their pencils. Dr. Robert Good began to speak and, after general remarks condemning

---

°° C. Chester Stock, Ph.D., Kanematsu Sugiura, D.Sc., Isabel M. Mountain, Ph.D., Elisabeth Stockert, D.d'Univ., Franz A. Schmid, D.V.M., George S. Tarnowski, M.D., Dorris J. Hutchison, Ph.D., and Morris N. Teller, Ph.D.

laetrile and its use, passed the microphone to one of his vice-presidents, Dr. C. Chester Stock. Dr. Stock, at sixty-seven, was the director of chemotherapy research at Sloan-Kettering, and head of its suburban Walker Laboratory. Originally an expert on insect control, he had switched to cancer research and for decades had supervised much of the animal testing of new drugs for Sloan-Kettering.

Stock attempted to explain some of the finer details of the testing, but as his voice droned on, the eyes of many turned toward another man to his left: a small, old Japanese scientist in a white lab coat, sitting upright and impassive, blinking at the lights through thick, rimless glasses.

When Stock finished and the conference was thrown open for questions, the first one was for this elderly gentleman, eighty-six-year-old member emeritus of Sloan-Kettering, Dr. Kanematsu Sugiura. Most of those present were aware of reports circulating for years that Sugiura had claimed positive results with laetrile in his animal experiments.

His presence on the dais this morning seemed, perhaps, to imply that he too now agreed with the negative verdict on laetrile.

"Dr. Sugiura," someone shouted out suddenly. "Do you stick by your belief that laetrile stops the spread of cancer?"

The television cameras swung in the old man's direction and began purring.

"I stick!" Sugiura shot back, in a voice startlingly loud and assertive. It was clear that rebellion still continued in the ranks of Sloan-Kettering on the emotional question of laetrile.

It is difficult to imagine a less likely rebel than Dr. Kanematsu Sugiura. Born in Japan in 1892, Sugiura had always been a grateful and loyal beneficiary of the establishment. He was brought to America by the railroad tycoon E. H. Harriman as a member of the first jiu-jitsu team ever to tour the United States. In 1905 he even performed at the White House for President Teddy Roosevelt. Sugiura proudly showed visitors pictures of himself as a handsome, athletic young man, standing barefoot in the snow in his *kendo* uniform (Sugiura, 1971).

After performing at many private homes and clubs, the entire team went home to Japan—all except young Sugiura, who chose to stay on as the house guest of Harriman's personal physician, Dr. William G. Lyle.

Although Sugiura was terribly homesick, he knew that this was the only way he would be able to get an education, since his father was a poor fencing master in Japan, and could not afford to send him to school.

Sugiura's interest in science began early. After his day's study at Townsend Harris Hall high school in New York City, a school which specialized in training gifted young students, he would go to work at Roosevelt Hospital, where he would wash instruments, scrub containers, and help doctors with their experiments.

In 1909 E. H. Harriman died of cancer and left $1 million to establish a cancer research laboratory at Roosevelt Hospital. Dr. Lyle became its director, and in 1911 young Sugiura became assistant chemist at the newly formed Harriman Research Laboratory.

In the next year, Kanematsu Sugiura began his first experiments in the chemotherapy of cancer with colleagues at Harriman and at Cornell University Medical College. At the time, he was only twenty years old and hadn't even begun college. In those days, cancer chemotherapy was a highly unusual and unorthodox procedure, frowned upon by the surgeons who then held surgery and radiation to be the only acceptable methods of treatment.

By 1917 Sugiura had received college degrees from the Polytechnic Institute of Brooklyn and from Columbia University, and was fully launched on his career as a cancer chemotherapist.[*] His lifetime in the field thus spanned the entire history of modern chemotherapy, and his work touched most of the chief areas of research and progress.

Sugiura's main influence was in developing the techniques of cancer research in rats and mice, and then in testing a wide variety of chemical and biological compounds in these mice to see if they had an anticancer effect. In the pre–World War I days, Sugiura and his colleagues tested various inorganic compounds on cancerous animals. They were able to demonstrate that such chemicals did have a small, but real, anticancer effect in laboratory animals. These findings helped overcome skepticism about chemotherapy in medical circles and spurred interest in finding even more active chemicals.

In 1917, however, the Harriman family suddenly lost interest in cancer research and turned to politics. (E. H. Harriman's son William Averell later became governor of New York.) The Harriman Research Laboratory closed its doors, and the various staff members were forced to seek positions elsewhere (ibid.).

On November 1, 1917, Dr. Sugiura came to Memorial Hospital, then under the direction of Dr. James Ewing, to work as an assistant chemist. (Before the founding of Sloan-Kettering Institute in 1945, both research and treatment were done at Memorial Hospital.) Rec-

---

[*] In 1925 he also received a doctorate in science from Kyoto Imperial University in Japan *(New York Times,* October 23, 1979).

ognizing Sugiura's talent, Ewing quickly sent him to the Crocker Laboratory of Columbia University to learn the new techniques of tumor transplantation being developed there.

In the early days of 1917, the question of diet and cancer was receiving a great deal of attention, spurred by the wide-scale malnutrition caused by World War I. Reports had also begun to reach the industrially developed countries that the peoples in underdeveloped areas of Africa, India, and the East Indian Islands rarely developed cancer. Sugiura, who maintained a lifelong interest in nutrition, began to perform research in this field. He fed mice which had received transplantable tumors a diet composed solely of bananas—since bananas formed the basis of some tropical diets. The tumors grew very slowly. However, when Sugiura added protein and yeast, the tumors grew at a normal rate.

Another interesting experiment involved keeping the mice on a starvation diet. Mice fed one-third the normal amount of food showed much less tumor growth than animals fed normal rations. These studies were then extended to mice which had first had their tumors removed surgically. Sugiura found that if he then underfed the mice, few new tumors occurred either at the site of the operation or elsewhere (ibid.).

This early work on diet and cancer was greeted with little enthusiasm by the surgeons and radiologists of Memorial Hospital. There were a few halfhearted tries at applying this knowledge in the clinic, but, by and large, doctors scoffed at the idea of "starving" an already weakened cancer patient. In fact, physicians who insisted that there could be a link between faulty dietary habits and the rising rate of cancer were looked upon as quacks (Sugiura, 1974).

A shy and retiring man, Sugiura never became embroiled in the controversies which raged over the link between diet and cancer. He remained aloof, and seemingly unaware of the larger issues involved. He was the laboratory scientist par excellence, content if he were left alone to do his work.

In the 1920s and 1930s, Sugiura studied the effects of such substances as coal tar–based dyes, hormones, and enzymes on cancer growth. He performed experiments which showed that butter-yellow dye caused cancer in experimental animals. This led to the dye's removal from the food supply. Again, however, he shunned the limelight, and was never involved in the fierce controversy over this concept.

Despite the fact that he had lived in this country for many decades, and had a daughter born in the United States, Sugiura was suddenly threatened with internment in a concentration camp with other Japanese after Pearl Harbor. Intervention by Dr. C. P. Rhoads,

Memorial's director, at the "highest levels of government" prevented this; Sugiura was "merely" placed under house arrest (*New York Times*, October 23, 1979).

Sugiura was therefore officially restricted to his apartment on the Grand Concourse in the Bronx for the duration of the war. He used to "wander" away, however, to do research at the New York Academy of Medicine or at the old, and by then largely abandoned, Memorial Hospital on 104th Street. Sixty-eighth Street, where the new hospital was located, was off limits to him (Sugiura, 1974).

After the war, the entire scientific structure changed at the Memorial Center, as it was then known. Whereas previously the scientific as well as the clinical work had been done at Memorial Hospital, most of the laboratory research was transferred to Sloan-Kettering Institute after 1945. Sugiura was transferred as well and was made an associate member (later, a full member) of Sloan-Kettering.

C. Chester Stock was put in charge of a massive campaign to test thousands of compounds in an empirical search for a cancer cure. Sugiura now worked under him. Various drugs currently in use were discovered during this period, including methotrexate and the antibiotic mitomycin C.

In 1962 Sugiura officially retired and became member emeritus. In 1965 Dr. Stock helped gather Sugiura's more than 200 papers into a four-volume *Collected Works*. His introductory remarks summed up world scientific opinion about Sugiura:

> Few, if any, names in cancer research are as widely known as Kanematsu Sugiura's. . . . Possibly the high regard in which his work is held is best characterized by a comment made to me by a visiting investigator in cancer research from Russia. He said, "When Dr. Sugiura publishes, we know we don't have to repeat the study, for we would obtain the same results he has reported" (Sugiura, 1965).

A decade later, Sugiura was a "fixture" at the Walker Laboratory of Sloan-Kettering Institute in Rye, New York. He had an office on the second floor, which he shared with scientist Isabel Mountain. Every day he arrived at the low-lying suburban building at 8:00 A.M. Every day at 5:00 P.M. he left for his home in a nearby Westchester town, where he lived with his wife and daughter and her husband, Sloan-Kettering scientist Franz Schmid.

Sugiura had lived a long and full life, had been honored by his peers, and was well known and respected in both his adopted and his native land. He had even received the Order of Sacred Treasure, third class, in 1960 from Emperor Hirohito of Japan for his contributions to medical research (*New York Times*, October 23, 1979).

By every indication, Sugiura would end his life as peacefully and quietly as he had lived it, content with his half-page niche in the National Cancer Institute–sponsored history of cancer research (Shimkin, 1977:404).

Instead, by 1973 Sugiura found himself unintentionally and uncomfortably the center of a furious controversy. Because he had merely done what he was told and recorded what he saw, he lived to see old friends desert and berate him, a close relative fail to support him, and former colleagues derisively question his sanity and competence.

What Sugiura did was to agree to test amygdalin (laetrile) in spontaneous animal tumors in the fall of 1972. In previous months, at the explicit request of the head of the President's Cancer Panel, Benno Schmidt, Sloan-Kettering had undertaken extensive tests of laetrile in transplantable tumor systems. The chemical failed to have any effects at all, thereby confirming all the statements and predictions made by orthodoxy about this "quack" remedy over a twenty-five-year period (*Science,* December 7, 1973).

But some scientists felt that transplantable tumors were not really similar to those which afflict the human cancer victim. What was needed was a more natural, spontaneous cancer that would simulate the clinical situation. Sloan-Kettering therefore obtained mice with spontaneous breast cancers from Dr. Daniel Martin of the Catholic Medical Center and gave them to its most experienced experimenter, Sugiura, for the testing of laetrile.

"Laetrile can't work on transplantable tumors," Dr. Sugiura said in 1974, in the course of a taped interview planned for the employee newspaper, MSKCC *Center News* (Sugiura, 1974).

"When I use it on a large spontaneous mammary tumor like this"—he made a circle with his thumb and forefinger about the size of a dime—"it has no effect. But a small tumor like *this*"—he made a tiny circle—"about one centimeter in diameter, laetrile stops the growth. Not permanently, but for a week, two weeks, three weeks. . . ."

"The most interesting part is metastases." (Metastases are secondary growths that come off the primary tumor and invade other areas of the body. Such secondary growths are often more lethal than the original tumor.) "When this mammary tumor grows to about two centimeters in diameter or more, about 80 percent develop lung metastases. But with treatment with amygdalin, it's cut down to about 20 percent" (ibid.).

"With all these positive results why is there all this controversy?" Sugiura was asked during the interview.

"Many people still doubt my work, and so I show them all my

work in this book—you see," and Sugiura took down from the shelf above him a volume, one in a long, uniform set of laboratory books, going back decades. "I keep records like this," he said, thumbing through the pages. "Here, amygdalin—"

The emeritus scientist pointed to pictures of small mice, each with an irregular circle on its breast—the outline of a tumor. The pictures were made with a rubber stamp Sugiura had used for over forty years. He used the stamped outline of a mouse, and drew in not only the size of a tumor but its location on the body, in the belief that the location of the tumor might influence the curative ability of the drug in question.

In addition, Sugiura said, the laetrile-treated mice definitely seemed healthier and friskier than the saline-treated control mice. These results seemed remarkably similar to the reports of tumor growth inhibition and pain relief then filtering across the border from Tijuana, Mexico. Sugiura was therefore asked what he thought of these anecdotal reports.

"I think there must be some benefit. Dr. Old believes it," Sugiura added quickly. Dr. Lloyd J. Old was, with Stock, one of the two vice-presidents of Sloan-Kettering Institute. "I think most people in this institution don't believe my work, although I show them results like this" (ibid.). Sugiura laughed sadly.

The senior researcher was asked if he had published any of these results.

"No, not yet." He hesitated, then said: "I'd like to, but it's up to the people 'downtown.' " (In Walker Laboratory parlance, "downtown" means SKI headquarters in Manhattan) "Dr. Old, Dr. Stock, if they want to publish it, they'll publish it." It would never have occurred to Sugiura to publish the results independently.

"Are you still doing work on amygdalin?" he was next asked.

"Oh, yes, I'm now doing work on prevention. In the first experiments [i.e., the first six treatment experiments] the mice already had tumors, see? But in the latest experiment the mice have no tumors. At four months old, with no tumors, I started to inject amygdalin to see whether or not mammary cancer develops. These are strains of mice that are sure to get cancer in about 80 to 85 percent of the cases, during a lifetime of from two to two and a half years. Now it's eighteen months and we've gone through three-quarters of their life span and I have found that the controls, receiving only saline injections, developed cancer in fifteen out of thirty cases. But the experimental animals, receiving laetrile, have developed only six tumors out of thirty mice, or about 20 percent."

"It would be interesting if it prevented it completely," Sugiura said, in a massive understatement. "One hundred percent prevention would be very interesting—then it would convince everybody. I never heard of anybody trying to repeat my experiment," he added. "Somebody should repeat my work," Sugiura said emphatically. "Not from this institution, somewhere else, a different institution."

Sugiura then drew a parallel between his own difficulties and those of William B. Coley, whom he had known at the old Memorial for twenty years.

"Nowadays, natural things are coming back, more and more," Sugiura said. "Dr. Coley was working before 1900 with toxins prepared from bacteria. Doctors used to laugh at Coley as 'nonsense.' Now it's no longer nonsense. Bacterial toxins contain polysaccharides, which inhibit the growth of tumors in animals. Japanese scientists are finding that polysaccharides prepared from mushrooms can destroy tumors in mice.

"Amygdalin, too—people now are laughing at that, especially the director of the National Cancer Institute [Frank Rauscher] and the American Cancer Society. They even wrote a book, *Unproven Methods of Cancer Management,* with chapters on Coley's toxins, laetrile, and so forth."

"Why are they so much against it?" Sugiura was asked.

"I don't know. Maybe the medical profession doesn't like it because they are making too much money" (ibid.).

Although Sugiura's experiments were unpublished, they were no secret to the leaders of Memorial Sloan-Kettering Cancer Center. The elderly scientist had first achieved positive results with the apricot-kernel extract in the fall of 1972. In the summer of 1973, these first results were "leaked" from Sloan-Kettering itself and used in a court case on behalf of Dr. John Richardson, then accused of violating the California antiquackery statutes *(Science,* December 7, 1973).

The positive results had been reported by Harry Nelson of the *Los Angeles Times* and Barbara Culliton of *Science* magazine. In the latter piece, Dr. Good had expressed an open-minded attitude toward the testing of all unorthodox methods, including laetrile.

Following the leak, the MSKCC Public Affairs Department had drawn up a cautious official statement for distribution:

The Sugiura report is preliminary and part of a broad ongoing scientific inquiry. It would be premature at this time to draw specific conclusions on the basis of the Sugiura report (MSKCC, 1973).

Nevertheless, the attitude of MSKCC leaders toward laetrile and its advocates was definitely open and inquisitive. In November 1973 the Institute sent Lloyd Schloen, Ph.D., a young biochemist then working on laetrile under the direction of Dr. Lloyd Old, to the International Medical Society for Blood and Tumorous Disease Congress in Baden-Baden, West Germany, to report on the positive laetrile findings. Cancer researchers from more than fifteen countries were present *(Madison* [Wisc.] *Capital Times*, November 3, 1973).

About six hundred health professionals listened as Schloen detailed Sloan-Kettering's success with laetrile. Characteristic of the relaxed atmosphere then prevailing, Schloen was accompanied by Dean Burk and Raymond Brown, M.D., an aide to SKI vice-president Old. Both of these men were considered advocates of unorthodox methods.

Schloen's statement to the congress, however, was a watered-down version of his original text. "Every hour on the hour [Schloen] was getting telephone calls from Sloan-Kettering to keep taking this out, and that out," Burk recalls. "There wasn't too much left when he got through" (Burk, 1977).

Despite this, enthusiasm for laetrile seemed to mount throughout 1973 and 1974. A "Laetrile Task Force" was created at SKI, and prominent members of the unorthodox community were welcomed on the thirteenth floor of the Howard Building—SKI headquarters. The minutes of one "meeting on amygdalin" (July 10, 1973) shows the following individuals in attendance: Dr. Old, Dr. Brown, New York Cancer Research Institute Fellow, Dr. Burk, Dr. Ernesto Contreras, the prominent Mexican laetrilist, Dr. Contreras's son, Dr. Raymond Ewell, a retired University of Buffalo professor interested in unorthodox approaches, Dr. Good, Dr. Vincent F. Lisanti, of the Council for Tobacco Research, Mr. Andrew McNaughton, sponsor of the laetrile movement, Mrs. Helen Coley Nauts, Dr. Morton K. Schwartz, a MSKCC biochemist, and Dr. C. Chester Stock. Dr. Old, the new vice-president, was chairman of the meeting, and believed to be the driving spirit behind this unprecedented reconciliation effort (Sloan-Kettering Institute, 1973).

Yet many at Sloan-Kettering were disturbed at Old's apparent drift toward unorthodoxy. "Had Good chosen Andrew Ivy, promoter of the discredited cancer drug Krebiozen as his deputy, the reaction of some members [of SKI] could not have been more categorically negative," says a former MSKCC official (Hixson, 1976a).

Simultaneously, advocates of other unorthodox approaches, such as Virginia Livingston, Eleanor Alexander-Jackson, Joseph Gold, and Hans Nieper, were also invited to Sloan-Kettering. The "Vatican of cancer research" also sent an observer to the convention of the International Association of Cancer Victims and Friends, a pro-laetrile organization (Schloen, 1973).

This détente with the unorthodox was a highly unstable affair from the beginning. It had no wide base of support at Sloan-Kettering, for relatively few scientists and staff members were invited to these meetings on the thirteenth floor of the Howard Building. Of those invited, some were disinterested or downright hostile, including those most closely tied to the current methods of treating cancer, such as the chemotherapists.

The main support for the new policy seems to have come from a few top administrators, especially Robert Good and his deputy, Lloyd Old. Not surprisingly, within about a year, the new policy had collapsed. The would-be innovators were back in the fold, condemning methods they once had greeted enthusiastically.

In retrospect, this change appears to have been the result of powerful economic and political forces which tended to discourage serious investigation of unorthodox approaches. At the time, however, a single incident triggered a retrenchment on the part of Sloan-Kettering's more innovative leadership.

In April 1974 the world was shocked by a scientific scandal at Sloan-Kettering Institute. Known as the "Summerlin painted-mouse affair," this bizarre story of cheating in high places raised serious questions about the conduct of cancer research in general, and about Sloan-Kettering's behavior in particular.

William Summerlin was a thirty-five-year-old dermatologist with a promising future. A protégé of Dr. Good's, (Good who had been appointed president of SKI only one year before), Summerlin had been brought in as a full member and made head of a clinical department at adjacent Memorial Hospital (Hixson, 1976a).

Most researchers spend decades working their way up the ladder until they became full members (the equivalent of professor). Dr. Sugiura, for example, had been at MSKCC *forty years* before attaining this honor. Summerlin's instant success stirred resentment at the Institute.

Dr. Summerlin's success was due to a novel application of a technique known as "tissue culturing." Using this technique, the young doctor claimed to be able to take skin, or other tissues, from one person and make them "stick" to another person. He backed up his claims with dramatic animal work: white mice which showed dark blotches of black skin, from unrelated other mice, on their backs.

Generally, skin from one animal will not make a permanent graft to another animal. After a temporary attachment, it becomes inflamed, ulcerates, and falls off. This is because the immune system of the receiver recognizes the new skin as foreign and rejects it. (The main exceptions to this rule are identical twins in humans and inbred strains in mice.)

By tissue culturing—first soaking pieces of skin in a special bath—

Summerlin claimed to be able to make these transplants "take" perfectly.

The implications of this work were revolutionary. At the present time, organ transplants are difficult and precarious, since the recipient's immune system will often reject the new organ as foreign in short order. To prevent this, the patient is given drugs to suppress the immune system. But these drugs have many drawbacks, one of which is heightening a patient's susceptibility to cancer. If Summerlin's technique were valid, organ transplants might have become relatively common and easy. Cancer patients, for example, whose disease had not spread beyond a single organ, could receive a suitable replacement—provided that replacement had first been soaked for a while in Summerlin's magic fluid. Burn victims would also be major beneficiaries of the new technique.

The Summerlin technique also had major theoretical importance. Cancer, after all, is a kind of foreign tissue in the body. If Summerlin had figured out what made the body accept a new piece of skin as its own, perhaps others could figure out why the body of a cancer patient accepts his tumor. Clearly, then, Summerlin had a big idea.

For Summerlin himself these ideas and claims had already taken him farther than most thirty-five-year-olds ever dream of getting: to a top post at a world-famous private research center.

Other scientists were watching Summerlin's ideas with great interest. Surgeons, for example, would benefit enormously by these new techniques. In fact, the entire medical world was buzzing with news of the imminent breakthrough at Sloan-Kettering.

But, above all, Dr. Good was at Summerlin's side, directing him, encouraging him, coauthoring his papers. Good had been brought in by the MSKCC trustees to make such breakthroughs and firmly reestablish SKI as *the* leading cancer research center, a position in jeopardy because of the government's recent largess to other institutes. What better way to prove his worth than with this startling finding?

It was no secret, either, that Good was hoping for a Nobel Prize in medicine. He had made several important discoveries in the field of immunology, but none of them seemed to warrant the prize. Sponsorship of Summerlin's work would have been a crowning achievement for the Minnesota pediatrician.

In 1973–74, at the same time that Lloyd Old was advocating the testing of unproven therapies, Good was trumpeting Summerlin's work. About this work, *Time* magazine wrote, in a cover story on the director, "No one appreciates [its] potential more than Good, . . ." who predicted that, as part of immunology, "it will enable us to understand the basic processes of life" (March 19, 1973).

In the middle of 1973, however, scientists began to write to Summerlin and Good that they could not reproduce the young dermatologist's techniques or results. Yet no one made these doubts public. Dr. Peter Medawar, a member of the SKI Board of Scientific Consultants, and a Nobel Prize winner, later explained why *he* had not said anything to contradict Summerlin, despite strong doubts at the time:

I simply lacked the moral courage to say at the time that I thought we were the victims of a hoax or a confidence trick. It is easy in theory to say these things, but in practice very senior scientists do not like trampling on their juniors in public *(New York Review of Books,* April 15, 1976).

Medawar certainly deserves credit for his honesty in admitting this. Nevertheless, it is quite revealing of the way frauds and cover-ups can be perpetrated in high places.

Good now put pressure on Summerlin to reproduce his famous results. This Summerlin could not do—perhaps because they were faked from the start, or perhaps because they were simply a one-time "fluke" which he didn't know how to repeat.

The showdown came on the morning of March 26, 1974. In the elevator of the Howard Building, on his way to Good's office, Summerlin quickly painted black splotches on two white mice with a felt-tip pen. The touch-up job escaped Good's notice. But an astute animal handler noticed the unusual patches while he was taking the mice back to their cages. Using a little alcohol, he removed the ink markings and immediately notified several young doctors working with Summerlin (Hixson, 1976a).

These doctors then went to Good and told him of the fakery. Good in turn informed Lewis Thomas, president of the Center. The recently appointed public affairs director, T. Gerald Delaney, was also brought in on the secret.

Suddenly, Summerlin's spectacular "breakthrough" had become a major problem for the new administration. Instead of confronting the issue head-on, however, the administration sat on the story for weeks.

"No written word about the trouble circulated within or outside the institution," wrote Joseph Hixson in his 1976 book on the scandal, *The Patchwork Mouse.* Delaney was simply given a short statement to read to the press "in case there was a leak."

As long as there was no leak, however, the administration said nothing, and there is no indication they ever intended to say anything to the public unless they were forced to do so. Finally, almost three weeks later, somebody tipped off the *New York Post*'s science reporter, who broke the story (ibid.).

A peer review committee was appointed by Good, made up of five long-time members of the Institute: Drs. Stock, Burchenal, Clarkson, Sonenberg, and Boyse. This committee issued a lengthy report which gave a detailed history of the facts of the case, seen from the administration's point of view.

The committee concluded, basically, that Summerlin was entirely to blame for the incident: "In several instances Dr. Summerlin did indeed grossly mislead his colleagues" (ibid.). They attributed Summerlin's fraud to such things as his personal "disarray," the "desultory conduct of his everyday affairs," and other aberrations. After lengthy consultations with lawyers, Summerlin was declared to be mentally unbalanced. He was dismissed, but given $40,000 severance pay (one year's salary) and told to see a psychiatrist (ibid.).

Summerlin is currently a practicing dermatologist in the South. Like former President Richard Nixon, he had "suffered enough" and never faced any charges from the medical society or the state.

The peer review committee exonerated Good of any guilt, although his name was on the fraudulent papers and shortly before Summerlin's downfall he had presented the young dermatologist's work at a scientific soirée thrown by the American Cancer Society's Mary Lasker (ibid.:106).

The only criticism of Good was for "prematurely" promoting the young researcher to full membership and for "undue publicity surrounding Dr. Summerlin's claims, unsupported as they were by adequate authenticated data." This criticism focused on individuals, but sidestepped the significance of such fraud for the "war on cancer," which was just then attempting to get into stride.

Prominent scientists noted at the time, however, that "the episode reflected dangerous trends in current efforts to gain scientific acclaim and funds for research, as well as the possible misdirection of research at Sloan-Kettering itself" (*New York Times*, April 17, 1974). It followed by only a year the Zinder Report, which had discovered evidence of financial irregularities in the government's virus program (see Chapter 1).

Science magazine pointed out that "Sloan-Kettering, these days, is not a happy place. It is rich and getting richer, but not happy. . . . It appears that a high-pressure environment that drives individuals to exaggeration and fosters hostility is not ideal for the kind of achievements in research that Good, like everyone else, would like to see" (May 10, 1974).

Summerlin himself later alleged there was a "pressure-cooker atmosphere" at SKI. He blamed his problems on the "frenetic situation" at the Institute and especially on the "extreme pressure put on me by the Institute director to publicize information . . ." (Hixson, 1976a:101).

The Summerlin affair was a major embarrassment for Sloan-Kettering, and especially for its new director. It put a damper on the enthusiasm for new research and reestablished the position of the conservatives who had viewed Dr. Old's ascent to vice-presidency with trepidation.

Laetrile testing thus got caught up in the Summerlin backlash. Good, who had said "we will test anything," became susceptible to pressure from outside and within to bring this open-minded policy to an end.

The evidence for such pressure is not merely anecdotal. In the course of researching a story on the unorthodox German Janker Clinic, Pat McGrady, Jr., son of the former ACS official, happened upon a revealing letter in the files on unproven methods at the American Cancer Society's headquarters. Before he could be stopped, he had copied the text and later reprinted it in a leading magazine. Written in January 1974 by ACS executive vice-president Arthur Holleb (a former Memorial Hospital breast surgeon) to Good, it appears to be an attempt to bring Sloan-Kettering under ACS's umbrella, at least on the question of the unproven methods:

I wish I knew how one could better control the unfortunate and premature publicity which links my distinguished alma mater to the promotional side of these unproven methods. We have both agreed that the public will be best served if tests are properly conducted in a prestigious institution, but the exploitation of the good name of the Sloan-Kettering Institute is becoming embarrassing. Perhaps your staff would be willing to consult with us and review our files before commitments are made (cited in McGrady, Jr., 1976).

There is no open threat here. Nevertheless, it could not have failed to escape Good's notice that ACS contributed almost $1 million a year to Sloan-Kettering at a time when MSKCC itself was suffering from what officials called a "disquieting deficit of $5 million" due to "expansion of research programs for which funding was simply not available" (MSKCC *Center News*, January, 1975).

On January 10, 1974, Dr. Good declared that "at this moment there is no evidence that laetrile has any effect on cancer." Most of Sugiura's highly positive results were already in the files, however. Shortly afterward, Dr. Holleb of the American Cancer Society told reporters at the ACS Science Writers' Seminar that "subsequent tests could not confirm the initial results" of Sugiura. The story was carried nationwide with such headlines as "Cancer 'Drug' Called Worthless" *(New York Daily News,* March 25, 1974).

Other establishment leaders also stepped up the attack on laetrile, completely ignoring the positive SKI data. "Every study to date has not found any evidence of efficacy" with laetrile, Dr. Alexander M. Schmidt, then commissioner of the FDA, told reporters on March 25, 1974. "If there was one shred of evidence from animal or cell systems I would issue an IND," that is, permission to test the substance in humans (Burk, 1974b).

A week later, Frank Rauscher, Ph.D., then director of the National Cancer Institute, said on the *60 Minutes* television show, "I would certainly not turn off laetrile if it had an iota of activity that we could pinpoint. Unfortunately, there's no evidence at all" (ibid.).

Dr. Jesse L. Steinfeld, former Surgeon General and an anti-laetrilist since the early 1950s, said, "There is no basis for the use of laetrile in man based on data derived from experiments in animals" (ibid.).

And Dr. Charles Moertel of the Mayo Clinic said, "Extensive animal tumor studies conducted independently at two outstanding cancer research centers—New York Memorial Sloan-Kettering and the Southern Research Institute—have shown this drug to be totally without evidence of anticancer activity" (ibid.).

How could Sloan-Kettering's leaders allow other prominent members of the establishment to so distort its own research findings? And how did these leaders get the idea that laetrile had, in fact, been proven ineffective? Was it the result of Dr. Good's January 10 statement, cited above?

No clear answers have emerged to these puzzling questions. One possibility, however, is that these statements coincided with MSKCC's difficulties with the Summerlin affair. Perhaps the New York leaders were unable to defend themselves at this critical juncture, and therefore the misleading or uninformed statements slipped by unchallenged.

In an apparent effort to set the record straight, however, a meeting was held at the Food and Drug Administration headquarters in Beltsville, Maryland, on July 2, 1974. According to the minutes of that meeting (obtained under the Freedom of Information Act by Representative John Kelsey of the Michigan House of Representatives), Sloan-Kettering leaders still maintained their belief in laetrile's effectiveness, as shown by Sugiura's studies (FDA, 1974).

The top leaders of MSKCC were present—Good, Old, Stock, and Lewis Thomas, president of MSKCC. In addition, a dozen other establishment leaders from the FDA and NCI were also in attendance.

Dr. Good emphasized that "studies on amygdalin are a *small* part of Sloan-Kettering's program" (emphasis in original), no doubt to correct the opposite impression circulating among the doyens of orthodoxy. Lloyd Old then presented the case for laetrile. He recounted his search for clinicians who had actually used the substance. According to the minutes:

Dr. Old has written to several world users of laetrile, including Drs. Contreras and Niepes [Nieper] and others. He found two groups: (1) Those who used it and found it of value [i.e., Contreras] and (2) Those who had *not* used it and did not believe in it (ibid.).

Old confirmed Sloan-Kettering's belief that laetrile had no effect on transplantable tumors but presented data, complete with accompanying charts, from Sugiura's studies to show that laetrile "inhibited metastases to the lung."

He even implied that laetrile might be useful against other chronic diseases:

It was mentioned that amygdalin may be useful in sickle cell anemia because of thiocyanate levels. The Sloan-Kettering group believe their results show that amygdalin used in animals with tumors show: a decrease in lung metastases; slower tumor growth; and pain relief. The Sloan-Kettering group are thinking of a study in man on pain relief (ibid.). °

After this buildup for amygdalin at the FDA meeting, it is rather curious to read:

Sloan-Kettering is not enthusiastic about studying amygdalin but would like to study CN [cyanide] releasing drugs (ibid.).

Such drugs could be patented and marketed in conventional channels and would have the additional advantage of unequivocally coming under the jurisdiction of the FDA, a point that would hardly need emphasizing in that company. Laetrilists had in fact postulated exactly such a scenario, in which laetrile's name and chemical structure would be modified by Sloan-Kettering in order to make it more acceptable to market forces (Griffin, 1975:464).

At the conclusion of the FDA meeting everything seemed encouraging. The final proposals indicated that the meeting and the presentation had been a success for SKI's leaders:

A discussion ensued on where we should go from here. Agreements: (a) Sloan-Kettering Institute and NCI will consider clinical trials aimed at treatment of cancer and for the relief of pain and will request consultation

° The idea of laetrile as possibly useful in sickle cell anemia was first proposed by Robert Houston in 1973, based on a hypothesis of Ernst T. Krebs, Jr. (Houston, 1974).

with ACS; (b) There are no regulatory policy problems preventing the study of amygdalin in man; (c) A standard scientific approach to studying amygdalin is recommended, meaning the drug should be worked up by standard approaches; (d) FDA will publicly endorse good research on amygdalin as in the public interest (FDA, 1974).

None of these proposals was carried through. It was to be four years before a new director of NCI called for clinical trials aimed at treatment of cancer and for the relief of pain. The FDA never came out for good research on amygdalin; on the contrary, it maintained its stand that laetrile has been adequately tested and found without an iota of value. Nor did the FDA declare publicly that there were no regulatory policy problems preventing the study of amygdalin in man. On the contrary, it maintained that such studies would be unethical.

How were these excellent proposals sabotaged, and by whom? There is a gap in our information here: we just do not know.

During the remainder of 1974 and 1975, in fact, the controversy only heightened. Sugiura continued to get positive results, this time adding the AKR system to his growing list of experiments. In these mice, doomed to die of leukemia, he saw a decided shrinkage of the swollen internal organs, the spleen, thymus, and the lymph nodes. This is normally taken as a sign of anticancer effects by cancer researchers (Kassel et al., 1977).

In preliminary tests, other SKI researchers, had also gotten highly positive results with laetrile. Dr. Lloyd Schloen, the same man whom SKI had sent as its spokesman to Baden-Baden, had reproduced Sugiura's results in Swiss albino mice. All of the mice receiving the highest dose of amygdalin were healthy at the time of "sacrifice" (death); all of those receiving lower doses, or only a saline injection, were sick. In addition, in one small experiment combining laetrile and an enzyme (after the manner of Hans Nieper, whom Schloen had visited in Germany), the young researcher got 100 percent cures. Dr. Elizabeth Stockert, another SKI researcher, got 25 percent cures in the same way (Second Opinion, 1977).

Stockert, however, entered the lists *against* Sugiura in March 1975, when she failed to confirm his experiments with the CD_8F_1 mice. Sugiura felt that she was unable to do so because she failed to follow the protocols of his experiments. In particular, Sugiura always used a microscope to examine the mice's lungs and considered microscopic evaluation the *sine qua non* of all such research. Stockert chose not to use a microscope at all and relied instead on gross visual observations (ibid.).

Another problem—at least early in the year—was the inability of another SKI researcher to duplicate Sugiura's work. This researcher was Walker veterinarian Franz Schmid, Sugiura's son-in-law, who also worked under Stock. In his first test, Schmid also did not use the microscope and was not able to confirm Sugiura's results. In this experiment, however, the treated mice lived somewhat longer than the controls.

In Schmid's second experiment, he used a dose which was one-fiftieth of Sugiura's. This dosage had been suggested by Dr. Stock, who felt that it was more analogous to the amounts being received by humans in the laetrile clinics. Again, there was no positive effect on metastases, according to Schmid's "eyeball" observations, but the laetrile-treated mice lived 50 percent longer. Nevertheless, the experiment was interpreted as a failure for laetrile, and no one outside the Institute knew that the treated mice had lived longer until a reporter extracted that information from Dr. Stock more than a year later. Nor was it generally known that Schmid had used a fractional dose (ibid.).

Far more serious a challenge to laetrile was presented by the appearance of Dr. Daniel S. Martin of the Catholic Medical Center, Queens, New York. Martin had supplied the mice for the early Sugiura experiments and had taken part in the first collaborative experiment which ended inconclusively.

In 1974 Martin had performed his own experiment with laetrile which, he claimed, had disproven Sugiura's contention. A study of this 1974 experiment showed that he changed a number of elements in Sugiura's original protocol (ibid.). Despite these changes, Martin publicly proclaimed that he had evidence that Sugiura was wrong.

Late in 1974, Sugiura traveled to Queens to take part in another collaborative test with Martin. Martin declared the experiment further proof that laetrile did not work. On the other hand, Sugiura pointed out that *even by visual examination,* there were twice as many metastases in the animals which did not receive laetrile as in those that did.

The issue might have been settled by recourse to a microscope—the most common way of determining whether or not secondary growths are present. But Martin did not believe in using the microscope to make such determinations. He relied on a relatively less common test called a "bioassay." * By this bioassay test, Martin claimed there was no difference between the treated and the control animals.

---

* In the bioassay, as was used by Martin, "All the lungs of each animal are shredded (by scissors) and injected subcutaneously into two male CD_8F_1 mice. . . . If a tumor subsequently arises at an injection site, it indicates that cancer cells (at least 10^5 cells) were present in the lungs" (Second Opinion, 1977).

One could hardly imagine a greater contrast than that which existed between these two scientists, Sugiura and Martin. Sugiura, who died on October 22, 1979, at the age of eighty-seven, was modest and deferential, a retiring scholar content to perform his humdrum tasks day-in and day-out for over sixty years. Martin, chairman of the Committee on Unorthodox Therapies of the American Society of Clinical Oncology, was outspoken and assertive. While Sugiura talked in hushed tones to his friends and colleagues, Martin blared his opposition to the world at scientific meetings, on the Op-Ed page of *The New York Times*, and in public debates.

"I flatfootedly and categorically tell you," Martin once said, "that laetrile is without activity against spontaneous tumors in mice—period" *(Medical World News,* October 26, 1975). "Laetrile has been found absolutely devoid of activity, period. It's just that simple" (MSKCC, 1977c). When *Science* magazine asked him if the Sloan-Kettering tests weren't addressed to scientists, he replied, "Oh, nonsense. Of course this was done to help people like [Benno] Schmidt and congressmen answer the laetrilists" *(Science,* December 23, 1977). Benno Schmidt is an investment banker who serves as vice-chairman of Memorial Sloan-Kettering Cancer Center and head of the President's Cancer Panel (see Appendix A).

Despite Martin's outspoken opposition, by 1975 Lloyd Old and others were back at work trying to push quietly forward with a clinical trial of laetrile. Two Mexican oncologists, Dr. Mario Soto de Leon and a colleague, went to SKI and arranged for the Institute to collaborate in a clinical trial of laetrile on Mexican government workers with cancer.

Old wrote Soto on January 24, 1975:

It was indeed a pleasure to have you and Dr. Sanen visit our Institute and share with us your clinical experience with amygdalin in cancer patients. I was pleased to hear from Dr. Sanen that our proposed collaborative controlled trials have the approval of your hospital. We are looking forward to a fruitful exchange of information (Committee for Freedom of Choice, 1975).

No such trials took place. Again, it is not clear who or what aborted this plan. However, the schism within orthodoxy was clearly growing. On March 4, 1975, another meeting was called, this one at the National Cancer Institute's headquarters in Bethesda, Maryland, "to decide on what further course of action should be undertaken with this controversial compound" (Stephen Carter, 1975).

Thirty-two top cancer establishment figures were present, including the director of the National Cancer Institute and eighteen of his assistants, six top leaders of MSKCC—this time including a surgeon and a chemotherapist—and officials of the FDA, the ACS, and the Mayo Clinic. Finally, there was Dr. Martin.

Once again, and for the last time as it turned out, Sloan-Kettering's leaders defended Sugiura's work. Lloyd Old summarized Sloan-Kettering's results:

(1) No tumor regression was observed.
(2) There is a variable slowing of primary tumor growth.
(3) There is a decrease in the incidence of pulmonary toxicity [i.e., metastases] from roughly 80% to 20%.
(4) There is no evidence of toxicity (Stephen Carter, 1975).

This time, however, unlike at the FDA meeting in the previous year, the opposition had found its voice. "Dr. Daniel Martin, of the Catholic Medical Center in Queens, New York then briefly summarized his results in the CD_8F_1 mouse system. . . . He has performed two experiments with Mexican amygdalin. . . . Both experiments were completely negative" (ibid.).

Sloan-Kettering officials contradicted this claim, calling Martin's results "limited data" and saying that only one of his experiments duplicated Sugiura's methods.

Dr. Old responded by citing the human, clinical data provided him by Soto and his colleague on their visit. "With one exclusion, there was a 46.6 percent objective response rate, with an objective response rate defined as a [greater than] 40 percent tumor shrinkage" (ibid.).

The Sloan-Kettering spokesman said that Soto was "going to undertake a trial of amygdalin in his hospital and would like to have help in the protocol design, if possible, and would welcome observation. Dr. Old felt that this was an opportunity to have a clinical trial of this compound undertaken, which might give us some believable data" (ibid.).

A "prolonged discussion" ensued in which two sharply divided sides emerged. One side, representing the views of SKI's top leadership, held that "the nontoxic nature of amygdalin made it a superb candidate for a double-blind evaluation"—it is taken for granted in all these discussions, that laetrile *is* nontoxic. It said that "the preclinical data are not that critical since the drug is being extensively used" (ibid.).

The anti-laetrile side countered that ". . . the preclinical data, only, clearly do not support a clinical trial being undertaken . . . there are no convincing clinical data to date [and] undertaken, a clinical trial in the U.S. would be fraught with many consequences on many levels." Unfortunately, the notes do not tell what those "consequences" would be.

After three hours of debate, the final consensus decision was to send a group of American cancer specialists to Mexico to help set up Dr. Soto's clinical trial there "and observe the results of any trial undertaken." Three doctors volunteered to participate in this study: Dr. Stephen Carter of NCI, Dr. Charles Moertel of the Mayo Clinic, and Dr. Irwin Krakoff, then of SKI (ibid.).

A trial in Mexico offered many advantages, and was an excellent way out of the dilemma. Principally, a Mexican trial would not have to be approved by the U.S. FDA, but if the test were supervised by three prestigious American doctors, positive results would certainly clear the way for a U.S. trial.

Again, however, this compromise plan was aborted. Sloan-Kettering wrote to Soto and Sanen and informed the Mexican doctors that the proposed collaborative trial was off.

This was followed by a dramatic turnabout on the part of the top MSKCC leadership. On April 2, 1975, Lewis Thomas told reporters at the ACS Science Writers' Seminar that two years of testing laetrile had demonstrated:

No protective effects against cancer.
Failure to provide any prolongation of life.
An inability to reduce the size of a tumor.
Failure to inhibit the growth of a tumor (*San Diego Evening Tribune*, April 2, 1975).

The story was circulated nationwide by the American Cancer Society's public information department.

One month later, *The New York Times* carried a front-page story, "Coast Ring Smuggles Banned Cancer Drugs" (May 26, 1975). It told how an Assistant United States Attorney was preparing grand jury indictments against the top leaders of the laetrile movement, including some of those (such as Krebs, Jr., McNaughton, and Contreras) who had been respectfully received at Sloan-Kettering not long before. Now they were accused of masterminding "an international smuggling operation" comparable, said the government official, to the Mexican brown heroin traffic.

Justification for the prosecution, said the *Times*, came from no less an authority than Memorial Sloan-Kettering and its respected president:

Dr. Lewis Thomas, president of Sloan-Kettering [sic], reported April 2nd while in San Diego, that the institute's study showed that laetrile had absolutely no value either in combatting cancer, prolonging life or inhibiting tumor growth (ibid.).

In July, Sloan-Kettering leaders amplified their beliefs in another front-page story in the *Times*. Sugiura's extensive results were now called "spurious" and the result of "the vagaries of experimental variation" and "unfamiliarity with the animals used." The CD_8F_1 system was, indeed, a relatively new system. But Sugiura had used the Swiss albino mouse system, in which he also saw positive results, since World War II.

Not only did Sugiura disagree with this new judgment on his work, but he now claimed, in August, that the most recent results, with the AKR leukemia system, confirmed his earlier findings. "No compound affects AKR about the same as amygdalin," he said in a private conversation. "There's something there" (Sugiura, 1975).

Sugiura himself said nothing in public, however, to refute or challenge the remarks of his superiors. He maintained his attitude that it was "up to downtown" what they would do with his results. His job was only to conduct research, not get involved in controversy. He emphasized that in sixty years no one had ever found cause to contradict his work.

In early August, Dr. Stock was interviewed by *Medical World News*, and he amplified the Institute's new position. "We have found amygdalin negative in all the animal systems we have tested," he said *(Medical World News*, August 11, 1975).*

Because this and the previous statements seemed completely out of line with the reality of laetrile testing at SKI, a number of the Center's employees privately decided to take action to counter the misstatements. (The author was one of these employees.) After failing to obtain a retraction through the normal channels, copies of Sugiura's laboratory notes—Xerox copies obtained from Sugiura himself—were sent to a number of writers.

By September, these notes and other documents had been reprinted by the Committee for Freedom of Choice in Cancer Therapy, Inc., a pro-laetrile group centered in California, under the title *Anatomy of a Cover-Up* (Committee for Freedom of Choice, 1975).

David Leff of *Medical World News*, who also had received a set of notes, was granted an interview with Sugiura; he was the first reporter who questioned the elderly Japanese scientist at length on his laetrile experiments. Sugiura repeated his belief in the validity of his results *(Medical World News*, October 6, 1975).

Before the leak, Memorial Sloan-Kettering officials had hoped to close the book on laetrile, and especially laetrile testing in humans. "Clinical trials?" Benno Schmidt, vice-chairman of MSKCC, had said in August. "No way! There's no way, I believe, that they can convince the people at Sloan-Kettering there's any basis for going further *(Medical World News*, August 11, 1975.)

The leak may have convinced the administration to perform fur-

* Stock claims to have been misquoted by MWN's David Leff. "I'll never live down the misquote I should have corrected," he wrote in 1977, after his statement had become a matter of public controversy (Stock, 1977).

ther tests, for a new trial was now called for. "He [Sugiura] will have another chance to check [his] belief, in a collaborative experiment with Dr. Schmid. . . . This time the two men are working together, with Dr. Schmid randomizing 15 controls and 16 experimental mice, Dr. Sugiura (who pioneered in tumor-transplantation techniques) doing the injecting, and both evaluating the grossly visible metastases. Results of this newest laetrile test are expected by late this year, depending on when the last animal dies (*Medical World News*, October 6, 1975).

This experiment differed from Schmid's previous ones in that the dosages given were the same as in Sugiura's experiments; the microscope was utilized; and Sugiura did the actual injecting of the mice, on the theory that results may be affected by the way in which the compound is given.

The results were a confirmation of Sugiura's work. According to Schmid's observations, there were 80 percent metastases in the control animals and 44 percent in the treated. Sugiura found 100 percent metastases in the controls and 38 percent in the treated. The Pathology Department of Memorial Hospital found 80 percent in the controls and 31 percent in the treated. All three sets of figures are what scientists call "statistically significant"—they show that the positive results were very unlikely to have been due to chance (Stock et al., 1978).

"A dramatic reversal of Dr. Schmid's previous tests" was what reporter Mort Young of the *San Francisco Examiner* called this experiment in a front-page story (November 12, 1975). Sugiura's enthusiasm dampened, however, when Schmid refused all comment on the test, wouldn't talk to reporters to confirm his findings, or even to people in the MSKCC Public Affairs Department.

Sugiura was confused and disappointed by this; the situation was made even more difficult by the close family relationship between him and Schmid. "The cooperative experiment came out my way," Sugiura said some months later. "Schmid's data confirmed my original contention. I try my best. I report what I see" (Sugiura, 1976a).

Instead of seeing these results as a confirmation of Sugiura, the administration scheduled yet another test, this one a "blind" experiment at Dr. Martin's Catholic Medical Center in Queens. Sugiura would not know which mice were receiving the laetrile and which were receiving only the saline solution. Only Dr. Martin would have the "key" and know which was which, and he would keep this secret from Dr. Sugiura.

In late November 1975 the plans for the blind test were made public. Apparently, though, Sugiura was told nothing about it, although he was the principal party concerned. "Maybe I'm supposed to do it," he said in mid-February 1976, "maybe somebody else.

Nobody has told me anything" (ibid.). By May 1976 the plans for the blind test were finalized by Stock and Martin. The experiments were to be performed in Dr. Martin's laboratory, under his supervision. Sugiura would travel to Martin's facilities in Queens several times a week to observe the mice.

This first blind test ended in bitter controversy. Sugiura had traveled from Rye to Queens each week, as planned, and had weighed the mice, measured their tumors, and observed their lungs, whenever possible, for secondary tumors.

In addition, bioassays were performed on the lungs of the sacrificed animals (those killed just before their natural demise, to prevent decomposition of their bodies before measurements could be taken).

In July 1976 Sugiura said privately that he was generally happy with the way the experiment was progressing. There were seventy mice, divided into fourteen cages, five to a cage. Four weeks into the test, Sugiura surmised that the first seven cages housed control animals (receiving saline injections) while the second group of seven cages housed the laetrile-treated animals (Sugiura, 1976b).

"There are seven new tumors in the first group of thirty-five," he said, "and only one new tumor in the second group. About 50 percent of the small tumors in the second group stopped growing, but far fewer in the first group. Nine animals are still alive in the 'control' group," he added, "and fifteen are alive in the 'treated' group. There is also a difference in the number of metastases" (ibid.).

"Couldn't Dr. Martin have mixed some of the laetrile-treated mice in among the controls?" he was asked.

Sugiura answered that in his opinion there would be too much chance of a mix-up in this way, it would be too difficult for the technicians to perform, without confusing the treated with the untreated and ruining the experiment. They would probably have to be arranged with each cage housing either treated or controls and the simplest way would be to form two distinct large groups (ibid.).

Sugiura added that he had seen Dr. Martin only once since the start of the experiment. He had wanted to speak to him because an unusual number of animals were dying suddenly, apparently from faulty injection procedures.

"I cannot criticize him," Sugiura said. "He's the expert. I can't ask to see his mice or feel them. But a funny thing: a couple of times I performed a bioassay procedure, and only three or four days later, when I came back, a tumor had already developed—much less time than normally. Very strange!" (ibid.).

Sugiura wrote into his interim progress report to Stock and Old that the first thirty-five animals were the treated animals and the second thirty-five animals were the controls. Was he right?

On September 9 Sugiura was jubilant. "Last Friday, Dr. Stock told me that I picked the controls and the experimental *correctly*. The first seven cages are the control group and the second seven cages are the laetrile-treated group. I don't have to rewrite my progress report" (Sugiura, 1976c).

According to his tally, there were 70 percent metastases in the controls and 30 percent in the experimental, a significant difference in favor of laetrile (ibid.).

Soon after Sugiura filed this progress report, the SKI administration declared the experiment invalid as a blind test. "We've lost the 'blindness aspect of it,'" Dr. Stock told reporters (Moss, 1976). He told *Science* the experiment "went badly because of clumsy injection procedures" *(Science,* September 10, 1976).

Consequently, another blind experiment was scheduled, this one to take place at SKI itself.

At around this time, Second Opinion began publishing a bimonthly newsletter of the same name at the Center. Second Opinion was composed primarily of employees and former employees of MSKCC, who had begun meeting in the fall of 1975 to discuss problems at the Center, including what they perceived as a cover-up of the laetrile results.

The group had sent a number of letters to MSKCC administrators asking them to release full details of the laetrile experiments and to publish Sugiura's results. To protect the anonymity of the MSKCC employees, only those Second Opinion members who had no affiliation with the Center signed these letters. The employees felt that they would be fired if they voiced criticism of the administration publicly.

The first issue of the newsletter *Second Opinion* (November 1976) contained the following characterization of the blind test:

Although the test was "blind" Dr. Sugiura surmised which mice were being treated with laetrile and which were receiving the inert saline solution. . . . As soon as Dr. Sugiura correctly surmised which group was which, his SKI superior, Dr. Stock, declared the entire test invalid!

According to the official Sloan-Kettering report on laetrile, however, this account is wrong, because Dr. Martin, who controlled the experiment, says that the animals never were grouped into two distinct sets of thirty-five. Rather, he says, the cages were randomly alternated between control and treated animals.

A four-month investigation by Richard Smith of *The Sciences,* a publication of the New York Academy of Sciences, was unable to unearth any proof that Sugiura had in fact guessed correctly or that the cages had later had their designations altered (Smith, 1978).

The second blind test was no less controversial. From the start, in private conversation, Sugiura had objected to the way in which the mice were to be arranged in their cages. He expressed fear that since the treated and untreated animals were to be put in the same cages, the technicians might inadvertently give laetrile injections to the control animals and saline injections to the treated animals. This would completely destroy the validity of the experiment. Since the animals were distinguished only by punch marks in their ears, and such holes can be torn in the course of an experiment, he felt that such a possibility was not at all farfetched (Sugiura, 1976c).

This is precisely how the administration decided to perform the test, however. "They must be smarter than me," Sugiura said ironically (ibid.). Although on this occasion Sugiura was vocal about his dissatisfaction with the setup, Stock later claimed he knew nothing about the senior scientist's reservations. "Sugiura never expressed to me dissatisfaction with the experiment," Stock later wrote. "I heard of it after the results were in, and not in confirmation of his own experiments" (Stock, 1977).

The second blind test also did not come out in Sugiura's favor, according to the SKI administration. A memo from the director of public affairs on January 26, 1977, stated:

> Stock insists the results from the experiment do not confirm the earlier positive findings of Sugiura. He further states that he has not found encouragement in the data to take laetrile to clinical trial . . . in general the results do not confirm Sugiura's earlier findings (Delaney, 1977a).

Sugiura was not only disappointed by these results, but upset by what he saw as discrepancies in the data. "There's something funny here," he said. "The small tumors stopped growing 40 percent of the time in the saline control group and only 27 percent of the time in the treated group. We people in chemotherapy use saline solution because it does *not* affect tumor growth. Now this happens. They must not forget to mention that there was more stoppage in the controls than in the treated. I won't give in to this" (Sugiura, 1977a).

One possible explanation for the discrepancy, he suggested, was that the technician had inadvertently given some of the control mice amygdalin, thereby causing temporary tumor stoppages, one of the three antitumor effects Sugiura had seen in his previous laetrile experiments. Another possibility was that the control mice, which are coprophagic (feces-eating), had ingested some of the amygdalin-laden wastes of their treated cagemates (ibid.).

In MSKCC public affairs, the professional staff was instructed to tell reporters who were carefully following the story that the second blind test had proven in general that the "results do not confirm

Sugiura's earlier findings" without telling them that Sugiura himself thought the experiment flawed and invalid (Delaney, 1977a).

At a Monday morning public affairs staff meeting, the author informed the director of public affairs that he could not give out that statement, since it failed to mention the inexplicable tumor stoppages in the control animals, and since it did not mention Sugiura's own reservations about the outcome of the test.

T. Gerald Delaney, director of public affairs, replied that the author could put that in a memo to Dr. Stock, but that he would probably be fired for doing so. All the other staff members present then agreed to be cosigners to this memo. As the author prepared to write it, Delaney modified his stand and agreed to talk to Stock about these omissions.

On February 1, therefore, Delaney issued an amended statement for the press. It included a new sentence: "Dr. Stock also points out that Dr. Sugiura continues to believe in the validity of his earlier findings" (Delaney, 1977b). Sugiura told reporter Mort Young pointblank, "The tests were not done to my satisfaction."

Five years of testing had ended in controversy and confusion—not a pleasing outcome for the leaders of the world's most prestigious private cancer center. Nevertheless, about twenty positive experiments with laetrile had been performed by three researchers: Sugiura, Schloen, and Schmid. Quite a few negative experiments had also been performed. In April 1977 Second Opinion issued an appraisal of the paths open to the Memorial Sloan-Kettering administration:

> If, on the one hand, they publish the truth about laetrile they will have to say something like this: we have been unable to reach any definitive conclusion on this substance. Dr. Sugiura, one of the most experienced researchers, has done many studies showing positive effects. Other researchers have claimed negative results. We think this issue can only be settled through a study on willing human volunteers with cancer, and we would like to conduct such a study here at Memorial.
>
> That would be honest, but it would also be disastrous from a fundraising point of view, since it would bring down the wrath of the American Cancer Society, and the National Cancer Institute, from whom MSKCC receives most of its research funds, not to mention the Food and Drug Administration. . . .
>
> The other choice is to publish a totally one-sided report. . . . This is the most likely prospect at the moment, but it too will bring down wrath and exposure—from tens of thousands of individuals around the country.

Sloan-Kettering took the latter course. In mid-June 1977 the aforementioned press conference was called and the public affairs office sent out a news release which summarized the ninety-page set of papers on the laetrile testing (reprinted in Zimmermann, 1977).

Despite Sugiura's "I stick!" the comments of all the other administrators were totally negative.

"We have no evidence that laetrile possesses *any* biological activity with respect to cancer, one way or the other," said Thomas (MSKCC, 1977c).

"We have found no reproducible evidence that amygdalin, or laetrile, is active," said Good (ibid.).

"Laetrile has been found absolutely devoid of activity, period. It's just that simple. It's all there in black and white if you take the trouble to read the paper," said Daniel Martin (ibid.). Meanwhile, MSKCC public affairs functionaries had been instructed by Delaney to hide copies of the paper itself behind a curtain in an adjoining room and give them out to reporters only if they explicitly asked for them. Only a handful did.

Laetrile's "failure" was carried on nationwide television that evening. Release of the report to the lay press, almost a year before its actual publication in the *Journal of Surgical Oncology*, coincided with the debate then raging on laetrile legalization in New York State. (The measure passed the legislature but was vetoed by Governor Hugh Carey.)

It also came less than a month before Senator Edward Kennedy's hearings, before the Subcommittee on Health and Scientific Research, on the "Banning of the Drug Laetrile from Interstate Commerce by FDA."

The Kennedy hearings were an unprecedented showdown between the pro-laetrile and anti-laetrile forces, after twenty-five years of skirmishes. It would have been embarrassing in the extreme if the pro-laetrile side had been able to present unpublished—apparently suppressed—documents from Sloan-Kettering showing that laetrile was indeed effective in some circumstances. This did not happen; Thomas came armed with a strongly worded anti-laetrile statement when he appeared before Senator Kennedy on July 12, 1977.

Thomas told the senators:

There is not a particle of scientific evidence to suggest that laetrile possesses any anticancer properties at all. I am not aware of any scientific papers, published in any of the world's accredited journals of medical science, presenting data in support of the substance, although there are several papers, one of these recently made public by Sloan-Kettering Institute, reporting the complete absence of anticancer properties in a variety of experimental animals (U.S. Senate, 1977).

In his prepared statement Thomas did not cite the many studies conducted worldwide showing laetrile's anticancer effects, nor did he mention Sugiura's work. Under questioning by Senator Richard Schweiker (R.-Pa.), Thomas admitted that "it did seem in Dr. Sugiura's experiment [laetrile] would inhibit the number of metastatic lesions in the lung." He claimed, however, that the number of mice involved in these tests was small and this observation was made only on "two or three occasions" (ibid.:19–21).

In the summer of 1977, a group of employees, including members of Second Opinion, met to discuss the latest developments in the controversy. It was decided at this meeting to write a counterreport to the official laetrile papers. In studying the Sloan-Kettering papers, the Second Opinion investigators decided that there were numerous errors in the SKI version. To err is human, of course. But one characteristic of these errors was that, big or small, they always seemed to be made to the detriment of laetrile and Dr. Sugiura.

One such error concerned the effect of various drugs on Dr. Martin's CD_8F_1 mouse. The SKI paper stated that the alleged failure of laetrile to stop the growth of cancer in these animals was highly significant, since other, conventional anticancer drugs were active against these tumors:

> Of those eight agents declared clinically active against human breast cancer by the National Cancer Institute, all eight agents also are active against this murine breast cancer. . . . Thus, the negative laetrile findings in this animal tumor model appear particularly significant (cited in Second Opinion, 1977).

Apparently, laetrile had failed where chemotherapy succeeded; an important charge, since the value of orthodox chemotherapy was also clearly at issue in the laetrile controversy. This point was emphasized a number of times at the June 15 press conference.

Research into scientific literature by the Second Opinion group in the summer of 1977 revealed that when chemotherapy was used in the same way that laetrile had been tested it, too, was ineffective against the primary breast tumors. Proof of this came from Dr. Martin's own papers, written between 1970 and 1975, which concluded:

> Cure has thus far been impossible to achieve by chemotherapy alone on large primary tumors. Hence, this most difficult methodology has been largely shelved. . . . (Martin et al., 1975).

Of the nineteen drugs and two immune-stimulating agents which had been "studied at length in the treatment of this tumor," all "proved to be quite resistant to influence by chemotherapy alone" and "ineffective in this spontaneous tumor system" (ibid.).

But this discarded method of testing drugs had been taken down from "the shelf" to test laetrile. When laetrile failed where other drugs had also failed, this was interpreted as "particularly significant."

The Second Opinion investigators also took issue with the manner in which SKI judged anticancer effects. According to the Second Opinion report:

In AKR leukemia, a recent publication by Robert Kassel [in a book edited by Robert A. Good] makes clear that while prolongation of life is the most certain sign of anticancer effects, it is very rare. Scientists therefore take a shrinkage of internal organs greater than 20 percent to be a sign of anticancer activity. While Sugiura saw such effects, and commented on them in memos, this is never mentioned in the text of the report.

Much was made at the SKI press conference about Martin's inability to reproduce Sugiura's results with lung metastases. Although it was admitted that Martin used a different method from Sugiura, the paper maintained that Martin's method, bioassay, was superior to Sugiura's method (visual gross observation plus microscopic slides).

Second Opinion found that Martin's method had not been adopted by many researchers. According to references in *Citation Index*, a standard bibliographic tool, no group other than his own had published papers on experiments employing his bioassay method. Between January 1976 and February 1977 there were eight articles dealing with the question of metastases in rodents in the journal *Cancer Research*. All but one of these used the macro-visual and/or microscopic techniques favored by Sugiura. The one that didn't was by Martin and his group (Second Opinion, 1977:8–10).

These are technicalities, but it was on technicalities such as these that laetrile had been condemned as totally ineffective.

On November 18, 1977, Second Opinion called a press conference at the New York Hilton and released its forty-eight-page report to the press. The author, who was part of the Second Opinion group from its inception, decided to makes his criticisms public and associate himself with the report. He was fired on the next working day for failing "to properly discharge his most basic job responsibilities," according to an official MSKCC statement (MSKCC, 1977d).

Two days later, Second Opinion received a letter from Sugiura, who had been sent a copy of the report. The elderly scientist wrote:

I read your paper in the Monograph [the report] with great interest. Your critical review of my positive results and negative results of three investigators at Sloan-Kettering Institute is very well done and accurate. Please accept my sincere congratulations (Sugiura, 1977b).

Others at Sloan-Kettering had a less positive evaluation of the report. At first the administration dismissed the charges as minor inconsistencies which an "irresponsible and malicious" group had "blown all out of proportion to their scientific significance" (MSKCC, 1977e).

The medical establishment realized it would have to take the charges more seriously when an article on the controversy appeared in *The Sciences* echoing the Second Opinion criticisms.

The president of the New York Academy of Sciences stated that the "misinterpretation by Dr. Martin was not excusable" *(New York Times,* December 13, 1977). Concerning Martin's claim that other drugs could cure breast cancer in the CD_8F_1 mouse, Stock told *The New York Times:*

We accepted the statement from Dr. Martin as submitted. I did not check the original publications to be certain of the appropriateness of the statement. It should not have been used in the context of this report, and therefore it has been deleted (ibid.).

The final version of the SKI paper, as published in 1978 in the *Journal of Surgical Oncology,* contains an addendum by Daniel S. Martin, C. Chester Stock, and Robert A. Good.

While clearly meant to refute unnamed critics who questioned the erroneous statements, the addendum threw fuel on the fire by stating that "the finding that laetrile is devoid of anticancer activity is particularly pertinent" and "laetrile's lack of anticancer activity in the CD_8F_1 animal tumor model is particularly significant" (Stock et al., 1978).

However, until his death Sugiura continued to hold to his original belief:

I still think my experimental results on the effect of amygdalin (with high doses) on spontaneous mammary tumors (adenocarcinomas) are correct—stoppage of growth of small tumors temporar[il]y; prevent the development of lung metastases 80 percent against 20 percent in control group (saline); delayed the development of spontaneous mammary cancers for three to four months (Sugiura, 1979).

In sticking by his own results, Sugiura is not unique in science. Experienced researchers, confident in their own abilities, often will hold out against a crowd of vociferous opponents—and often they will be vindicated in the end.

Nobel Prize–winner Sir Peter Medawar, who serves on Sloan-Kettering's Board of Scientific Consultants, has related a similar instance in his own career:

. . . several people tried to repeat our work and failed. There were, however, always good reasons why they did so; either they had introduced into our techniques little "improvements" of their own, or they were too clumsy or something. These failures did not disturb us in the very least: we knew we were right—and we were—so we did our best to tell those who were struggling with our techniques how best to carry them out (*New York Review of Books*, April 15, 1976).

But the establishment does not want to hear any more about Sugiura's laetrile experiments, nor does it want the public to hear. In 1979 reporters seeking to interview the elderly researcher were told by him: "I am not allowed to talk about laetrile" (Pressman, 1979).

Thus ended the most extensive study ever carried out on an unorthodox method of treating cancer.

10

Hydrazine Sulfate: Unorthodox Chemotherapy

Since the end of World War II, the battle between the orthodox and unorthodox "camps" in cancer has often centered on the controversial question of chemotherapy.

To the orthodox scientists, pure chemicals are the most desirable forms of therapy, since each batch of these drugs is identical to the preceding one, and dosages can be set as precisely as the rads of a cobalt beam. To the unorthodox, however, such chemical treatments are anathema since, it is claimed, the human body has not evolved to handle substances so completely foreign to its normal metabolism as methotrexate or 5-FU.

This is the general outline of the debate. Nevertheless, there are certain exceptions to this rule. Some drugs, highly unnatural by anybody's standard, are scorned by the establishment and embraced by many advocates of unorthodox therapy. One example is the simple, off-the-shelf chemical hydrazine sulfate.

Unlike most anticancer agents, which have been discovered by trial and error, hydrazine sulfate's use was the end result of a series of logical deductions—a rational quest for a specific type of therapy.

In 1968 Joseph Gold, M.D., of Syracuse, New York, published a scientific paper in which he proposed a new departure for cancer chemotherapy (Gold, 1968). Chemotherapy was still a relatively new field, but it had become apparent, even by this time, that the principle upon which it was based—toxicity—limited the ability of these agents to kill cancer cells without also damaging the healthy cells of the body.

Perhaps it was not necessary to kill cancer cells directly with poisons, Gold suggested. Possibly the same or even better results could be achieved if scientists were able to block the cancer cells from inflicting damage on the patient's body.

Gold had studied the work of Otto Warburg, winner of the 1931 Nobel Prize in physiology and medicine for his discovery of a respiratory enzyme. One of Warburg's most controversial theories concerned the nature of cancer cell metabolism—the way in which such cells obtained their energy. Warburg's work formed the theoretical underpinning of Gold's innovation (Warburg, 1930).

Normally, human cells obtain their energy through respiration—taking in oxygen and giving off carbon dioxide and water. This is a complex—but highly efficient—way of generating energy. There is, however, another, far more primitive and wasteful way of generating energy: fermentation. This type of energy production is common to some simple forms of life, such as the bacteria which cause milk to sour or the yeast which makes bread rise.

There are times, however, when our human cells also employ fermentation. One is when the muscles or brain require a quick burst of energy. Another, said Warburg—and this is the essence of his controversial theory—is in cancer. According to Warburg, all cancer cells live by fermenting sugar in what are essentially "airless" (anaerobic) reactions. Find a way of stopping this fermentation, and you might have a way of stopping cancer.

Warburg's theory was eclipsed in the 1950s, but in the following decade, before Gold began his work, Dr. Dean Burk and others at the National Cancer Institute had attempted to iron out some of the problems and restore the credibility of this aspect of Warburg's contribution. Burk himself won a scientific prize for his demonstration that, in at least some cases, Warburg's proposal that cancer ferments had been correct (Burk, 1965).

Warburg's theory has remained controversial over the years. "Unfortunately," wrote Pat McGrady, Sr., "Warburg was only partly right; some tumor cells, to a great or small degree, can adapt to a respiration mode of life, and some normal cells have fermenting mechanisms." A drug which blocked fermentation, oxalic acid, was tried as a cancer treatment but was toxic and gave only mixed results (McGrady, Sr., 1964).

"The relation between the Warburg effect and transformation [of normal cells to cancerous ones] is still unclear," the Science report noted in 1975. "Warburg's theory does not account for the aberrant properties of tumor cells" (Maugh and Marx, 1975).

Gold took Warburg and Burk's studies as his starting point, but then attempted to pursue this concept further than anyone had yet done in the practical application of these ideas to cancer. He reasoned as follows:

A prime cause of death in cancer is the weight loss and debilitation often seen in the disease. This is known medically as cachexia. If cancer cachexia could be interrupted, the disease itself might be brought under control, much as diabetes is controlled by a daily injection of insulin.

But what causes cachexia—a frightful condition which often reduces the dying patient to skin and bones, while his tumor grows with apparent vigor? Orthodox science had no answer. Gold's research indicated that cachexia was the result of cancer's ability to "recycle its wastes," but at the energy expense of the body. It thus imposes a severe energy drain on the body, eventually resulting in emaciation.

Specifically, Gold pointed out, cancer uses glucose (sugar) as its fuel but only incompletely metabolizes, or combusts, it. The waste product of this incomplete combustion is lactic acid. This lactic acid then spills into the blood and is taken up by the liver and kidneys (normal noncancerous tissues). But the body must now expend a great deal of energy from these normal tissues merely to reconvert this lactic acid back into glucose.

Ironically, the body then returns an ever-increasing amount of this new glucose back to the tumor for fuel, and the process is repeated over and over again, to the great benefit of the cancer, and the great detriment of the normal tissues of the body. "The net result is a loss of energy from normal body energy 'pools,'" says Gold. "As the cancer grows, its production of lactic acid grows, imposing on the body a condition in which the normal body energy 'pools' become more and more depleted" (Syracuse, 1979).

Eventually, the body reaches a point where it can no longer keep up with these constant energy losses. The result is rapid weight loss and debilitation—in other words, cachexia.

Gold reasoned that

cachexia is but the end result of an insidious process—unrecognizable at first, but slowly taking its toll of the body's reserves until a "point of no return" is reached. Cachexia begins with the very first cancer tissue. What we need is a way to stop the vicious cycle and thereby put a halt to the leading cause of death in cancer: cachexia (Gold, 1968).

Armed with his theory, Gold now went in search of a drug that could interrupt this "sick relationship" which had developed between the liver and the cancer. He toyed with various drugs, diets, and compounds, including the amino acid tryptophane. In the early 1970s, however, he found a scientific paper which stated that hydrazine sulfate could block a key enzyme in the liver which allowed lactic acid to be converted into glucose.

Before beginning clinical trials, Gold put hydrazine sulfate through a battery of animal tests. In four different transplantable tumor systems, hydrazine sulfate performed well. It also appeared as if the chemical was working according to Gold's innovative theory. For one thing, the drug did *not* damage cancer cells in the test tube, yet it did destroy them in the animal's body. This suggested that the drug worked by some indirect mechanism. Second, examination of the animals' tumors suggested that the cells were, in fact, not directly poisoned, as in conventional forms of chemotherapy (Gold, 1971a, 1973).

Gold also found that hydrazine could be used to enhance the effectiveness of most of the major cell-poisoning drugs in tumor-bearing animals (Gold, 1971b, 1975a).

The toxicity studies also seemed promising. A very high dose could certainly kill the animals. But at the optimal dosage, anti-cancer effects were accompanied by a minimum of side effects (Gold, 1975a).

Shortly after Gold's first animal studies were published, he gave a talk about his new concept at the New York Academy of Sciences. After the talk, a doctor came up to the Syracuse physician and said, "Dr. Gold, I have a patient who will certainly die in three or four days. I would like to try hydrazine sulfate on her." Gold and the doctor exchanged information on probable dosages and routes of administering the compound. Shortly afterward, according to Gold, the woman experienced a remarkable change in her condition. Within a few weeks she was up and about, greatly improved. A number of other patients also appeared to experience dramatic remissions (Wayne Martin, 1977).

By August 1973 there were about twenty or thirty patients taking hydrazine sulfate in different parts of the country. By the middle of September, there were about two or three hundred. And by October there were over one thousand.

When hydrazine sulfate at the optimal dose had been shown to be relatively nontoxic and effective in animal studies, the Food and Drug Administration cautiously began to give out a few Investigative New Drug (IND) permits to a handful of doctors. For example, they granted an IND to the Medical College of Virginia to study the substance. Another permit went to the California drug company Calbiochem, Inc. But the number of INDs granted was very few, and many individuals began to obtain the drug on their own and treat themselves. The American Cancer Society and the National Cancer Institute officially maintained silence, but Gold began to experience difficulties in his requests for funds from NCI.

However, not everyone at NCI was negative. Dr. Burk, then the head of cell chemistry at the government's cancer center, was understandably enthusiastic over Gold's work. Since the death of Warburg in 1971, one author has written, "Burk could well be called the world's greatest biochemist, and he has borne the torch of Warburg's life work since then" (ibid.). Gold's finding seemed to vindicate Warburg and Burk's work on cancer cell metabolism.

Burk declared hydrazine sulfate to be "the most remarkable anticancer agent I have come across in my forty-five years of experience in cancer." He predicted that the FDA would make hydrazine freely available to cancer patients, but added, "it would make little difference with hydrazine sulfate if the FDA wanted to balk, because this material is so cheap—and it is cheap because it is made by the trainload for industrial purposes" (Burk, 1974a).

In mid-August 1973, Burk met with top officials of Sloan-Kettering Institute in New York to tell them about hydrazine's successes. Burk thus presented his case:

Let me tell you this perfectly true story. There is nothing mystical or poetic about it—and I could give you many [such stories]. A woman with Hodgkin's disease who had been flat on her back for seven weeks, who had no appetite and who had lost all her weight—a "paper-thin" patient—took hydrazine sulfate. One week later she was shopping in the grocery store with her own bag; five days later she was spending most of the day in her garden. I don't give you that as any miraculous story—it is simply the plain truth (ibid.).

According to Burk, some of the leaders of Sloan-Kettering were highly enthusiastic about the early reports on hydrazine sulfate. Some of them were immunologists, who considered themselves the heirs of Dr. Coley. But hydrazine sulfate was no immune-stimulating natural agent, like Coley's toxins, but a drug, pure and simple. Because of this, hydrazine sulfate was given to the chemotherapists to evaluate. In general, the chemotherapists were far less receptive or enthusiastic about innovative approaches, especially those advocated by "mavericks" such as Dean Burk.

Hydrazine sulfate was immediately put into clinical trials, an unusual step since most other drugs have first been subjected to extensive animal testing at Sloan-Kettering itself before human tests have been started. A meeting was held between Gold and his colleagues and the Memorial Sloan-Kettering leaders in September 1973. Shortly afterward, the public affairs department at MSKCC issued a press release which stated that a "joint effort" was being undertaken by the two institutions (MSKCC and Syracuse Cancer Research Institute) to test the new substance in terminal patients. It appeared to many as if the two camps were finally coming together for serious study, for the benefit of all cancer patients.

However, according to Gold, SKI immediately reneged: "Once

the study began, no person at Sloan-Kettering responsible for this study ever got in touch with me. No information was released. No data were volunteered. No questions were asked" (Gold, 1974).

Thirty-two patients were given hydrazine sulfate, patients on whom no other form of therapy any longer had any positive effect. Several of these patients died before the test could even begin, in violation of the agreed-upon protocol that each patient put in the study have a life expectancy of at least two months. An SKI chemotherapist later claimed that hydrazine had failed to have an effect in *these* patients—literally true, since they were already dead at the time the test began (ibid.).

The two research centers had agreed at several meetings that the patients would start with a dosage of 60 milligrams a day. Instead, Gold said, the Sloan-Kettering chemotherapists took it on themselves to change this to 1 milligram on the first day, then 2 milligrams on the second day, and so forth, until they reached a dosage of between 20 and 30 milligrams per day—still a fraction of the adequate amount (ibid.).

An emergency meeting was convened between Gold and Memorial Sloan-Kettering doctors Lewis Thomas, Robert Good, Lloyd Old, Raymond Brown, Irwin Krakoff, and Manuel Ochoa, who was supervising the clinical trial. The latter agreed—for the third time—to abide by the optimal dosage: 60 milligrams for the first three days, 60 milligrams twice a day for the next three days, and 60 milligrams three times a day thereafter "with the option of allowing the patient to remain on 60 milligrams [twice a day] if there was a continuing good response" (ibid.).

After hearing nothing from his Sloan-Kettering collaborators, Gold came to New York and paid a surprise visit to the cancer clinic, accompanied by Raymond Brown, then an aide to SKI vice-president Lloyd Old. Four of the seven patients' records they examined showed strong subjective responses to the new therapy, Gold claimed; the patients were eating more, feeling more alert and stronger. This was documented in the progress reports and the nurses' notes (ibid.).

At this point, instead of going on the twice-a-day schedule, as agreed upon, however, the chemotherapists gave each patient a massive, single dose of approximately 120–190 milligrams, "which quickly wiped out whatever good response they were beginning to show," according to a letter of protest which Gold sent to SKI's Ochoa (ibid.).

The SKI chemotherapist told a relative of one of the first patients that he had "no enthusiasm or interest in" hydrazine sulfate and that the drug was "worthless" in the treatment of cancer, Gold said (ibid.).

After treating the patients in this way, the chemotherapists then concluded that not only was hydrazine sulfate not effective, but that it caused dangerous side effects, such as "serious central nervous system toxicities." Ochoa brought up these alleged shortcomings at an open discussion of Gold's paper at the March 1974 meeting of the American Association for Cancer Research in Houston. "You should know by virtue of your training," Gold told Ochoa, "that in critically ill patients it is quite easy to produce serious toxicities with any anticancer drug by overdosing" (ibid.).

In response to repeated public requests for information on the new drug, the public affairs department of MSKCC drew up the following statement in mid-1974:

In September 1973 MSKCC began clinical trials on the drug hydrazine sulfate, after published reports indicated that it seemed to have effectiveness as an anticancer agent.

This project was carried out under the directorship of Dr. Manuel Ochoa, Jr., M.D., Associate Member of Sloan-Kettering Institute and Attending, Solid Tumor Service at Memorial Hospital.

Dr. Ochoa now reports that he has adequately treated 29 patients at Memorial with this drug. The results have been that (1) *none* of these patients responded positively to hydrazine sulfate, and (2) some of the patients developed neurotoxicity [nerve damage], apparently due to the administration of this drug.

Based on these findings, therefore, MSKCC is no longer treating patients with hydrazine sulfate, nor are we conducting any further experiments with it at the present time (Moss, 1974).

Gold strongly disputes this statement. First, he says, Sloan-Kettering never *adequately* treated twenty-nine patients, or even one patient: the correct dosages, which were worked out over a period of years, were never used. Second, the statement fails to mention the subjective responses of patients to initial treatment with the drug. These subjective effects are included in the published paper of the Sloan-Kettering group (Ochoa, 1975). Third, the nerve damage mentioned occurred only when the patients were overdosed.

In reviewing his experience with SKI, Gold has said: "I've heard of cancer politics, but I've never seen anything like this in my entire life. In fact, I wouldn't believe it, if I hadn't seen it with my own eyes." He feels that there are "several different Sloan-Ketterings," since while the official statements on hydrazine have all been as negative as the one above, several top officials at SKI have privately conveyed to him their continuing interest in the compound, and their inability to influence the actions of the chemotherapists (Gold, 1975b).

The "failure" at Sloan-Kettering was one in a number of setbacks for hydrazine within the cancer establishment. Dr. William Regelson of the Medical College of Virginia also claimed to see no benefit in patients using hydrazine in a double-blind study. But neither did he see any toxicity. It was, in his view, totally inert. However, Regelson's study was never published. It was rejected by *Cancer Treatment Reports* (an NCI publication), says Gold, because of the paucity of patients and because the limited data were impossible to interpret (Gold, 1979).

Another doctor reporting negative results was Dr. Harvey H. Lerner of the Department of Surgery at the Pennsylvania Hospital in Philadelphia (Lerner, 1976). His negative one-page article was published in *Cancer Treatment Reports,* despite the fact, says Gold, that the referees, who read the paper for accuracy, argued that it should not be published unless *all* the data upon which the conclusions were based were included.

Gold objects to the Lerner study on the grounds that it used only outpatients, who may have been using alcohol, tranquilizers, and barbiturates at the same time as receiving hydrazine. Any of these substances is incompatible with and inhibits the action of the new anticancer drug.

The Syracuse physician soon countered with a clinical report of his own, published in the international cancer journal *Oncology.* In it he analyzed data gathered by many doctors under an IND granted to Calbiochem, Inc., the California drug company which was once interested in the new substance (Gold, 1975c).

Gold found that out of eighty-four advanced patients treated adequately, 70 percent had subjective improvement, such as increased appetite, weight gain or cessation of weight loss, increase in strength, and decrease in pain. In addition, 17 percent also showed objective improvement, including tumor regression, disappearance of cancer-related disorders, or more than a year-long stabilization of their condition. The length of time this improvement lasted varied from patient to patient, but in some cases it had lasted years and was still continuing when the paper was published (ibid.).

Under treatment with hydrazine sulfate, a dentist with Hodgkin's disease who had not responded to either radiation or chemotherapy was able to return to work after only two weeks on hydrazine. He remained working, in good health, for a number of years (Wayne Martin, 1977).

A forty-five-year-old man with prostatic cancer which had already spread throughout his body, and who was racked with pain, was freed from his agony and enabled to resume a normal life (ibid.).

A sixty-two-year-old woman with cancer of the cervix, in the last stages of cachexia, began to gain weight, got out of bed, and was finally discharged from the hospital, to the amazement of her doctors. Most remarkable was the complete disappearance of a secondary tumor the size of an orange (ibid.). Hydrazine sulfate appeared to be relatively nontoxic when given correctly, but at its worst the side effects were transient and mild, especially when compared to the harrowing effects of standard chemotherapy. Some individuals (about 2 percent, after long-term high dosage administration) did experience a feeling of pain or weakness in their limbs, but this condition was quickly controlled by reducing the dosage and administering vitamin B_6. A few others experienced nausea, dry skin, dizziness, and drowsiness. Most importantly, in no cases did hydrazine sulfate therapy depress or destroy white blood cells or bone marrow, as standard chemotherapy often does. This is important because the bone marrow produces many of the cells which comprise the patient's immune system, which many scientists believe is crucial in the fight against cancer (Gold, 1975c).

Gold's paper concluded with a plea to his medical colleagues to keep an open mind on the new therapy:

> Hydrazine sulfate therapy is a new type of chemotherapy. Its clinical use at present represents a *beginning*. Whether a study with any new drug is positive or negative, it must always be evaluated in terms of the "state of the art." Hydrazine sulfate represents the *first* of a class of new agents designed to interrupt host participation in cancer. Other agents in this class now in development may prove to be far superior to hydrazine sulfate. . . . It must be emphasized that the clinical potential of hydrazine sulfate-like drugs in cancer has only just begun to be explored (ibid.).

Gold's plea fell on deaf ears within the establishment. Even Calbiochem, Inc. soon dropped out of the picture. A spokesman for the company attributed this action to the fact that hydrazine was in the public domain and thus unpatentable. "We saw absolutely no place to go with it," he allegedly remarked (quoted in Rorvik, 1976).

In March 1976 the establishment made its condemnation official: the American Cancer Society added hydrazine sulfate to its unproven methods list.

The ACS spoke only of the negative results with hydrazine sulfate, such as the Sloan-Kettering study, and included the tests which had been rejected by a scientific journal. On the other hand, it failed to mention Gold's positive clinical data, or the important foreign data which were then emerging. So erroneous were the statements attributed to Sloan-Kettering's chemotherapists that they were later retracted by Sloan-Kettering itself under threat of "troublesome repercussions" by Gold's lawyer (Grauer, 1975).

The ACS also made what appears to be a personal swipe at Gold himself: it claimed that he was in "full-time practice" in Syracuse. This seemed to imply that cancer research was a sideline avocation in which he dabbled. The opposite is the case: Gold has been involved in cancer research since graduation from Upstate Medical Center of the State University of New York in Syracuse in 1956. He has published numerous papers on the disease, and is anything but a dilettante.

After the ACS condemnation was made public, however, many newspapers automatically reprinted the thumbs-down verdict with stories entitled, for example, "Tests Show Drug Useless for Cancer" (*Long Beach* [Calif.] *Independent*, May 19, 1976).

Gold's funding dried up. From 1973 to 1976 the Syracuse group received NCI support for its basic scientific research. "Once hydrazine became clinical, and once it was placed on the ACS unproven list," he has said, "we could not get a renewal by hook or by crook" (Gold, 1979).

Despite this, hydrazine sulfate's prospects have hardly been diminished. First, as Dean Burk noted, hydrazine sulfate is so readily available that it is virtually impossible to stop anyone from taking it, or marketing it. It is extremely inexpensive. Burk estimated that one year's supply of the drug, in pill form, would cost between $25 and $50, mainly "to cover the expense of the man who makes the pills" (Burk, 1974a).

Second, Soviet researchers have opened another front in the cancer war, and some of them appear to be impressed with hydrazine sulfate and the rationale behind its use.

Workers at Lenigrad's N. N. Petrov Research Institute of Oncology of the USSR Ministry of Health, a large Soviet cancer center, have supported Gold's concepts. These investigators are part of the joint U.S.–USSR cancer program.

Soviet scientists seem to grasp the philosophical basis of Gold's new approach better than his own countrymen. They have written:

Almost all research in the field of experimental and clinical chemotherapy of malignant neoplasia [cancer] up to the present time, one way or another, reflects the principles of a direct . . . attack on growth and multiplication of cancer cells. However, there may well be other means of medicinal influence on the progress of neoplastic growth. One of these includes Gold's hypothesis (Seits et al., 1975).

The Soviet team then went on to confirm the following claims for hydrazine therapy.

Hydrazine stops the growth of animal cancers: Soviet scientists found that hydrazine definitely retards the growth of cancer in experimental animals. In Walker carcinosarcoma in rats, for instance, they were able to demonstrate a 97.4 percent inhibition of tumor growth with a high dose of hydrazine given orally. Other types of experimental cancer also showed moderate responses to the drug (ibid.).

Hydrazine works by stopping gluconeogenesis: This, at least, was the most likely explanation of the drug's action. Microscopic examination of tumor remnants in cured rats showed "well-preserved tumor tissues." This means that hydrazine destroys tumors without directly poisoning cancer cells by some "indirect mechanism of inhibition of tumor growth" (ibid.).

Hydrazine is relatively nontoxic: In animals, there was no damage to the liver of the treated animals, and little weight loss, especially at lower dosage levels. Most important, in humans there was no damage to the blood-making cells, although the Soviet doctors saw the same minor side effects as Gold noted, such as limb weakness and nausea, in a minority of patients (ibid.).

Hydrazine controls cancerous growths in humans: This is, of course, the bottom line of any cancer therapy. Forty-eight patients were given hydrazine as a last resort "in all cases after exhausting possibilities of surgical, X-ray treatment or other types of chemotherapy." In other words, these were patients on whom nothing else would work—patients with debilitated bodies, doomed to die within a few months (ibid.).

The Soviet scientists carefully followed Gold's suggestions for dosages. They noted that the usual criteria for evaluation of the effectiveness of a drug—especially tumor shrinkage—may not be applicable in this case "in view of the unusual action of hydrazine sulfate." Nevertheless, in these forty-eight very sick, terminal patients the Russians achieved the following results.

Objective anticancer effects in over one-third of the patients tested: This included "objective regressions of tumor mass" in 20 percent of the cases and an additional 15 percent whose cases were stabilized; i.e., whose cancers stopped progressing.

Subjective anticancer effects in 58 percent of the patients: This included complete disappearance or marked reduction of bone pain, increase in appetite, and an unexpected desire to get out of their beds and walk around. In short, there was a "sharp improvement of general well-being" in over half the terminal patients (ibid.).

The Soviet scientists found that hydrazine was not simply a painkiller in the ordinary sense, but induced a sense of euphoria in many patients. Suddenly, people who were in the doldrums, waiting to die, became active, cheerful, optimistic, wanting to live. The Soviet doctors noted hydrazine sulfate's "peculiar influence on the psyche," particularly a "sharp improvement of mood in a significant portion of the patients . . . to the point of euphoria" (Danova et al., 1977). This was so even in cases where no objective regression of the cancer could be seen.

The Leningrad researchers singled out two cases treated in 1974 with the new therapy. The first was a man of forty who was suffering from the last stages of Hodgkin's disease. He had already been through a succession of ten treatment sessions, with practically every known anticancer agent, such as steroid hormones, cyclophosphamide, vinblastine, and leukeran.

Several times these drugs had succeeded in putting him into remission for a year or more, but each time the cancer had returned. The last time his doctors attempted to treat him with a combination of vinblastine and a hormone, but with no effect.

Since his symptoms were progressing, the doctors decided on hydrazine therapy. "After one week," they report, "the first indications of curative effect were noticed in the form of diminution of weakness, lowering of temperature." Remarkably, after one and a half months, "the symptoms of malignant disease completely disappeared." The lymph nodes and the liver decreased in size and "there was noticed a gradual but steady improvement in the blood picture."

This lasted four months, and then moderate signs of cancer began to reappear. At this point, the specialists took him off hydrazine and back on vinblastine and the hormone. But, unlike before, these treatments were now successful, and the patient went back into complete remission of his cancer (Seits et al., 1975).

This case indicates not only the value of hydrazine itself, but its possible use in conjunction with standard forms of chemotherapy. In some cases, as in the animal studies, hydrazine sulfate appeared to make the cancer more vulnerable to the cellular poisons.

Another case the Petrov Institute scientists reported in depth was that of a sixty-three-year-old woman with cancer of the lungs, as well as secondary growths in the lymph nodes. This patient had difficulty in swallowing food, due to the progressive growth of the tumor, a loss of appetite, and a coughing-up of blood. She was losing weight steadily.

On July 22, 1974, the Soviet doctors started her on hydrazine sulfate and within two weeks "a pronounced subjective effect was observed—marked diminution of weakness and coughing, restoration of appetite, disappearance of hemoptysis [spitting of blood]" (ibid.).

X rays revealed that the tumor was shrinking in the left lung, and there were other signs of cancer regression. The woman continued to improve as of the date of the report. Neither she nor any of the other patients showed any signs of damage to the vital immune system.

The Soviet report emphasizes that these observations were not flukes "but rather typical in those cases in which hydrazine sulfate was basically effective and as a rule did not cause side effects."

How has the American cancer establishment reacted to these Soviet studies? In general, quite negatively. NCI published an abridged and, Gold feels, watered-down version of one of the Soviet papers in 1976. But they coupled it with a negative American study. ACS editorialized about them both as follows:

> The July issue [of the NCI publication] contains two important reports on the lack of clinical effect of hydrazine sulfate. This compound received considerable publicity in the lay press prior to confirmation of clinical utility. Lerner and Regelson report no clinical effects in 25 evaluable cancer patients, and Gershanovich et al. (Petrov Research Institute of Oncology, Leningrad, USSR) report a minimal objective effect (greater than 50 percent tumor regression) in two of 95 evaluable patients. . . . Thus, the weight of clinical evidence has failed to confirm the early enthusiastic reports by Gold (ACS, 1976).

That ACS officials can consider the Soviet studies, summarized above, to be reports "on the lack of clinical effect of hydrazine sulfate" certainly defies logic. But such a version maintains the line that there are three—and only three—"proven" forms of cancer therapy, and that chemotherapy must be highly toxic to be effective.

Despite this type of official negativism, the interest in hydrazine sulfate has continued to grow in both the United States and the Soviet Union.

In the United States, Gold estimates that about 5,000 patients are being treated with hydrazine sulfate by hundreds of physicians (*Medical Tribune,* October 4, 1978). Many of these doctors have written or telephoned their favorable impressions of hydrazine. In many cases, hydrazine sulfate lacked cell-killing ability, but promoted subjective effects. Gold bristles at those who criticize his compound on these grounds.

"This is like faulting Babe Ruth for being a poor football player," Gold observes. "Baseball was the Babe's game—subjective response is hydrazine's game" (ibid.).

Many doctors are unwilling to allow their names to be mentioned in the same breath with hydrazine sulfate, lest their professional standing suffer. But others told of positive experience with the drug.

Timothy P. Ahmadi, a Mobile, Alabama, internist, reported favorably on Gold's work in *Medical Tribune*. He had used hydrazine sulfate to treat his wife, who had a form of brain cancer; she had already undergone brain surgery and treatment with radioactive cobalt.

Mrs. Ahmadi had a rapidly growing tumor of the type which the patient usually survives only several months after diagnosis. "Following the use of hydrazine sulfate," he said, "my wife felt better, her headaches decreased. She survived for two and a half years, as against the usual few months" (ibid.).

Dr. R. O. Bicks, clinical professor of medicine, University of Tennessee, and chief of gastroenterology, Baptist Hospital, told *Medical Tribune* he had used hydrazine sulfate in the treatment of two male patients with inoperable cancer of the pancreas:

I had the clinical impression that they survived longer than expected. In my experience these patients usually last four or five months. They survived nearly a year, with objective changes in the size of liver metastases, and with relative well-being. There were no cardiologic, renal, or hematologic side effects.

"And then," the Memphis physician recalled, "the FDA got in touch with me and was very upset. They said the drug causes bone-marrow toxicity [a statement that has no basis in fact, Gold counters]. We'd have continued using hydrazine if the FDA hadn't raised hell" (ibid.).

In September 1978 the National Cancer Institute announced that it was looking for research into "host/tumor competition–cachexia metabolism" as part of its expanded Diet, Nutrition and Cancer Program. The description of the project in the National Institutes of Health's *Guide for Grants and Contracts* sounded remarkably like Gold's work:

Further work is required in the area of carbohydrate, lipid, protein and overall energy metabolism of the cancer patient. Mechanisms of accelerated protein and fat depletion in these patients require further elucidation. Ineffective utilization of dietary carbohydrates with energy wasting metabolic pathways must be further clarified with the eventual aim being therapeutic intervention. . . . (National Institutes of Health, 1978).

Gold, who had had his grant renewal application turned down after the ACS "unproven method" story appeared, wrote again to

NCI and suggested that his work might qualify for a new NCI grant.

Daniel L. Kisner, M.D., special assistant for nutrition at the Institute's Division of Cancer Treatment, wrote back saying that "more extensive human biochemical work would be required before the Division of Cancer Treatment could invest the considerable sums of money necessary to test hydrazine sulfate as an anti-cachexia agent."

What sort of information was needed?

> There is no information with regard to dietary intake in the patients treated. Hydrazine sulfate may have been an appetite stimulant. There is no information as to whether the weight gain was in the form of body muscle, fat, or fluids. The meaning of this weight gain then is also left open to question. The exact metabolic effects of the drug in humans are unknown. . . . More basic biochemical rationale is not presented. Without that biochemical rationale, I believe the existing empirical data would be inadequate (Kisner, 1978).

Such an investigation would tax the resources of a major laboratory, of course, and the Syracuse Cancer Research Institute is a relatively small operation. It would also require "considerable sums of money"—but NCI was requiring Gold to perform this work *before* it would give him any financial support. This appears to be a classic double-bind situation: one must do more research before getting a grant—but in order to do that research, one must have a grant.

This is similar to NCI's treatment of Linus Pauling, who was also told he must do more laboratory work before his method could be tested in humans, but was then been turned down five times in his request for funds to do that research (see Chapter 11).

Yet, surprisingly, at the end of his letter NCI's Dr. Kisner had some encouraging words for Gold:

> Please do not misread my comments. As I have stated to you in prior correspondence and phone conversations, we are indeed interested in hydrazine sulfate as a potential anti-cachexia agent. The section on cachexia metabolism in the grants program announcement published September 25 [cited above] was written with hydrazine sulfate specifically in mind. I will continue to try to stimulate grant proposals that will answer the basic metabolic questions surrounding this agent in humans. I, too, would like to see the development of a chemotherapeutic approach for interrupting the aberrant metabolism of the cancer patient (ibid.).

Hydrazine sulfate obviously has some friends, then, in high places. Even more encouraging was the fact that NCI, in early 1979, invited Dr. Michael L. Gershanovich, director of medical oncology, Petrov Research Institute of Oncology, Leningrad, to come to the

United States and describe his four-year study of hydrazine sulfate.

Dr. Saul A. Schepartz, deputy director, Division of Cancer Treatment, stated, "We have an interest in seeing Dr. Gershanovich's report," which detailed positive results with 225 patients in the Soviet cancer center. In addition, in a cable to the Soviet scientists, NCI offered "to arrange for seminars" at which Gershanovich could present his data (Medical Tribune, May 16, 1979).

In March 1979 Gershanovich arrived at NCI headquarters in Bethesda, Maryland, as part of the annual meeting between Russian and American scientists under the U.S.–USSR Cancer Agreement.

In addition, Gershanovich was scheduled to speak at the American Association for Cancer Research (AACR), which met in New Orleans in May 1979. A summary of his paper, "Hydrazine Sulfate in Late Stage Cancer: Completion of Initial Clinical Trials in 225 Evaluable Patients," was duly printed in the Proceedings of the American Association for Cancer Research as abstract #969. Gold was scheduled to introduce the Soviet scientist.

Suddenly, however, the cancer research group denied Gershanovich a place on the program. AACR chairman, Dr. Bayard Clarkson, a Memorial Sloan-Kettering chemotherapist, said:

> Dr. Gershanovich's abstract was reviewed like any other, and, as I recall, it did not receive a high enough rating from the review committee. In any case, the important way to present data to the profession is through publication (Medical Tribune, May 16, 1979).

Asked by a reporter whether consideration should not have been given to the fact that the Soviet trial was the first large-scale test of this controversial agent, and claimed to show significant benefits from its use, Clarkson replied, "Our decision is final. The Gershanovich paper is not going to be presented, and that's it." °

Since the abstracts had already been printed, however, it appears that Gershanovich's summary will remain in the AACR Proceedings. It not only gives the relevant statistics cited above, but concludes that "initial studies thus indicate hydrazine sulfate to be clinically effective in reversing cachexia and producing disease stabilization in late-stage cancer patients."

A schism appears to have developed within the top circles of cancer orthodoxy on how to deal with hydrazine sulfate. On the one hand, certain forces within orthodox medicine may favor developing hydrazine. At the moment this group consists principally of those

---

° According to MSKCC Center News, shortly before this conference Dr. Clarkson and another researcher received grants totaling $123,000 from the American Cancer Society (March 1979).

within NCI who are most responsive to public pressure. As *Medical Tribune* noted:

A turn of events began shaping up for Dr. Gold's concepts as pressures from Capitol Hill forced the NCI to take a closer look at the role of nutritional factors in cancer (ibid.).

On the other hand, there are powerful forces that wish to maintain the ban on hydrazine sulfate. These include those conservative forces more isolated from such pressure, including the American Cancer Society, which has already committed itself through the unproven methods list, Memorial Sloan-Kettering chemotherapists, whose own work is directly contradicted by the Soviet studies, and apparently the leadership of AACR, which is committed to the highly toxic forms of chemotherapy.

In late January 1979 an NCI official told a United Press International reporter that the Institute was

interested in the research and would consider supporting additional tests in humans if the Soviet results—*which have not yet been officially reported to the scientific community*—show that the drug has an effect against cachexia (Frank, 1979).

The AACR's refusal to allow the Soviet scientist to present those results at its meeting has therefore blocked for now NCI-sponsored testing of the drug. It still "has not yet been officially reported to the scientific community," although twenty-five papers reporting positive results have been published by Gold and the Soviet scientists, and many physicians' reports are available for analysis.

Had Gershanovich been allowed to present his paper at one of the most prestigious forums in the cancer field, however, it would have become nearly impossible for the conservatives to continue their blind opposition to hydrazine sulfate's use.

The crack in orthodoxy's solid front on the hydrazine sulfate question is significant. It accompanies similar divisions on laetrile, vitamin C, the treatment of breast cancer, and the nutritional and environmental approaches to cancer.

Nevertheless, Gold cautions against premature optimism:

As of now, hydrazine sulfate seems to be swinging toward the realm of being accepted. However, one mustn't delude oneself. I think the effect of the Russians' seminars and presentations has been not to decrease opposition to the drug, but rather to polarize it. There is still a long row to hoe (Gold, 1979).

11

Vitamin C and Other Nutritional Approaches

In 1976, readers of the *Wall Street Journal* were startled to see, amid the Amex reports and notices of bond offerings, an unusual advertisement. Dr. Linus Pauling, professor emeritus at Stanford University and the only person ever to win two solo Nobel Prizes (chemistry, 1954; peace, 1962), was offering to sell "1,000 mice with malignant cancer" to readers of the *Journal* for $138 apiece in order to raise funds.

Our research [the ad read] shows that the incidence and severity of cancer depends upon diet. We urgently want to refine that research so that it may help to decrease suffering from human cancer. The U.S. government has absolutely and continually refused to support Dr. Pauling and his colleagues during the past four years (Von Hoffman, 1976).

What was behind this unprecedented public appeal from an eminent researcher, a man who is generally considered one of America's greatest chemists and one of the outstanding scientists of this century?

Basically, Pauling had stepped over that invisible but very real line separating orthodoxy from heresy. He was to suffer for his sin.

For decades, the California scientist had made contributions to chemistry, especially those chemical processes underlying life. He had helped elucidate the nature of DNA and proteins, including hemoglobin and antibodies, and had played a major role in deciphering the riddle of sickle cell anemia.

Despite the fact that Pauling was a political activist, who won his second Nobel Prize for initiating a massive peace petition during the cold war, he had never lost the support of the scientific establishment. This was because his research work was abstract and, to most laymen, arcane. In April 1966, however, Pauling entered the field of medical controversy. Since he was not a medical doctor, some of his critics implied that he was unqualified to speak on the subject of cancer or even disease in general.

A century before, Pasteur suffered a similar fate. A biographer has written that "at every incursion on the domain of medicine, he was looked upon as a chemist . . . who was poaching on the preserves of others" (Vallery-Radot, 1924).

The campaign against Pauling culminated in 1973 when one of his papers was rejected by the *Proceedings of the National Academy of Sciences,* even though he was a member of the Academy. Pauling has commented that "it was the first paper with a member as an author that had been rejected in the fifty-eight years that the *Proceedings* had existed" (cited in Null, 1979).

Pauling's involvement came about initially because of a letter from biochemist Irwin Stone. Stone had done pioneering work with ascorbic acid, ortherwise known as vitamin C, and had evolved a theory that mammals required very large amounts of this vitamin every day in order to maintain optimal health. Because of a genetic mutation, he said, man was unable to synthesize his own supply of this vitamin, as almost all of the earth's animals can. We therefore have to obtain our supply from outside, from our food (Stone, 1972).

A study of other mammals revealed that they produced substantial quantities of vitamin C, especially when they were under stress. These quantities, translated into human dimensions, meant that we needed *grams* of ascorbic acid. However, the National Academy of Sciences had declared that humans need only a tiny fraction of that amount—about 75 *milligrams* (thousandths of a gram) to remain healthy.

The reason for the glaring discrepancies between the conventional belief and Stone's is that it takes only milligrams to prevent the clinical signs of scurvy. Scurvy, a disease marked by fatigue, anemia, and bleeding gums, had been a scourge of Europe until scientists discovered that fresh fruit and vegetables could prevent and cure it.

But, argued Stone, vitamin C does more than just prevent scurvy. In fact, the scientific literature was filled with reports of vitamin C having a beneficial effect in other conditions, including, Stone believed, the common cold.

Pauling and his wife decided to pursue Stone's high ascorbic acid regimen for a while. They had both been particularly susceptible to colds. "We noticed an increased feeling of well-being," Pauling said later, "and especially a striking decrease in the number of colds that we caught, and in their severity" (Pauling, 1971).

Pauling began to tell others about this personal finding and soon was being quoted in the press as "pro-vitamin C." This brought a quick response from established figures in nutrition, especially Frederick J. Stare, a Harvard nutritionist.

Stare declared, "Vitamin C and colds—that was disproved twenty years ago." He then cited a 1942 study claiming that vitamin C did not prevent colds whereas, says Pauling, the study showed the opposite. Pauling comments:

I gradually became aware of the existence of an extraordinary contradiction between the opinions of different people about the value of vitamin C in preventing and ameliorating the common cold. Many people believe that vitamin C helps prevent colds; on the other hand, most physicians deny that this vitamin has much value in treating the common cold (ibid.).

Medical men, in general, refused even to consider the possibility that vitamin C had this effect. Pauling proposed two reasons for their refusal.

First, doctors, drug companies, and government bureaucrats are looking for drugs that are uniformly effective in treating an ailment, such as the antibiotics. "In the search for a drug to combat a disease the effort is usually made to find one that is 100 percent effective," Pauling says.

"Another factor," he adds, "has probably been the lack of interest of the drug companies in a natural substance that is available at a low price and cannot be patented" (ibid.).

Pauling found a discrepancy between the facts and the medical opinions on vitamin C and the common cold. For example, researchers who achieved *positive* results in preventing colds with vitamin C sometimes reported those tests as *negative* in their summaries.

These inaccurate summaries were then reported uncritically in news articles, editorials, and reviews, which both laymen and doctors depended upon for information and opinions.

When Pauling's book *Vitamin C and the Common Cold* appeared and sold briskly, this seemed to sharpen the resistance of the medical conservatives, despite the many arguments and detailed analyses of data in that slim volume. Apparently these doctors had made up their minds about vitamin C. "The negative attitude of the medical establishment has continued to the present time," Pauling noted in an updated edition of his book (Pauling, 1976).

The commissioner of the Food and Drug Administration now

launched an attack, calling Pauling's arguments "ridiculous." Pauling wrote several letters to the commissioner, Charles C. Edwards, and finally this official telephoned and invited the California scientist to a meeting in Washington. But when Pauling informed Edwards he was ready to come Edwards withdrew the invitation.

A double standard was used to attack Pauling's arguments. These critics, wrote Abram Hoffer, a well-known Canadian physician,

use two sets of logic. Before they are prepared to look at Dr. Pauling's hypothesis, they demand proof of the most rigorous kind. But when arguing against his views, they refer to evidence of the flimsiest sort for the toxicity of ascorbic acid (Pauling, 1971).

But Pauling's troubles with orthodoxy were only beginning. To be sure, the "common cold" can be a serious health problem. But when Pauling turned his attention to cancer, he entered an area of medical controversy unprecedented in its bitterness.

It is difficult to say exactly where or how the belief that vitamin C might benefit cancer patients originated. Juices containing vitamin C have long been used as folk remedies. Its use may have originated among North American Indians, who drank brews made from ascorbate-containing plants as a kind of "miracle drug" to treat a variety of ailments (Bailey, 1972:14). A sailor on the ship of the English explorer Captain James Cook, who introduced the use of limes for the British "limies," wrote exuberantly:

> We were all hearty seamen, no colds did we fear
> And we have from all sickness entirely kept clear.
> Thanks be to the Captain, he has proved so good
> Amongst all the Islands to give us fresh food
> (Quoted in Pauling, 1971:10).

Over the years, a number of prominent doctors have abandoned surgery and radiation and introduced nutritional therapies for cancer (Morris, 1977). In retrospect, it can be seen that many of these dietary regimens were high in vitamin C.

From the time of its discovery, in fact, vitamin C has been studied in relation to cancer. Early experiments were not promising. One of the first investigations on the effect of ascorbic acid on experimental animals was carried out by Kanematsu Sugiura and K. Benedict in the 1920s. They reported that "the vitamins A, C, D and E are not essential for the growth of transplanted neoplasms" (cited in Hoffman, 1937).

In the 1930s German physicians began to use vitamin C in one- and two-gram doses in the treatment of human cancer. According to

Irwin Stone, W. G. Deucher (1940), Von Wendt (1949), and L. Huber (1953) all had some success with this method (Stone, 1972).

Richard Passwater noted in his book *Cancer and Its Nutritional Therapies* that researchers found that cancer patients had "lower than average amounts of vitamin C in their blood plasma and white blood corpuscles" (Passwater, 1978). This laboratory finding supported epidemiological studies which seemed to correlate a lack of vitamin C with a high death rate, including a high cancer death rate. A study was initiated in 1948 when 577 older residents of California's San Mateo County were interviewed. When scientists followed up these interviews eight years later, they found that the death rate for those receiving the highest amount of dietary vitamin C was only 40 percent of those with much smaller amounts of the vitamin (ibid.).

In 1954 the Canadian physician W. J. McCormick found that "the degree of malignancy is determined inversely by the degree of connective tissue resistance, which in turn is dependent upon the adequacy of vitamin C status" (ibid.). McCormick's work received little scientific attention but was widely reported by the health food movements. All of this research pointed in the direction of an attempt at using large doses of the vitamin in a systematic study of cancer. A few years later, in the mid-1960s, Ewan Cameron and Linus Pauling entered the investigation.

Settling the question would not seem to be very difficult, since vitamin C is a chemically well-defined substance, unlike some other proposed anticancer agents such as Krebiozen, Coley's toxins, or Burton's vaccine (see Chapter 12). Instead, the investigation has turned into a bitter controversy.

To understand the reason for this, it is necessary to look at the broader context of the debate. Orthodox spokesmen have always reserved their greatest scorn for the "quacks" and "food faddists" who put "great stress on the special dietary value of various 'wonder' foods" (Young, 1967). Since 1929, the Food and Drug Administration in particular has kept up a running battle with the health food movement (ibid.:336).

"There is no diet that prevents cancer in man," Dr. Morris Shimkin wrote in an NCI primer. "Treatment of cancer by diet alone is in the realm of quackery" (Shimkin, 1973:112).

"To stress the nutritional approach to cancer," historian Nat Morris has written, "eventually became the surest way to become branded a quack" (Morris, 1977:44).

The biggest battle of the 1940s and 1950s raged over the work and theories of Dr. Max Gerson. In 1946 the German-born Gerson was called to testify before a United States Senate committee investigating cancer. Gerson brought with him five patients who had had some of the most common forms of cancer in the United States. He also came armed with X-ray photographs, pathology reports from leading hospitals (including Memorial), and testimonials from many other patients and relatives of cancer victims.

Gerson's credentials were respectable. He had graduated from a prominent German medical school between the wars and had studied with noted neurologists and physiologists. At the time of his appearance before the committee of Senator Claude Pepper (D.-Fla.) Gerson was affiliated with Gotham Hospital in New York and had a private practice on Park Avenue. He was the author of approximately fifty articles in medical journals (Haught, 1962).

What made Gerson controversial was his method—entirely dietary and natural. This included fresh fruit and vegetable juices, a vegetable broth, fresh liver juice, and foods high in potassium to counterbalance what Gerson considered the oversalting of modern foods. One unusual aspect of Gerson's regimen for cancer patients was a daily coffee enema to cleanse the body. This eventually became a source of jollity within the establishment—"With cream or sugar?" they invariably asked.

But Gerson's patients were articulate witnesses, and Senator Pepper's committee was not unfriendly to the unorthodox physician.

The Pepper hearings were convened at the request of the American Cancer Society. Pepper himself was politically in the ACS's debt.° Although Gerson received much favorable publicity because of his Senate appearance, Pepper's committee did not follow his recommendations for a dietary-preventive approach to cancer.

Gerson and his dietary method were gaining in credibility and prestige just at the moment that chemotherapy also sought public acceptance. Orthodox forces in the cancer field were not slow in responding to this challenge. Their ire was heightened by the publicity given Gerson in the newspapers and on radio, and in John Gunther's best-selling memoir, *Death Be Not Proud*, in which Gerson's method is credited with a temporary remission in his son's brain tumor (Gunther, 1949).

Gerson was reviewed twice in *JAMA*, the journal of the American Medical Association, and both times it was concluded that his method of treating cancer "was of no value" (ACS, 1971b).

In 1947 a committee of the New York County Medical Society

° The *Miami Daily News* had supported Pepper for the Senate in 1944 in exchange for his support for holding hearings on medical research. Mrs. Daniel (Florence) Mahoney, Mary Lasker's friend and colleague in the ACS, was an owner of the newspaper. Mrs. Lasker chose and briefed many of the witnesses before the Pepper hearings, including C. P. Rhoads (Strickland, 1972).

reviewed the records of eighty-six patients, but claimed to be unable to find any scientific value in Gerson's treatment. Gerson was not allowed to defend himself before these investigative boards (Haught, 1962).

Gerson's medical privileges at Gotham Hospital were revoked, and he was unable to find an affiliation with any other hospital in the city. In 1953 his malpractice insurance was discontinued. Refusing to give up his innovative approach, after the authorities had ruled it invalid, he opened a sanatorium of his own. On March 4, 1958, he was finally suspended for two years from the New York Medical Society. The leaders of the surgery, radiation, and chemotherapy approaches to cancer gathered at the New York Academy of Medicine and condemned a colleague who claimed to live by Hippocrates's dictum "Above all, do no harm." Gerson died a year later, and his method (documented in 1958 in the book *A Cancer Therapy*) was never subjected to the kind of double-blind test that could have established its true worth.

Upon Gerson's death, Albert Schweitzer, the Nobel Prize–winning physician and missionary, and a patient of Gerson's, issued the following statement:

I see in him [Gerson] one of the most eminent medical geniuses in the history of medicine. Many of his basic ideas have been adopted without having his name connected with them. Yet he has achieved more than seemed possible under adverse conditions. He leaves a legacy which commands attention and which will assure him his due place. Those whom he cured will now attest to the truth of his ideas (Haught, 1962).

Gerson's daughter, Charlotte Gerson Strauss, has kept Gerson's ideas alive. She runs a health retreat in Mexico which employs the Gerson method in the treatment of cancer, and frequently speaks at "health food" conventions on her father's approach (*Cancer Control Journal*, Vol. 3, Nos. 1–2, 1975). A popular book on Gerson's work (*Has Dr. Max Gerson a True Cancer Cure?*) has reputedly sold almost a quarter of a million copies. Some physicians today have quietly incorporated Gerson's ideas into their practice: a number of the latest developments in cancer research appear to owe a debt to Gerson "without having his name connected with them."

But to the "cancer establishment," Gerson is still the refugee quack with the coffee enemas.

It was controversies such as this over "food faddism" which set the stage for Linus Pauling's entrance into the cancer controversy. In 1971, Ewan Cameron, M.D., at the Vale of Leven District General

Hospital in Loch Lomondside, Scotland, working with Pauling, began to give terminal cancer patients high doses of vitamin C on the theory that ascorbic acid was not (in Pauling's words) "a special anticancer wonder drug" but could "bolster up the body's natural protective mechanisms."

Most of these patients had first received standard methods of treatment—surgery, radiation, and hormones; only a few had received cytotoxic drugs. When at least two doctors decided these methods had failed and nothing further could be done, in other words when the patients were terminally ill, high-dose vitamin C therapy was begun.

Dr. Cameron had arrived at vitamin C therapy by a different route from Pauling's A clinician as well as a cancer researcher, Cameron had studied the biochemistry of cancer cells and found that cancer spread by invading healthy normal tissue in its vicinity. To do so, it was known, the cancer cell produced an enzyme, hyaluronidase. This enzyme attacked the intercellular ground cement, the material that holds cells together in tissues. In 1966 Cameron published this theory in a book called *Hyaluronidase and Cancer*. From that point on, the Scottish surgeon searched for a substance—he thought it would be a hormone—which could strengthen the intercellular cement and slow the growth of the tumor. Success came not from a hormone but from vitamin C, which other researchers had shown was a powerful builder of this "cement."

Cameron was well situated to undertake a large-scale study of cancer. Scotland has the dubious distinction of being the cancer capital of the world—more people die of the disease, per hundred thousand, than in any other country. In fact, the Scottish cancer death rate is more than *nine times* that of some countries, such as the Dominican Republic or Mexico (ACS, 1971a). The exact reasons for this are not known but it is generally assumed to have a great deal to do with environmental factors, including diet (Fraumeni, 1975:206).

In the Loch Lomondside area, near Glasgow, about 90 percent of the cancer patients are sent to the Vale of Leven hospital, whose surgical unit is under Cameron's control. Cameron's clinical research work is supported financially by Scotland's Secretary of State and the Linus Pauling Institute.

The vitamin testing began in 1971 and, as Pauling recently related, the doctors were startled by the results:

Dr. Cameron first noticed that the patients felt well when they received 10 grams a day or more of vitamin C. They developed good appetites, increased energy, got up from the hospital, went home, went back to work and got along much better than with conventional therapy. Patients who were on morphine for pain could be taken off their morphine in five days (quoted in Newbold, 1978).

In order to put these results in a scientifically provable form they began a detailed study of 100 terminal cancer patients—terminal being defined as a situation in which continuance of any conventional form of treatment would offer no further benefit according to two independent physicians.

A biostatistician, Dr. Frances Meuli, went through the records of cancer patients at Vale of Leven and matched each experimental subject with ten other patients who had the same kind of cancer, and were of the same sex and approximately the same age (plus or minus five years). In the records of each there was a notation that treatment had been abandoned because the patient was considered terminal. Meuli then computed the survival time for each of these 1,000 patients, who had been treated by conventional means, and compared this to the patients receiving vitamin C under Dr. Cameron's care.

The results were striking. Patients receiving 10 grams a day of vitamin C lived, on the average, four times as long after having reached the terminal state than those who received only conventional therapy. They also experienced the improvements in life quality already mentioned. What was even more interesting, a minority of the vitamin C patients—about 16 percent—experienced a dramatically marked increase in survival time. While the mean control group survival was only fifty days, these individuals all lived more than a year. Some of them, declared terminal in the early 1970s, are still alive today.

One woman, who was terminally ill with breast cancer, is now said to be healthy and free of cancer. Another patient, a truck driver on the Glasgow–London route, was cleared of all visible signs of cancer within four to five days of starting on vitamin C. As with many patients, however, once he was cured his physician stopped his "medicine," the vitamin supplements. His fever returned and soon he was back in the hospital with cancer. It took somewhat longer the second time, but after vitamin C therapy the cancer disappeared again. The trucker remains in good health (Passwater, 1978).

Cameron continues to treat terminal cancer patients with vitamin C, and he soon expects to have 4,000 cases in his records. The results appear to be better when the treatment is started earlier, however. "We surmise," Cameron and Pauling wrote in their 1976 *Proceedings of the National Academy of Sciences* article, "that the addition of ascorbate to the treatment of patients with cancer at an earlier stage of development might chang[e] life expectancy . . .

from, for example, 5 years to 20 years" (Pauling and Cameron, 1976).

"With the proper use of vitamin C for cancer," says Linus Pauling, "we could cut the death rate by 75 percent. It is probably wise for every cancer patient to receive vitamin C" (Passwater, 1978).

In some cases Cameron has used 20 or 30 grams a day on patients, by intravenous drip. "The results were really quite astounding," says his California colleague (quoted in Newbold, 1978).

In the United States, the cancer experts responded with suspicion and hostility to Pauling, Cameron, and vitamin C therapy.

They refused to accept foreign clinical accounts, but insisted that animal work be started from scratch before clinical trials in the United States could begin. This could take years, but Pauling consented to do it, and applied for a modest $30,000 grant from NCI. The government then refused him the money.

Five times this well-known scientist, author of more than 400 scientific papers, requested funds from NCI, and five times he was rejected. In fact, in some ways the lines seem to be hardening. When Pauling first applied for funds, the application was technically approved, but with "low priority," and it was never funded. But after the 1976 National Academy of Sciences paper came out, the chief of diagnosis and treatment at NCI wrote in his summary statement, "Based on evaluation of scientific merit of this application disapproval must be recommended" (Passwater, 1978).

Pauling replied:

The National Cancer Institute is not operated in such a way as to favor the discovery of new methods of controlling cancer. . . . In my opinion the NCI does not know how to carry on research nor how to recognize a new idea (cited in Houston, 1978).

Instead of funding Dr. Pauling, the NCI set up a study of vitamin C at the Mayo Clinic in Rochester, Minnesota. Terminal cancer patients received vitamin C while others received only a placebo. According to an NCI press handout:

Subjective data about relief of symptoms is being collected from all of the patients, and survival times are being recorded. Results are expected to be available in 1979. In addition . . . NCI has tested vitamin C in animal models used to screen drugs for anticancer activity. These tests are continuing, however, results thus far have not been encouraging (Cancer Information Service, 1978).

In September 1979, Mayo Clinic researchers announced that they had found large amounts of vitamin C ineffective in curing cancer or in alleviating pain in patients with advanced cancer (Creagan, 1979). The majority of these patients had first received chemotherapy and radiation. The researchers themselves granted that it was "impossible to draw any conclusions about the possible effectiveness of vitamin C in previously untreated patients" (quoted in *New York Times*, September 27, 1979).

In a press release dated September 28, 1979, Pauling disputed the validity of the Mayo test, claiming that the results of the study had been "misrepresented by the Mayo Clinic investigators and in newspaper articles" (Hoefer–Amidei, 1979).

The release stated that the Mayo test was intended to be closely modeled after the work of Dr. Ewan Cameron. But Pauling earlier, on August 9, 1978, had warned the Mayo scientists that the "patients studied by Dr. Cameron had not received chemotherapy. The cytotoxic drugs damage the body's protective mechanisms, and vitamin C probably functions largely by potentiating these mechanisms. . . . You should be careful to use only patients who have not received chemotherapy. . . . Otherwise, the trial cannot be described as repeating the work of Cameron" (ibid.).

Furthermore, the Mayo oncologists claimed that 50 of the 100 ascorbic-treated patients in the Scottish study had received chemotherapy and high-energy radiation, "whereas in fact," says Pauling, "only 4 had received chemotherapy and only 20 had received high-energy radiation" (ibid.).

Pauling and Cameron have called on NCI to do another controlled clinical study on patients with advanced cancer who have not received treatment with chemotherapy, but the prospects for such a study seem slight.

Some doctors are now using vitamin C megadoses along with other nutrients in the treatment of cancer. One such nutrition-oriented doctor is H. L. Newbold of New York City. Trained as an internist and a psychiatrist, Newbold now treats many ailments with nontoxic approaches. For cancer he favors the use of vitamin C.

For skin cancer, Newbold uses a combination of about 15 grams a day by mouth and a topical vitamin C ointment applied to the tumor itself, five or six times a day. "It's very effective in treating skin cancer," he has said. "I've had three or four of those who have done very well, and I've talked to doctors who have had many more" (Newbold, 1979).

In other kinds of cancer Newbold tries to get the dosage up as high as he can. "By mouth you can seldom go to more than 50 or 60 grams a day." He also generally gives 50 grams by the intravenous route. "I had one patient I gave 50 grams to for two months, six days a week. There were no serious complications."

"If I had cancer, that's what I would do," he added. "I'd take that for three months, and as much as I could get by mouth also" (ibid.).

One patient received an extraordinary 105 grams a day of vitamin C, starting in December 1977. To put this in perspective, the Food and Drug Administration says humans need only 60 *milligrams* of this nutrient. Newbold is therefore giving almost *two thousand times* the government's recommended dosage.

This woman had a deadly "oat cell" carcinoma of the lung. More than a year later the woman was back on her job and feeling fine. The tumor, however, is still there. "It's a pretty good remission," says Newbold. "I'm sure she would have been dead long ago [without vitamin C]" (ibid.).

Other forms of nutritional therapy are also generating interest after many years of neglect. For example, there is increasing evidence that vitamin A has anticancer properties. In 1976 the NCI announced clinical trials with a chemical substance related to vitamin A. But the empirical use of vitamin A–containing foods for cancer goes back much further than the NCI—in fact, it goes back at least to the eighteenth century.

Bernard Peyrilhe (1735–1804), professor of chemistry at the École Santé and professor-royal at the College of Surgery in Paris who is remembered as the winner of a 1773 prize from the Academy of Lyon on the subject "What Is Cancer?" (Shimkin, 1977), advocated the use of carrot juice in the treatment of cancer. Carrot juice is one of the best sources of vitamin A: it figured in Gerson's diet, as well.

The rationale for the use of vitamin A in cancer is that this oil-soluble vitamin nurtures and protects the epithelial (lining) cells of the body. A lack of vitamin A will lead to night blindness as well as to many kinds of skin diseases, retarded growth, and a susceptibility to infection.

In the 1920s Japanese scientists showed that stomach cancer could be produced in rats by simply depriving the animals of this life-sustaining nutrient (Hixson, 1976b).

In the 1930s scientists in Cambridge, England, showed that vitamin A was essential for the proper differentiation—or maturation—of epithelial cells. A majority of lung cancers occurred when these same cells in the bronchi of the lungs failed to mature (ibid.).

Experiments at Memorial Hospital in the 1940s showed that there is often a deficiency of this vitamin in the blood of cancer patients. (The same observation has been made for vitamin C.) At the time, this deficiency was related to an impairment of the liver, which stores and distributes vitamin A throughout the body (*New York Journal-American*, November 17, 1941).

Although heralded at the time as a discovery of "capital significance," vitamin A was forgotten or scorned when chemotherapy came to the fore. In the 1960s, some interest in vitamin A was revived. Dr. Umberto Saffioti, now a government cancer researcher, found that vitamin A inhibited the development of lung cancer in experimental hamsters. Unsupplemented animals, however, developed lung cancers "remarkably similar" to the human kind when they were dosed with a by-product of cigarette smoke (Hixson, 1976b).

This discovery, too, was widely heralded as a breakthrough which could "possibly lead to results of practical significance for the prevention of lung cancer," according to the scientist. Ten years later, however, Saffioti resigned in protest as head of NCI's entire prevention program, charging that there was "inadequate support for . . . cancer prevention" (*Cancer Letter*, May 7, 1976).

This has not stopped some clinicians from using vitamin A against cancer. To increase their resistance to the disease, Newbold gives his patients this vitamin in dosages tailored to their individual needs. To some patients he gives as much as 200,000 International Units (I.U.) of the vitamin. Vitamin A in high doses can be toxic. If this dose produces signs of toxicity, he lowers it. By orthodox standards, this is an extraordinary amount, since 50,000 I.U. is supposed to be the threshold for toxicity (Newbold, 1979).

Some German cancer specialists have long been using a special form of vitamin A called "A-mulsin" as part of an overall treatment of cancer. They have found a way to emulsify it so that it is supposedly no longer harmful, even when given daily in colossal (up to 3,000,000 I.U.) dosages.

In early 1976, *Esquire* magazine prepared to publish a controversial story on cancer by science writer Pat McGrady, Jr. McGrady, the son of the former ACS official, hailed the use of this therapy at Germany's Janker Clinic. Using a combination of agents unavailable in the United States, the Janker Clinic, he said, got full or partial remission in 70 percent of the 76,000 patients it has treated since 1936. Yet the Food and Drug Administration had banned A-mulsin, the NCI was uninterested in it, and the ACS "prides itself on keeping the Janker techniques out of the United States" (McGrady, Jr., 1976).

In March 1976, as the *Esquire* article approached publication date, the National Cancer Institute suddenly announced a clinical trial with a vitamin A–like compound of its own. The "breakthrough" was given wide publicity and made banner headlines across the country. Yet, as Joseph Hixson pointed out, "The timing of the . . . revelation was curious. It came while the April issue of *Esquire* was still on the presses" (Hixson, 1976b).

The NCI did not choose to use carrot juice or plain vitamin A for its trial, much less the "unproven" A-mulsin. It chose instead a synthetic variant, a chemical called the "13-cis isomer of retinoic acid." This form of retinoic acid is manufactured by the Swiss pharmaceutical giant Hoffmann–La Roche. Actual clinical trials did not begin until the summer of 1978, and only about a dozen patients have been studied at this writing, all of them with premalignant lesions which may develop into bladder cancer. According to doctors at Massachusetts General Hospital, who are directing the study, they hope eventually to enroll about seventy people in the program. Results were to be announced in 1980 (*New York Post,* June 28, 1979).

What gives the question of vitamin A some urgency, however, is that about 30 percent of the American public does not receive even the dosage recommended by the Food and Drug Administration: 5,000 I.U. a day. And many nutrition-oriented doctors believe that the optimal dosage, especially for smokers, is three to six times that amount.

Not long ago, the cancer experts rejected any suggestion of a link between food and malignancy, and generally pointed with pride at the "great American diet." Because of this attitude, throughout the 1960s and much of the 1970s, NCI spent virtually nothing on nutrition research. The same held true of other centers, such as Memorial Sloan-Kettering, which avoided the topic almost entirely.

In 1974, under pressure from the parents of children with cancer, Congress *forced* NCI to devote a part of its budget to nutrition. Even so, this amounted to just 1 percent of its total funds, and even this amount was not always spent (Chowka, 1978b).

A turning point came, however, when Senator George McGovern's (D.-S.D.) Senate nutrition subcommittee issued a report, "Dietary Goals for the United States," which indicted the fatty, overprocessed American diet for the high incidence of cancer and other degenerative diseases. Despite screams of "insufficient evidence" from the AMA and other bastions of cure-oriented medicine, McGovern's report was influential *(Los Angeles Times,* January 24, 1978).

Federal health officials depend on Congress for their jobs and appropriations; they could not afford to ignore what McGovern was saying. National Institutes of Health director Donald Frederickson now testified before McGovern's committee that of the estimated 75 percent of human cancers due to environmental causes, *most* may be related to food. NCI director Arthur Upton, Ph.D., declared, "A large fraction of the cancer burden may be related to diet" (quoted in Houston, 1978).

Upton hastened to add, however, that this is "still only a hypothesis and the leads must be nailed down."

"To a cross," added Robert Houston sardonically.

12

Burton's
Immunological Method

Since the early 1970s, immunology has been one of the great hopes of the cancer establishment. The basic principle of cancer immunology is to find natural factors which will attack cancer cells in the same way that our native immune system attacks bacterial, viral, or parasitic invaders.

The existence of such immune mechanisms was postulated in the 1950s by such prominent scientists as Sir MacFarlane Burnet and Dr. Lewis Thomas.

They argued that cancer cells are different from normal cells. Ordinarily, the immune system recognizes these cells as foreign and destroys them before they reproduce and get out of control. But if the defense mechanisms are weak, they cannot do away with the mutant cancer cells. They therefore run wild, invade normal tissues, and ultimately, if they are not destroyed, kill the host (Burnet, 1970).

Animal experiments to corroborate this thesis were encouraging. But when scientists attempted to carry this work into the human, clinical situation, they ran into a number of problems. In 1976 Dr. Peter Alexander, head of tumor immunology at the Chester Beatty Research Institute in Surrey, England, said that cancer immunotherapy had been on the wrong track for at least a decade (*Medical World News*, November 1, 1976).

No procedure, he told a combined American Cancer Society–National Cancer Institute meeting, has proved clinically effective against human cancers. The reason for this "failure to translate immunotherapy from mouse to man" was that researchers were unable to simulate in their laboratory the actual human situation, in which patients die most often of secondary growths.

Dr. Donald Morton, chief of oncology at the University of California, Los Angeles, agreed with Alexander's assessment. In recent years, he said, "over-enthusiastic" newspaper reports raised hopes that immunotherapy might provide a "cure" for cancer. "It was doomed not to live up to that type of expectation," he said. "With present-day knowledge it is unlikely immunology will reverse the tide and make the patient disease-free" (ibid.).

Yet, as fund-raising time rolls around, newspaper reports about immunology's great promise begin to pick up once more. This leads to an upsurge of hope in the desperate and, probably, an increase in donations to the cancer fund-raising agencies. More often than not, however, these reports speak of distant promise rather than present-day clinical accomplishments.

At least one immunologist has attempted to break out of the confines of the laboratory and directly apply his mouse techniques to suffering, often dying, human patients. This scientist is Lawrence Burton, Ph.D. In doing so, he has incurred the wrath of his former colleagues and the medical profession, and alienated himself from the established centers of power.

Burton's background seems orthodox enough. Born in the Bronx, New York, in 1926, he attended Brooklyn College and New York University, from which he earned a Ph.D. in 1955. Burton held various research and teaching positions at the California Institute of Technology, New York University, and St. Vincent's Hospital, where he was a senior investigator in the Hodgkin's Disease Research Laboratory.

In the mid-1950s, Burton and another researcher, Frank Friedman, Ph.D., managed to extract a factor from the larvae of fruit flies which induced tumors in noncancerous insects. Burton and Friedman, fresh out of graduate school, published this work in *Science* and then went together to the California Institute of Technology for postdoctoral research (Burton and Friedman, 1956).

Back in New York, in the late 1950s, Burton and Friedman joined with Dr. Antonio Rottino, M. L. Kaplan, and Dr. Robert Kassel, in extracting, through trial and error, a tumor-inhibiting factor. The original purpose of these experiments, says Burton, was not to find a treatment for malignancies, but to speed up cancer experiments and thus save money. The group received research grants for this purpose from the Damon Runyon Memorial Fund for Cancer Research and the National Cancer Institute (Kassel et al., 1963).

The group now extended these fruit-fly findings to mice. Using similar techniques, they extracted a factor from mouse blood which caused long-term remission of cancer in mice (Burton et al., 1959).

Actually, this prosaic description cannot convey the excitement of the St. Vincent's group at what they had discovered. The animals' cancers within a matter of hours would begin to *disappear*. According to Rottino, it was new, original, and dramatic (Rottino, 1978). Eventually, the cancer would return, but an exciting empirical observation had been made about the relationship between normal blood and the defense against malignancy. The tumor-inhibiting factor could also cross species lines. Thus a factor derived from fruit fly or mouse could trigger anticancer effects in human cells and vice versa. This finding "strongly suggests that the inhibitor system in the human may be directly comparable to that demonstrated in the mouse," the scientists wrote later in the *Annals of the New York Academy of Sciences* (Kassel et al., 1963).

In the early 1960s the St. Vincent's team came to the attention of the cancer establishment. Sloan-Kettering Institute dispatched Dr. John J. Harris to Burton's laboratory to learn the new techniques. After several months, Harris coauthored a paper with the St. Vincentians in which his name, quite properly, was listed *after* those of the original discoverers (ibid.). Burton claims that the SKI administration put pressure on Harris.

For example, Harris received a reprimand from Frank Horsfall, the director of Sloan-Kettering Institute, for publishing with the St. Vincent's team; Horsfall told him that Sloan-Kettering scientists never allowed their names to be listed in papers after those of scientists at "lesser" institutions.

Harris died on April 27, 1978, at the age of fifty-four, but his widow confirmed Burton's account of the episode. According to Mrs. Harris, when her husband published with his name listed fourth on the 1962 article,

Horsfall couldn't take this. If anything, Sloan-Kettering should be first. But my husband didn't see it that way. He and Horsfall had several disagreements.

My husband was enthusiastic about what Burton and Friedman were doing, and pushed them along. Horsfall tried his best to hamper my husband in every way. He finally left. He had had it. They pressured him quite a bit (Bertha Harris, 1979).

Another Sloan-Kettering scientist was given what Burton calls "the office treatment":

They put him in a room—no telephone, no lab, no work. "You're here nine-to-five, you can bring all the newspapers you want. No secretary, no visitors." He lasted about a year and a half and then he couldn't take it anymore (Burton, 1978).

"But they weren't through," Burton recalls heatedly. "They sent us contracts. They said they'd give us all the wonders of the world, all the credit, if we would work with them." The St. Vincent's scientists turned down the offer. "What the hell do we need them for?" they asked (Burton, 1978). "Then the fun started," Burton says. "We were on a Public Health Service grant. Termination. We had the largest Damon Runyon grant at St. Vincent's. Termination. We couldn't understand what hit us. We were naive" (ibid.).

Brought to their knees financially by this sudden withdrawal of their support, the researchers decided to offer their techniques to Sloan-Kettering after all. SKI now dispatched Dr. Aaron Bendich, one of its senior scientists, a person as outspoken and blunt as Burton himself. When the SKI scientist heard the offer, Burton recalls, he told the young researchers, "It's got to be a pile of crap if you're offering it to us for nothing" (ibid.).

The St. Vincent's group desperately started reapplying for government grants. Each time, however, they were turned down, on the recommendation of a Sloan-Kettering chemotherapist who was sent to make a site visit for the National Cancer Institute.

On the advice of another scientist who said, "Let 'em look at bumps," the St. Vincent's team switched from leukemic mice to animals with spontaneous breast cancers, similar to those used in Sugiura's laetrile experiments. The strain of mice they chose was designated $C_3H(t)$, (t) for Dr. Albert Tannenbaum, director of the Department of Cancer Research at Michael Reese Hospital in Chicago, who supplied the strain.

Injecting their mouse-derived tumor-inhibiting factor into animals with rock-hard breast tumors, the St. Vincent's scientists watched in amazement as the growths became soft, spongy, and disappeared within a day or two. "We achieved tremendous results," Burton says, with no false modesty. "It was dramatic to see how the tumor would undergo necrosis," says Rottino, a scholarly research physician not given to overstatement. "That is important, and it is something very fundamental that should be studied" (Rottino, 1978).

In 1966 Patrick McGrady, Sr., happened to be a patient at St. Vincent's. He asked Burton for an on-the-spot demonstration of his techniques. "I saw him perform miracles on these mice," McGrady recollects. "He'd make the tumors disappear while you watched. There's no question in my mind that this was authentic" (McGrady, Sr., 1979).

McGrady was well aware that no form of orthodox treatment had an equivalent effect on these tumors. Since he had originated and controlled the selection list for the ACS Science Writers' Seminar, he invited Burton and Friedman to Phoenix that March to demonstrate their new technique.

As prominent scientists and reporters watched, Burton picked up four mice with big, bulging tumors and injected them with what he called a "de-blocking" agent. An hour later, the assembled doctors and writers, many of them skeptical of the whole procedure, approached the demonstration table.

According to David Cleary, science writer for the *Philadelphia Bulletin* who was present at the meeting, "The two gentlemen from St. Vincent's Hospital demonstrated before our very eyes that injection of a mysterious serum . . . caused the disappearance of massive tumors in mice within a few hours" (cited in Houston, 1979b).

Here was the stuff scoops are made of. Reporters suddenly rushed from the room and fought for telephones to be the first ones to break this story. By the end of the day, banner headlines in Los Angeles and other major cities proclaimed, "15-MINUTE CANCER CURE FOR MICE: HUMANS NEXT?" (Anderson, 1974). Burton has since claimed that the American Cancer Society made $4 million from the public as a result of favorable publicity generated by his work (Houston, 1979b).

Many of those present reacted with hostility and suspicion. A rumor even began to spread: "The mice were switched!" Five top scientists, including a leading New York cancer virologist, formed a committee and scheduled a news conference to denounce Burton as a fraud and his method as quackery. At the last minute, McGrady and others at the ACS managed to dissuade them (Burton, 1978).

Within a year there was a repeat performance at the conservative New York Academy of Medicine. Burton once again injected the mice with the "de-blocking" factor and once again the tumors began to melt away. "The immediate reaction was that it was a fake," Rottino recalls (Rottino, 1978).

One researcher said, "That's very interesting, but since I didn't do it, I can't really say that it works" (Anderson, 1974).

Rottino shrugged it off with philosophical comments about "human nature." But Burton lashed out publicly at his accusers and detractors. With obvious sarcasm, he told the gathering that he had hypnotized them en masse during the performance and then substituted fresh, healthy mice for the tumorous ones.

By the early 1970s the researchers, principally Burton and Friedman, had elaborated a theory on how the mysterious injections worked. It involved the interaction of blocking protein, de-blocking protein, tumor antibody, and tumor complement.

These terms are foreign to the public, and it is beyond the scope of this discussion to greatly elaborate on their meaning. They are fairly familiar to orthodox cancer researchers (see Maugh and Marx, 1975:58–61). Tumor antibody is Burton's term for a form of gamma globulin (IgG) as well as related proteins (IgA and IgM). Blocking factors are now common scientific concepts. Similarly, unblocking, or de-blocking, factors, such as the alpha-2-macroglobulin, which Burton claims caused the sensational remissions in mice, have also been frequently posited by scientific researchers (ibid.).

Unorthodox cancer scientists are sometimes accused of inventing outlandish scientific vocabularies simply in order to amaze and befuddle the nonprofessional. The American Cancer Society has suggested that "the proponents of new or unproven methods of cancer management . . . are often inclined to use complex jargon and unusual phraseology to embellish their writings" (ACS, 1971b). In Burton's case, at least, the novelty does not lie so much in the arcane terminology as in the way the terms are put together to formulate a theory of cancer.

The greatest challenge for a research scientist is to see his work applied to the human situation. As Dr. Peter Alexander indicated, this is often the moment of greatest disappointment as well. Laboratory conditions are usually far different from clinical conditions.

In 1974 Burton was offered a chance to test his approach on human patients. With the help of wealthy supporters, he and Friedman left St. Vincent's after more than fifteen years and founded the Immunology Research Foundation in Great Neck, New York.

Burton administered an immuno-competence blood test to determine the levels of blocking protein and the other factors, and medical doctors affiliated with the new foundation began to treat cancer patients with a sequence of the various blood components.

In July 1974 *New York* magazine ran a front-page story on the two Long Island researchers titled: "The Politics of Cancer—Why Won't the Medical Establishment Pay Attention to These Two Men?" The cover of this widely read magazine showed Burton and Friedman, in full color, holding out a $C_3H(t)$ mouse for the inspection of the general public (Anderson, 1974).

Suddenly Sloan-Kettering seemed interested again. This was the period of liberalism toward unorthodox approaches at the New York cancer research institute, the period of laetrile and hydrazine sulfate. According to nutritionist Carleton Fredericks, Ph.D., Sloan-Kettering even sent a small number of patients to Burton's clinic for treatment at this time. (A relative of Fredericks was treated with Burton's method and apparently underwent a remission of his cancer, but he died of other causes.) (Fredericks, 1978).

For a brief period the following year, it looked as if Burton and Friedman were about to be accepted back into the establishment fold. They applied for an Investigative New Drug permit from the Food and Drug Administration. Dr. William Terry and other National Cancer Institute officials visited the Great Neck laboratory and told *Modern Medicine,* a magazine for doctors, "Anything that can control tumor growth is significant" (Yasgur, 1975).

Modern Medicine also reported that

eleven New York–area doctors, including some physicians at Downstate Medical Center, have expressed great interest in participating in a clinical protocol if the IRF [Immunology Research Foundation] request is approved, and it is possible that trials may have begun by the time this article appears (ibid.).

That was January 1, 1975. But trials never began. There are radically different versions of why human tests of Burton's method did not come to pass. According to an official National Cancer Institute release, Burton was simply asked to answer several questions by the Food and Drug Administration. "No response to these questions was ever received. Consequently, Immunology Research Foundation's IND application was not accepted by the FDA and was withdrawn at the request of IRF on March 8, 1976" (NCI, 1978).

Burton tells a different story. First, the FDA sent back his request with three questions. Burton answered the questions and then prepared for trials to begin. But the FDA responded with more questions, three pages of them, single-spaced. "It became apparent that the FDA regulations and the National Cancer Institute (NCI) protocols would take too long" (Cameron/Friedlander, 1979).

Furthermore, Burton considered the kind of clinical trial proposed by the NCI to be unethical. According to a press release prepared for him:

The NCI protocols would have required Dr. Burton to treat a certain number of terminal patients—half of which would have to be a control group and would in actuality receive no treatment. "It's not humane to keep human controls. Why should some people get the 'good' treatment and others get none?" (ibid.).

Burton therefore took a very radical step for a laboratory scientist: in 1977 he moved to the Bahamas and established a research-treatment center at the Rand Hospital, Grand Bahamas. The clinic is a new, one-story building within the grounds of the hospital, with a modern waiting room, treatment rooms, and several spacious laboratories where the blood fractions are prepared and animals are tested.

Burton's method in the Bahamas is basically the same as it was in Great Neck, but on a larger scale. Burton administers the blood tests, using a computer to keep track of the patients' "blood profile." His physician colleague, Dr. Frederick Weinberg, then administers blood fractions, derived from normal human blood (serum) flown over from the mainland. (Friedman did not join Burton in his Bahamian venture.) Burton claims to offer these fractions "only after they have been fully tested for toxicity and efficacy in the strain of spontaneous tumor mice" (ibid.).

How successful has Burton been in the Bahamas?

It is impossible to give a definite answer to this question. Burton's follow-up of patients is understandably poor, since patients come from—and return to—places all over the United States, and even the world. What is more, Burton has not published any clinical results; in fact he has not published anything since the mid-1960s, a point to which we shall return.

Burton claims to be having success with his treatment, however, and a number of other physicians and patients back him up on this. Burton calls some of these effects "miracles." He modifies this by adding that he does not have all the answers. "We don't have a cure-all," he hastens to add (Burton, 1978).

So far, the best results have been in cases of prostate cancer, malignant melanoma, bladder cancer, and some head and neck tumors. Burton claims, for instance, that nine cases of metastasized prostate cancer "have improved and gone home." A person who came at the same time that Hubert Humphrey was dying, with the same diagnosis and the same prognosis, "is completely free of the disease according to an oncology center in Atlanta, Georgia" (ibid.).

Of the 186 patients treated between 1974 and 1977 (presumably in Great Neck), Burton claims that 30—or 16 percent—had what he calls "miracle remissions—they exhibit no sign of cancer." Some 80 others experienced tumor regression, and there was at least a partial stoppage of tumor growth in 60 percent of those treated. Only 8 of these 186 individuals were *not* deemed "terminally ill" at the time of treatment with Burton's method.

Twenty advanced patients were sent to Burton by John Beaty, M.D., of the Greenwich Hospital, Greenwich, Connecticut, who also teaches medicine at Columbia University's College of Physicians and Surgeons. Beaty told science writer Robert Houston that ten of the twenty underwent tumor regression. "All ten," he says, "owe their very survival to Dr. Burton's treatment. . . . They also show tumor shrinkage, appetite improvement, weight gain, and loss of pain. I believe this is a breakthrough in the treatment of cancer—the single best frontier in cancer therapy today" (cited in Houston, 1979b).

A number of other individuals familiar with Burton's work concur. One of these is Dr. R. J. Clement, president of the Bahamian Medical Association. Clement was born in England and studied at London's St. Thomas Hospital. He practiced medicine for five years before going to the Bahamas in 1965.

This physician spoke highly of Burton and his work. He claimed to see many of the American's patients for their non-cancer-related problems. "I'm all for it," he said, simply, in an interview. "I go by the patients I've seen." He then recounted many anecdotes of Burton's apparent success. "If I get cancer, I know where I'm going," he added (Clement, 1978).

Others complain that Burton's treatment is inordinately expensive. In 1978 Burton requested a $7,500 donation to his not-for-profit foundation, now called Immunology Researching Centre, Ltd., before treatment could begin. In 1979 this was lowered to $300 for an evaluation, $2,220 for the first four weeks of therapy, and $300 for each week thereafter (Immunology Researching Centre, 1979). Patients must also come with a companion and make their own living arrangements on the island. Burton justifies the expense by the cost of the treatment itself and the difficulty in obtaining research support (Burton, 1978).

Burton's most serious problem concerns publication or, rather, his lack of it. From 1956 to 1963 Burton and his colleagues published regularly in prestigious journals such as *Cancer Research, Science,* and the *Annals of the New York Academy of Sciences.* Between November 1962 and February 1963 they published four papers on their work and methods. At that point they began to experience great difficulty in getting their work published. After one last attempt to publish, in a South American pathology journal, Burton simply gave up in disgust on his critical colleagues. He has published nothing since that time.

In *Modern Medicine,* Burton invoked the authority of the late Dr. Sidney Farber, who was one of the most prominent cancer chemotherapists, for his decision not to publish:

We visited Sidney Farber at his laboratory, and he said, "Look, you're 10 to 20 years ahead of your time. You've got three options. First, you can keep repeating the same work over and over.

"Or, second, you can keep rewriting and resubmitting your papers. Or, third, you can keep chopping wood—just keep on working and forget what's going on around you." Contrary to what our peers would have advised, we chose the last one (cited in Yasgur, 1975).

Critics offer a less charitable explanation of Burton's reticence. "By nature he's secretive and paranoid," Rottino says. "His great fear was that other people would steal his ideas and he wouldn't get the credit for it" (Rottino, 1978). (A sign on the bulletin board in the Bahamas clinic reads, "Even paranoids have enemies.")

Others maintain that Burton is less than candid about the way he derives his blood factors, that for all his apparent openness, there may be some secrets to the method which Burton is reluctant to part with at this point.

In the 1960s, for example, a prominent Israeli researcher sought to duplicate Burton's methods. According to one account:

. . . there were a few steps that puzzled him, but he thought it was an exceedingly interesting project and definitely worth pursuing. He even asked for a flow chart to try running their program in his own lab in Jerusalem (Anderson, 1974).

But Burton and Friedman refused to send him instructions for isolating the fractions of blood serum—apparently the key step in the whole process and the one most difficult to arrive at empirically. "What if something went wrong?" Burton asked. "We'd be hung without a trial" (ibid.).

Instead of staying in the United States, attempting to publish his ideas, and battling with the government—a process that could admittedly take years—Burton has attempted to shortcut the entire process by going to the Bahamas.

In the summer of 1978, Burton tried to gain the cooperation of the new director of the National Cancer Institute, Dr. Arthur Upton. Wealthy sponsors, he wrote, had agreed to put up $1 million for Burton to treat 1,000 patients. The patients would be chosen by NCI itself and certified by them to have advanced cases of cancer. They would then be sent to the Bahamas and after their treatment would return to NCI for evaluation. NCI-appointed scientists could then decide for themselves whether these patients had benefited from Burton's techniques.

But NCI rejected the offer, once again hammering at Burton's weak spot, his conspicuous lack of publications, especially relating to his clinical work. In a letter dated August 11, 1978, Upton replied:

The question of collaboration is not as simple as it may appear. . . . In other words, we cannot force our intramural staff to work on a problem in which they have no interest.

In order to determine possible interest, I believe it will be necessary for you to provide us with written reports of the studies already carried out. . . (Upton, 1978).

Almost a year later Upton confirmed his stand on Burton's proposal. "Since we have never received the reports of Dr. Burton's studies that I have requested, I would state that our position at this time is the same as it was one year ago. . . ." (Upton, 1979).

If NCI scientists have "no interest" in Burton's techniques, Sloan-Kettering researchers appear to be working on a similar research project with great enthusiasm.

In 1977 Sloan-Kettering announced that it had assigned several of its most experienced researchers to investigate a substance then called "tumor necrosis factor" (TNF). This was described as "a substance, derived from animal's blood, which has the ability to swiftly and dramatically destroy some animal tumors." They claimed it was discovered by accident at Sloan-Kettering in 1971. "One afternoon we injected this serum into mice growing transplants of Meth A tumors. When we walked into our laboratory the next morning, we couldn't believe our eyes. All the Meth A tumors had turned black, had just shriveled and died" (cited in Moss, 1977).

One of the two scientists who made this discovery was Robert Kassel, Ph.D., now a Sloan-Kettering researcher, but from 1953 to 1963 a member of Burton's team at St. Vincent's (ibid.).

In March 1979, amid much fanfare, another Sloan-Kettering researcher, Saul Green, Ph.D., announced the discovery of a similar substance in human blood. Green called this substance "NHG," or "normal human globulin." NHG destroyed human cancer cells in the test tube as well as human tumors growing in mice. Green made his announcement at the American Cancer Society's annual Science Writers' Seminar in Daytona Beach, Florida, and the discovery was promptly announced to the world and carried by the wire services and the tabloid *National Star* (April 17, 1979).

Green drew an enthusiastic picture of NHG's potential. If his experiments were correct, he said, and the human factor does have antitumor effect, then large-scale tests in humans would be justified. It also might be possible to increase the normal production of NHG by the liver, the apparent site of its synthesis. Also, a test might be devised to detect deficiencies of NHG in the blood of individuals with a high risk of developing cancer (Cameron/Friedlander, 1979).

Shortly thereafter, Burton hired the public relations firm of Cameron/Friedlander, Inc., Fort Lauderdale, to issue a press release on his work. Not surprisingly, the release claimed that "experimental evidence announced at an American Cancer Society seminar during March corroborates" Burton's work and that "Dr. Burton is now a man whose early work has been vindicated by this latest paper delivered by Dr. Green before the American Cancer Society seminar" (ibid.).

Some scientists would undoubtedly turn up their noses at a scientist who "publishes" through a press release. Burton's defenders point out, however, that Green also did not publish his work before announcing it, in dramatic fashion, at the American Cancer Society affair.

Burton's work appears to have reached an impasse. In the Bahamas, he may have the freedom to treat cancer patients, but he is almost completely isolated from his scientific colleagues and the general public, as well. Having been stung by what appears to him to have been unreasonable rejection in the past, he now refuses to publish his methods or his results on principle.

Although his facilities on the island are modern, it is questionable whether any single individual can develop both a new scientific concept and a methodology for treating cancer on his own. Rottino explains:

> He can't see it through, because he doesn't have the physical capabilities nor the knowledge of the basic sciences. He's a biologist, but the basic science is very deep and broad. No one man can encompass it all. You need a National Cancer Institute to take a concept like this and really go into it in depth (Rottino, 1978).

The National Cancer Institute has "no interest" in the matter, as Dr. Upton said. Sloan-Kettering, on the other hand, displays no official interest in Burton's technique, while pursuing research projects which are strikingly similar in their basic concepts and goals.

It has been two decades since Burton and his colleagues at St. Vincent's discovered the growth-inhibiting factor, and more than a dozen since they demonstrated the effects of this factor at the American Cancer Society seminar. It has been half a dozen years since Burton branched out on his own and initiated the treatment of patients with blood components. Yet today the cancer establishment still shows little interest in giving Burton credit for anything more than troublemaking.

A great deal is said and written about immunology, which is struggling to become a "fourth modality" of cancer therapy, beside surgery, radiation, and chemotherapy. In the eyes of some people, however, the orthodox immunologists are simply borrowing freely from the unorthodox innovators, and especially from Lawrence Burton.

13

*Livingston
and the Cancer Microbe*

In the late nineteenth and early twentieth centuries, it was widely believed that cancer was caused by a microorganism, a germ. In fact, this idea was as much a dogma as the belief today that it cannot be caused by a microbe. According to an NCI-sponsored history of cancer:

it appeared to have been a question, not so much as to the infectious origin of cancer, but rather as to which of the many parasites was the real causative agent (Shimkin, 1977:176).

James Ewing, later medical director of Memorial Hospital, listed thirty-eight different kinds of bacilli, molds, spirochetes, and protozoa which were candidates for the title in 1907 (ibid.). The director of research at Roswell Park Memorial Institute, Buffalo, and many other prominent scientists were firm believers in the microbial theory.

Scientific thinking changed rapidly, however. "By 1910," wrote the historian Michael Shimkin, M.D., "scientific consensus was for a noninfectious nature of cancer" (ibid.). Those who continued to believe in the role of an infectious organism were branded "quacks." [*]

In the 1922 edition of *Neoplastic Diseases*, Ewing summed up the controversy as follows:

The parasitic theory is the oldest hypothesis of the origin of cancer. It appealed to the ancients, was tacitly accepted throughout the Middle Ages, was definitely argued by modern observers, and reached the height of its popularity as a scientific theory around 1895, but during the last fifteen years it has rapidly lost ground, and today few competent observers consider it as a possible explanation (Ewing, 1922:113).

[*] "The theory that cancer is of germ or infectious origin" was attacked on the grounds "that it was supported by 'quacks' who thrive on the gullibility of the public" (Coley, 1926).

At an international cancer research conference held at Lake Mohonk, New York (September 20–24, 1926), Ewing went so far as to claim that the microbial theory itself was the greatest hindrance to progress in the study of the control of cancer, according to William B. Coley, who reported on the meeting for a medical journal (Coley, 1926).

Only "feeble voice[s]" were raised in defense of the theory. Yet the perceptive Coley warned his readers:

Until it is settled beyond the shadow of a doubt that cancer is not due to a microorganism, we believe that every effort should be made to stimulate to the utmost cancer.research along these lines rather than to attempt to hinder or to discredit it (ibid.).

One of those scorned by the establishment was Peyton Rous, a medical researcher at the Rockefeller Institute (Now Rockefeller University). Rous claimed to have discovered an infectious agent in fowl in 1910, but his findings were ignored. Furthermore, Rous claimed that his agent would pass through the smallest filter known.

It was only with the development of virology—the study of submicroscopic organisms—that scientists took a second look at Rous's once-heretical theory. In 1966, at the age of eighty-nine, Peyton Rous was awarded a Nobel Prize for this work.

The discovery of viruses and unraveling of the genetic code led to a new enthusiasm for the infection theory of cancer. The first director of the National Cancer Program, Dr. Frank Rauscher, was a young virologist, and hundreds of millions of dollars were spent on the search for a cancer virus.

While viruses have been shown to play a part in numerous animal tumors, and to be involved in two forms of human cancer, Burkitt's lymphoma and nasopharyngeal carcinoma, they do not appear to be the cause of most forms of the disease (*Immunology Tribune,* April 30, 1979).

Enthusiasm for the viral theory appears to be waning. Even Dr. Howard Temin, who won the 1975 Nobel Prize for his work on cancer virology, commented:

We can now say that infectious viruses like those that cause many human diseases do not cause most human cancer. Therefore, we cannot hope to develop a vaccine against a virus to prevent most human cancer. . . . We do not have the fundamental knowledge to prevent or cure most human cancer (cited in Harper and Culbert, 1977).

At the same time, the bacterial (as opposed to the viral) theory of cancer has never died in this country or abroad (Boesch, 1960). In fact, some of the fiercest cancer controversies of this century have concerned proposed treatments for the cancer "germ" (ACS, 1971b:79 ff).

Today, a small number of scientists keep alive this theory. The leader of this school of thought is Dr. Virginia Wuerthele-Caspe-Livingston-Wheeler—Dr. Livingston, for short—who believes that major breakthroughs have already been made into the cause, prevention, and cure for human cancer.

Scorned by the establishment for several decades, in the last few years some of Livingston's ideas have received surprising support from scientists at Rockefeller University, Princeton Laboratories, the University of Pittsburgh, and other well-known institutions.

Livingston is currently president of the Livingston-Wheeler Medical Clinic in San Diego, California. Her husband, Owen Webster Wheeler, M.D., is vice-president. Dr. Livingston is a graduate of Vassar College and received her medical degree from New York University. She was the first woman to be a resident physician in a New York City hospital (the Contagious Disease Hospital), and in the course of her long career has been associate professor of biological sciences at Rutgers University, New Jersey, director of the Laboratory of Proliferative Diseases at Presbyterian Hospital in Newark, New Jersey, and a research associate at the San Diego Biomedical Institution. In addition to running the Livingston-Wheeler Clinic, with its staff of twenty-four, Livingston is also an associate professor emeritus-in-residence at the University of San Diego.

What makes Livingston controversial is not her background or credentials, but her ideas: essentially that a hitherto-unsuspected microbe is virtually the source of life (conception) and death (cancer) in many vertebrate species, including man.

Livingston's first encounter with this microbe was in 1946 when she treated a nurse in the New Jersey public schools for scleroderma, a condition sometimes called the "hidebound disease." Orthodox medicine recognizes no known cause of this condition, but Livingston found a swarm of unidentified microbes deep inside skin specimens taken from this patient.

With the help of a pathologist, she injected these microbes into laboratory chicks and guinea pigs. The chicks died, but the guinea pigs developed a scleroderma-like disease. "The involvement of a lifetime can start with a very simple observation," Livingston has said. "All of my life's work started with the desire to help a school nurse who had ulcers of her fingertips and a perforated nasal septum" (Livingston, 1977:8).

Livingston named this microbe *Sclerobacillus Wuerthele-Caspe* (*Sclerobacillus*, meaning the "scleroderma-causing organism"; *Wuerthele-Caspe* was then her surname). She published a paper on "a probable cause of scleroderma" with two other physicians in 1947 (Wuerthele-Caspe et al., 1947).°

At the same time, Livingston noted that some of the guinea pigs developed cancer, an exceedingly rare occurrence among these animals. Working with staining techniques utilized by Eleanor Alexander-Jackson, Ph.D., of Cornell University Medical College, Livingston began to examine cancer specimens from many animals, including man. In more than fifty tumors she found a particular microbe present. This microbe, which is now called *Progenitor cryptocides*, was similar to the *Sclerobacillus* organism she had identified a year before.

In fact, Livingston noted in 1947, "the disease entities of tuberculosis, leprosy, generalized sclerosis, and cancer have certain features in common. All four diseases are characterized by a simultaneous process of production and destruction of tissue and by a progressive, systemic involvement of the host" (Livingston-Wheeler, 1977a:18).

At this point, Livingston invoked a concept also employed by Dr. Alexander-Jackson in her work on tuberculosis: pleomorphism. This means that the organism is not fixed eternally in a single size or shape, but can radically change both of these. Livingston now formulated a remarkably fluid and dynamic view of the microscopic world, a view perhaps too radical for her more conventional colleagues:

> Instead of a bacillus being a bacillus, *ad infinitum*, it can and does change into numerous other forms dictated by its need to survive or stimulated to greater productivity by an unusually favorable environment. Since man exists in a sea of microorganisms his ability to withstand them and their urge to survive often leads to a stage of symbiosis, that is, they live together. This can be on a competitive basis where the human keeps the bugs in check so that they are latent or resting. In some cases the captive microorganisms may play a useful role (Livingston, 1972).

In the early 1950s, Livingston appeared on the way to gaining acceptance for her ideas. She was appointed director of the Laboratory for Proliferative Diseases. She collaborated with prominent scientists at leading laboratories. She received grants from the Damon Runyon Fund, the Rosenwald Foundation, Reader's Digest Associates, Chas. Pfizer & Co., Lederle Laboratories, Abbott Laboratories, and even the American Cancer Society. Much basic work on the microbiology of cancer and other diseases was done at this time. For

---

° Livingston's observations on the *Sclerobacillus* have since been confirmed by a number of groups, including N. Delmotte and L. van der Meiren (1953) and Alan R. Cantwell, Jr., M.D., and Dan W. Kelso of Los Angeles (1971).

instance, the Newark researchers decided they were dealing with organisms that formed part of the Actinomycetales order, a family of germs which dates back to the Precambrian era, hundreds of millions of years ago (Livingston, 1972).

They attempted to fulfill Koch's four postulates, the four laws laid down by Robert Koch (1843–1910) for establishing the microbial origin of any disease. By the early 1950s, they believed they had done so: they could show, Livingston says, that the cancer organism was present in every case of the disease which they examined; could be cultivated outside the host animal in an artificial medium; inoculation of this culture produced the disease in a susceptible animal; and the germ could be reobtained from the inoculated animal and cultivated once more.

At that time, Virginia Livingston had a large tumor service at Presbyterian Hospital in Newark, where she cared for twenty to thirty cancer patients daily. She obtained her cancer specimens from these patients. Using cultures of human blood from cancer patients, the incidence of cancer among guinea pigs could be increased from the natural rate of 1 in 500,000 to 1 in 4 by injecting microbes derived from human patients into these animals. The "cancer microbe" crossed species lines, Livingston said. Animals could catch it from man; and man, she believed, could catch it from animals—specifically by eating the contaminated flesh of fowl and other animals.°

Livingston had not yet begun to *treat* cancer with any unusual methods. Nonetheless, her work came to the attention of the leaders of cancer research and began to meet resistance. This was at the time that chemotherapy was being promoted as *the* answer to cancer. Sloan-Kettering Institute dominated the drug-testing field, at least until 1955, and not surprisingly, the strongest opposition to Livingston and her Newark colleagues came from the leader of the Sloan-Kettering chemotherapists, C. P. "Dusty" Rhoads. In her autobiography, Livingston recalls Rhoads and Sloan-Kettering in the early 1950s:

> Many of the large research centers, such as Sloan-Kettering . . . under Dr. Cornelius P. Rhoads, were dedicated largely to finding a chemical or group of chemicals that would destroy the cancer cell. He would brook no competition or interference from any one who disagreed with his concepts. He considered us an upstart group. This included our collaborators as well.

° Cancer in America's chicken flocks has been called a "nightmare" by the *Wall Street Journal* (cited in Livingston, 1972). Livingston claims to have found a large degree of infection with *Progenitor cryptocides* in chickens, and therefore considers them particularly dangerous. (See Livingston, 1972, and Livingston-Wheeler, 1977b for full discussion of this controversial point.)

He was often heard to say, "When the cause and cure of cancer are found, I will find it." He died a disappointed man (ibid.).

Rhoads proved to be a determined and powerful opponent. For example, says Livingston, he opposed Dr. Irene Diller, a Philadelphia scientist who collaborated with the Newark group. His opposition seemed to increase after Diller's work was featured in a mass circulation magazine. (Rhoads himself had been on the cover of *Time,* June 27, 1949.) In 1950 Dr. Diller attempted to set up a symposium at the New York Academy of Sciences to present a number of papers on the infectious nature of cancer.

Rhoads managed to kill this meeting, says Livingston, by charging Diller with having "commercialized" her work. Diller had received several ultraviolet sterilizing lamps from a company, with no strings attached. But the charge appeared serious enough—and its source powerful enough—for the meeting to be canceled. This charge was ironic, Livingston noted, coming from the head of a center with millions of dollars in grants from giant corporations and individuals financially interested in the cancer field (see Appendix A). The meeting was not finally convened until well after Rhoads's death, twenty years later *(Annals of the New York Academy of Sciences,* vol. 174, October 30, 1970).

In her autobiography, Livingston includes many other instances of the way in which Rhoads and other establishment figures attempted to block the free development of her research approach (Livingston, 1972). For example, in the early 1950s, amid much publicity, Livingston's laboratory at Rutgers was awarded a bequest of $750,000 from the Black-Stevenson Cancer Foundation for excellence in cancer research. These funds were never conveyed to the microbial researchers, however, but instead were used to build a new wing on the hospital to house a giant cobalt machine. Among other factors, this misappropriation, as Livingston calls it, forced her to close the Laboratory for Proliferative Diseases. "Dusty" Rhoads appears to have been involved in convincing a trustee of the Black-Stevenson fund, then a patient at Memorial Hospital, to divert the money away from the "upstarts." "It was the long arm of Dr. Cornelius P. Rhoads that closed the Newark laboratory," says Livingston (ibid.).

In 1953 the Newark researcher and her colleagues traveled to Rome to present some of their findings to the Sixth International Conference on Microbiology. Livingston presented a summary paper, "Microbiology of Cancer: Neoplastic Infection in Man and Animals" (Livingston-Wheeler, 1977a:53). The expenses for this journey were paid for by Livingston's then-husband, Dr. Joseph Caspe, who was a chemist working as a consultant to the British leather and fur industries. Upon returning to the United States, however, they found that they had been attacked in the press by the president of the New York Academy of Medicine. Soon after this, the Internal Revenue Service, acting on an informer's "tip," began to question Dr. Caspe about the source of his revenue and how he had paid for the European trip. Livingston was told that the informer was "someone high up in New York in cancer" (Livingston, 1972).

Eventually, Caspe was cleared of all suspicion, but the experience was an embittering one. The couple decided to resettle in California. In the early 1960s Dr. Livingston did little work; she struggled with personal illness and problems, including a divorce; but she did manage to speak at a few conferences and pursue a small amount of research.

In 1966 Pat McGrady, Sr., invited Virginia Livingston and Eleanor Alexander-Jackson, who had joined her as a full-time researcher before the closing of the Newark laboratory, to speak at the American Cancer Society Science Writers' Seminar. This was the same Phoenix meeting at which Lawrence Burton demonstrated his "fifteen-minute cure" for mouse cancer. Livingston attempted to keep her presentation on a theoretical plane, but questions naturally arose about the practical application of her work: how did she *treat* cancer?

Actually, although both she and her second husband, Afton Munk Livingston, M.D., were practicing physicians, they shied away from cancer therapy:

We were reluctant to enter the field of cancer therapy since we believed that present-day methods of treatment were seldom effective. In the past, observations on animal models led to the conclusion that the very methods used to treat cancer were carcinogenic in themselves, that is, that radiation and chemotherapy not only induced cancer but also destroyed immunity to cancer (Livingston-Wheeler, 1977a:9).

Nevertheless, Livingston conceded that some colleagues had begun to make attempts to immunize cancer patients, based on her earlier animal experiments with the microbes. Some reporters immediately blew this out of proportion and believed she was claiming another "cure for cancer." The furor surrounding a different unorthodox technique—Burton's blood fraction—may have spilled over into the Livingston controversy.

When Alexander-Jackson returned to New York from this meeting, she discovered that she had been abruptly terminated from the Institute of Comparative Medicine at Columbia College of Physicians and Surgeons, where she had gone to work after the Newark laboratory had closed. Both women believe the American Cancer Society instigated the firing.

In 1968 "the Livingston Vaccine" took its place in the ACS's *Unproven Methods* book. After "careful study," the American Cancer Society did not find evidence that "the treatment with the Livingston Vaccine resulted in objective benefit in the treatment of cancer," nor that it could be used as a diagnostic tool.

An interesting fact about the so-called Livingston Vaccine, evident from the ACS book, is that at that time Livingston herself had never used a vaccine to treat cancer. The "careful study" was a report of Livingston's speech at the aforementioned ACS seminar, at which she said that other doctors had treated approximately fifty patients with an anti–*Progenitor cryptocides* vaccine. Of these, Livingston said, thirty-seven had died, but the others had improved. In particular, ACS quotes her as having said, three patients "with far advanced cancer had received no treatment except the vaccine, and these were reported to have survived for more than eighteen months and to be still improving" (ACS, 1971b).

What sort of investigation was conducted of Livingston's method before it was included on the list? None—no examination of patients, materials or methods, no study of case records, of objective or subjective effects, much less a single- or double-blind test. The "investigation" consisted of the fact that "at the Science Writers' Seminar, the findings of Drs. Livingston and Alexander-Jackson were strongly criticized" by a Sloan-Kettering scientist, among others (ibid:150).

The scientist Dr. Jørgen Fogh has even said, "You realize that the agents they [Livingston and Alexander-Jackson] claim to work with probably don't exist. I think they are imagining them" (Fogh, 1979).

The establishment's condemnation does not seem to have daunted Dr. Livingston. Perhaps it even goaded her into activity, for the past dozen years have been among Virginia Livingston's most productive.

In 1968, under a Fleet Foundation grant at the Biomed Laboratory of San Diego, it was shown that the "cancer microbe," when filtered and put into tissue culture, produced the degeneration of cells under certain conditions and the proliferation of cells in others. The study of several hundred cultures showed that the specific microbes were sensitive to some antibiotics when they were outside cells, but markedly less or not at all when they nestled inside the human cells (Livingston-Wheeler, 1977a:12).

In 1970, working under Fleet and Kerr grants at the University of San Diego, Livingston showed that the "cancer microbe" produced an antibiotic (actinomycin) as well as toxic materials which enhanced the incidence of cancer in mice. In the same year, the New York Academy of Sciences finally held a symposium to air the views of the microbial school. It was at this symposium that the microbe received its present name: *Progenitor cryptocides,* the hidden, ancestral creator and killer.

In 1972, Livingston reexamined the various phases of the microbe through the use of the dark-field microscope. The dark-field microscope has a special condenser and other attachments which make light scatter from the object observed, with the result that it appears bright on a dark background, instead of the other way around. It is a superior method of viewing *Progenitor cryptocides.* Using it, Livingston was able to describe the entire life cycle of this complicated, ever-changing germ, and name it according to modern usage.

It was in the same year that Livingston made what some scientists are now calling a major breakthrough in the cancer field. She found that this same organism is capable of producing a *human* hormone—HCG (human choriogonadotrophin)—in the test tube (Livingston-Wheeler, 1979).

For the average layman, of course, this finding may not appear earthshaking. But there are several important features to this discovery. First, until this time, no microbe had ever been found to produce a human hormone. The implications of this were intriguing for scientists, especially those concerned with the topical field of recombinant DNA research.

Second, this particular hormone—HCG—has long been associated with cancer. The test for HCG is, in fact, not only the standard pregnancy test, but an accurate monitor of at least one type of cancer (choriocarcinoma), and a fair barometer of many other types as well. Many theories have been propounded to account for this unnatural—or "ectopic"—production of what is essentially a growth hormone by a cancer cell.°

Livingston's lifelong research may provide a more fruitful explanation of why HCG appears in so many cancer cells and in the blood of many cancer patients. According to her theory, the "cancer microbe" produces it. The hormone, in turn, may "transform" (turn cancerous) normal cells whose immune functions are inadequate or when "essential nutritive elements become deficient" (Livingston-

° Technically, HCG (also called CG or CGH) is a glycoprotein with a carbohydrate fraction composed of galactose and hexosamine, and has traditionally been thought to be produced by placental trophoblastic cells. In pregnancy, it appears to stimulate the ovarian secretion of estrogen and progesterone required for the integrity and survival of the embryo during the first trimester of pregnancy.

Wheeler, 1977a:11). Thus, HCG may be the "hidden killer' which is secreted by the ever-changing, mysterious microbe to kill the deficient cell.

Yet, Livingston emphasizes, this microbe has two names: one redolent of death, the other full of life. It is also a "progenitor," a life-giver. Recent experiments suggest that the microbe is also present in normal sperm and may enter the newly conceived human at the union of sperm and egg. Once inside, it multiplies and provides the embryo with its HCG, a hormone without which life certainly would not be possible.

Although not yet a proven certainty, parts of Livingston's theory have already received confirmation from surprisingly orthodox institutions, and have created a stir among major research groups. Livingston published her finding on HCG in 1974 in the *Transactions* of the New York Academy of Sciences (Livingston and Livingston, 1974). Two years later, Herman Cohen and Alice Strampp of the Princeton Laboratories confirmed the "bacterial synthesis of a substance similar to human chorionic gonadotrophin" (Cohen and Strampp, 1976).

In 1978 another research group, headed by Hernan F. Acevedo, Ph.D., of the William H. Singer Memorial Research Institute, Allegheny General Hospital, Pittsburgh, confirmed the fact that *Progenitor cryptocides* produced the human growth hormone. Acevedo believed that a number of different bacterial strains isolated from the tissues of cancer patients also produced the hormone.

A research group at Rockefeller University, headed by Samuel Koide, M.D., Ph.D., is also studying the microbe, and has confirmed the fact that it produces a gonadotrophic hormone which appears to be identical to that of the human. This group is looking at the germ from the point of view of a new approach to birth control. Since the hormone is apparently present in normal sperm, it might be possible to use it to prevent pregnancy (Koide, 1979).

Within a few years in the late 1970s Livingston appears to have gained the respect of at least some established researchers, and the attention of many more. While none of these scientists has become an open convert to the bacterial theory of cancer, Livingston is doubtlessly correct when she states that the discovery concerning the HCG hormone "immediately gave credence and stature to the entire microbial theory" (Livingston-Wheeler, 1977a:7).

An indication of Livingston's new stature can be gleaned by this comment from Acevedo's 1978 paper:

The impact of these findings in the fields of oncology, bacteriology, epidemiology, genetics and molecular biology is so great that a detailed description will be beyond the scope of this communication. . . . It is apparent that this phenomenon exposes the need for a new approach to the analysis as well as to our current concepts of cancer (Acevedo, 1978).

Livingston now believes she has such a new approach, and is applying it in the treatment of cancer patients at the Livingston-Wheeler Clinic.

Livingston has also discovered a natural substance present in many foods, abscisic acid, which neutralizes the HCG and thus should have an anticancer effect. Although difficult and expensive to purify for laboratory experiments, abscisic acid, similar to vitamin A, is plentiful in nature (see Table 7). Animal experiments showed it to be a powerful anticancer agent (Livingston-Wheeler, 1977b).

In 1969 Livingston and her husband opened the Livingston Medical Clinic in San Diego and began immunization treatment of cancer patients. "My studies had led me to the conclusion that cancer is an immune deficiency disease based on infection by a definite etiological agent, the *Progenitor cryptocides*. On the basis of treating an immune deficiency in man, we began to accept cancer patients."

The treatment included a vaccine to fight the *Progenitor cryptocides*, antibiotics, antisera, immune stimulants such as BCG,° and a health food diet. In addition, like many unorthodox practitioners, Livingston urged her patients to adopt a new, more relaxed way of life:

It is ideally hoped that your whole foods will be grown in a naturally fertilized and composted home garden. Relaxation, plenty of rest, exercise and fresh air are as much a part of your new life as the food you will eat. They are all contributing towards your recovery. Most important is proper attitude. Negative emotion and its by-products waste much precious energy. A positive attitude taken with this change in life style will allow your new way of life to become a happy and rewarding experience (Livingston-Wheeler, 1977b).

In 1972, the Livingstons received as a patient a fellow physician, Owen Webster Wheeler. Suffering from malignant lymphoma of the neck "the size of a tennis ball," Wheeler made the "momentous decision" to be treated by immunization alone, without conventional therapies. The deadly lymphoma, Livingston says, was completely gone in six months, and Wheeler remains cancer-free and in good health eight years later.

After the death of Dr. Afton Munk Livingston, Virginia Living-

° Bacillus *Calmette-Guérin*, the antituberculosis vaccine used as an immune stimulator in both orthodox and unorthodox clinics.

ston and Owen Wheeler were married, and the clinic was renamed the Livingston-Wheeler Clinic.

With the recent discoveries concerning the HCG hormone and abscisic acid, the treatment at the clinic now routinely includes a heavy emphasis on the ingestion of food containing the vitamin A-like substance. Like many unorthodox practitioners, Livingston does not believe that the average American diet is adequate to maintain health:

In a society commercially oriented toward the profit system, mass production of cheap food, preservatives to prolong shelf life, exploitation of taste over quality, convenience, attractive packaging, the trusting and unsuspecting individual can become lost in a jungle of incomprehension, leading to poor health and general deterioration. . . . (Livingston-Wheeler, 1977b).

The great hope of Livingston and her followers, however, is to produce a really effective, universal anticancer vaccine. This may seem like a wild dream, but Livingston is presently hard at work on this project. In fact, in the late 1970s, she sent a colleague, John Majnarich of the BioMed Research Laboratories in Seattle, to Japan to learn firsthand the techniques of a Japanese immunologist, Dr. Chisato Maruyama. Livingston and her colleagues hope to use this new technique with the *Progenitor cryptocides* to produce a vaccine which will be an effective form of cancer prevention, and possibly a cure (Livingston-Wheeler, 1979).

At the same time, Alexander-Jackson, on the East Coast, continues to prepare autogenous vaccine for patients—that is, a vaccine derived from samples of their microbes. About a dozen physicians commission Alexander-Jackson to grow these microbes from patients' urine, and then a medical laboratory prepares the vaccines. She claims that these vaccines are useful in the treatment of cancer if the patient is in the early stages of the disease, if radiation and chemotherapy have not destroyed the immune system, and if the patient has a proper diet and receives other nontoxic forms of therapy.

Although Sloan-Kettering claimed to be unable to find the *Progenitor cryptocides* microbe when Alexander-Jackson worked there temporarily as a visiting scientist in 1973, she is adamant that the microbes are real, have been correctly described, and can form the basis for an effective treatment.

"Will there be a shot against cancer? Someday . . . probably yes!" This optimistic appraisal of the chances for a cancer vaccine comes not from Livingston or one of her colleagues but from an American

Cancer Society press release (New York City Division, February 2, 1976). It would be ironic indeed if such a "shot" came not from a beneficiary of ACS funds, but from scientists long considered deluded and incompetent by the cancer establishment.

TABLE 7
Foods Containing Abscisic Acid
(Information from Livingston-Wheeler, *Food Alive*)

Fruits

Mangoes
Grapes
Avocados
Pears
Oranges, with the white underpeel
   and pulps
Apples, whole with the seeds
Strawberries

Fruit Blossoms and Leaves as Tea

Peach Flowers
Strawberry Leaves
Cherry Flowers
Apple Blossoms

Vegetables

Pea Shoots
Lima Beans
Potatoes
Peas, Dwarf
Yams
Sweet Potatoes
Asparagus
Tomatoes
Onions
Spinach

Root Vegetables °

All Root Vegetables–especially
   Carrots

Seeds and Nuts

Seeds and Nuts of all kinds

Leafy Vegetables

Mature Greens

° All seeds, nuts, fruits, root storage vegetables, and fresh vegetables with their mature greens seem to contain abscisic acid.

PART THREE
Prevention

14

Preventing
Prevention

Can cancer be prevented? This question has split the cancer field as profoundly as the debate over unorthodox methods of treatment, and perhaps more profoundly, for an effective program of prevention would render all methods of therapy—orthodox and unorthodox—obsolete.

The traditional establishment answer to this question has been that only a small percentage of cancers can be prevented. According to the American Cancer Society:

> Some cancers, not all [can be prevented]. Most lung cancers are caused by cigarette smoking, and most skin cancers by frequent overexposure to direct sunlight. . . . These cancers can be prevented by avoiding their causes. Certain cancers caused by occupational/environmental factors—for example, bladder cancer in the dye industry workers—have been prevented by eliminating or reducing contact with carcinogenic agents (ACS, 1979:4).

In a 1962 poll of 1,400 physicians a researcher associated with the American Cancer Society reported in *JAMA*, the journal of the American Medical Association, that

> the idea of preventing cancer seemed vague and doubtful to the [physician] audience as a whole. Added to this discouragement is the fact that not one idea, lead or theory on cancer prevention was suggested by the entire professional audience (McGrady, Sr., 1964:394).

Today the situation is somewhat better, and many doctors urge their patients to stop smoking. But beyond this largely ineffective measure (the lung cancer rate continues to rise), little is done to stop the incidence of cancer before it occurs.

A small, but growing, number of scientists have maintained, however, that cancer is a preventable disease. The pages of health magazines such as *Prevention, Herald of Health,* and *East West Journal* have been filled with their claims. Often, they have urged a return to a more simple, organic diet as a way to prevent what has been called the "disease of civilization."

Others, working in the laboratory, or compiling statistics on cancer's victims (epidemiology), have proposed evidence that shows a link between chemicals encountered at home or at work and the rising rate of cancer.

What are these chemical factors, or carcinogens?

Scientists have pinpointed at least two dozen that are known to cause cancer in laboratory animals and almost certainly contribute to cancer in man. These include tobacco and particularly its smoke, which can cause not only lung cancer, but tumors of the mouth, throat, and bladder; smoked foods, which have been implicated as a cause of stomach cancer; alcohol, suspected of being a co-carcinogen, potentiating other cancer-causing substances; various drugs, including those used to treat cancer itself; female hormones; food colorings; pesticides; and nitrosamines, formed by a combination of nitrites or nitrates and amines in the body (Fraumeni, 1975).

Industrial chemicals which cause cancer may afflict workers on the job, people who live in the vicinity of factories, or even consumers of products containing such chemicals. These carcinogens include asbestos, benzene, cadmium, arsenic, nickel, vinyl chloride, and beta-naphthylamine—the dye chemical alluded to in the ACS description above (ibid.). As everyone is now aware, the list of suspected carcinogens grows steadily, almost with every passing day.

An effective strategy for dealing with cancer might be to reduce or eliminate exposure to these chemicals and environmental pollutants. Some physicians, familiar with the poor record of conventional treatments, believe this is the *only* effective way to fight cancer.

Minnesota pediatrician Ronald J. Glasser, has warned: "We are not doomed to die of cancer—unless we persist in dooming ourselves . . . unless we take steps right now to defend ourselves, the incidence [of cancer] will continue to rise in the decades to come" (Glasser, 1979:172).

Giulio J. D'Angio, M.D., then chairman of the Department of Radiation Therapy of Memorial Sloan-Kettering Cancer Center, expressed a similar sentiment after many years of treating cancer with radiation:

> It is natural for physicians to focus on treatment. A far better focus is prevention. The recent identification of environmental oncogenic [cancer-causing] factors, some of them prenatal, some of them found even in the household, and their elimination are obvious and totally effective ways of curing cancer, before it develops (D'Angio, 1975).

The elimination of these cancer-causing substances might, at first sight, appear a simple and rational way to reduce the incidence of cancer. It may be rational but it is certainly not simple. Critics charge that the main obstacle is the powerful force of industry to hinder such changes:

Today, more than ever before, the price of health is vigilance, and this vigilance means that we must recognize not only the poisons in our environment but also the efforts on the part of industry to resist, in the name of profit, the removal of these carcinogens and mutagens, as well as government tolerance of these efforts (Glasser, 1979:173).

In a recent exhaustive study of environmental carcinogens, *The Politics of Cancer,* Samuel S. Epstein, M.D., professor of occupational and environmental medicine at the School of Public Health, University of Illinois, attempts to dissect the eight-part strategy which industry uses to prevent the prevention of cancer (Epstein, 1978):°

(1) *Minimizing the risk:* Industry will try to downplay the importance of a particular compound, and chemicals in general, in the causation of cancer. For example, Exxon Corporation and the industry trade group the Manufacturing Chemists Association claim that although benzene may cause leukemia, this is no longer an environmental problem. Scientific reports show, however, that chemical workers are still exposed to dangerous levels of this substance (ibid.:132–33).

(2) *Diversionary tactics:* Industry spokesmen will attempt to drag a red herring across the scene to divert attention. For example, they will demand a degree of precision which they know is impossible to achieve. Or they will call for more research into a known hazard. This has been a favorite tactic of the tobacco lobby.

(3) *Propagandizing the public:* With tremendous resources at its disposal, industry has been able to confuse the public about the risk of cancer-causing substances. In fact, historian David F. Nobile has called this "the corporate ideology of the 1980s" (Nobile, 1979). Mobil Oil, he reports, spent $3.2 million on "grass-roots lobbying" in 1978; Monsanto is spending $5 million a year on television spots, newspaper ads, and pamphlets for school children; and Union Carbide has formed a communications department to "engage in public policy dialogue on issues that affect our business" (ibid.; Epstein, 1978:394).°°

° Much of the information which follows is derived from Epstein's useful book.
°° William S. Sneath, Union Carbide president, is a member of MSKCC's board of overseers.

Recently, as Nobile explains, there has been a shift in corporate strategy:

In the past when regulators identified a chemical as carcinogenic, that charge alone was enough to alarm the public. . . . Today, corporations like Union Carbide have begun to shift the very nature of the debate. They now readily concede that their products are carcinogenic, but blandly insist that the acknowledged risk of cancer be put in "perspective," that it be compared with other risks and traded off against product benefits. Life, after all, is risky (Nobile, 1979).°

(4) *Blaming the victim:* Industry will sometimes claim that cancer is not really caused by chemicals, but is the fault of the person who gets the cancer. Thus industry spokesmen have postulated a "hypersusceptible worker" who is genetically predisposed to contract the disease. This has been a favorite concept with the asbestos industry, says Epstein (1978:94).

(5) *Controlling information:* While independent scientists have gathered quite a bit of information on carcinogens, most of the public's and Congress's information about chemicals and their effects must necessarily come from the manufacturers.

This situation leaves the door open for distorted presentations or even outright fraud. The *Congressional Record* of July 30, 1969, cites numerous instances of data manipulation with such drugs as MER/29, for which executives of Richardson-Merrell Company were convicted of criminal charges; Dornwall, for which Wallace and Tiernan Company were found guilty of submitting false data; and Flexin, about which McNeil Laboratories failed to submit toxicity data on drug-related liver damage, including eleven deaths, in their reports to the FDA (cited in ibid.:303–04).

(6) *Influencing policy:* Even if a substance is proven carcinogenic, it is a long way from being regulated, controlled, or banned. It took more than half a dozen years of consumer lobbying to gain passage of the Toxic Substances Control Act of 1976. But not only did the Manufacturing Chemists Association manage to tone down that once-promising legislation, through daily conferences with con-

___

° Similarly, when critics charged that the American Cancer Society–National Cancer Institute breast screening program would *cause* as many deaths through radiation-induced breast cancer as it would save through early detection, ACS vice-president Arthur I. Holleb, M.D., replied in identical fashion: "From the moment of birth we face innumerable risks that not only threaten our existence, but also carry the potential of temporary or even permanent infirmity. To avoid most risks one would have to take to the bed—a considerable circulatory risk in itself—and shun normal activities" (Holleb, 1976). Thus, women should ignore the risk of breast cancer and take their mammograms. Despite this, an NCI panel ruled against the routine use of mammography in women under fifty (see Chapter 2).

gressmen and their staffs, but little has been done since then to enforce the control of toxic substances.*

(7) *Exhausting the agencies:* The regulatory agencies often show little inclination to control industry. But if they ever do, industry is able to overwhelm the would-be regulators with legal paperwork. One or two major cases, such as Shell's protracted defense of its cancer-causing pesticides aldrin and dieldrin, can totally exhaust the resources of a government agency.

Even when Shell finally lost its aldrin/dieldrin case, it used the *identical* arguments and tactics in the almost *identical* chlordane/ heptachlor pesticide case. Industry has insisted that every case must be argued separately, on its own merits, instead of on the basis of commonly agreed-upon cancer principles. Thus, a would-be regulator of industry is in the same plight as Sisyphus, in Greek mythology, whose punishment in Hades was to roll a giant rock to the top of a hill, only to have it constantly fall back to the bottom again.

(8) *The flight of the multinationals:* If all else should fail, the giant corporations can pick up their operations and move to regions or countries more receptive to "dirty" industries. With the passage of the Occupational Safety and Health Act of 1970, such runaways within the United States have become more difficult. But the manufacturers of asbestos, benzidine dye, pesticides, plastics, and copper have moved their carcinogenic processes out of the country.

It should hardly shock anyone that industry will use a wide variety of tactics to protect its investments. What is more surprising is the degree to which leaders of the cancer field have also helped to obscure the need for prevention.

Memorial Sloan-Kettering Cancer Center, which has often been the pace-setter for other institutions, has done surprisingly little in the field of prevention. Some research was conducted on the link between tobacco and cancer in the 1950s and 1960s, but this almost entirely came to a halt when Dr. Ernst Wynder left the Center in 1969.** Some other work on chemical carcinogenesis was carried out at the Walker Laboratory of Sloan-Kettering. But this work was of a rather abstract nature and never entered the public debates on the cause of cancer.

The tone for Sloan-Kettering was set by its leaders, and these men were fully in accord with the view of industry that cancer was not caused, to any appreciable degree, by products of industry.

---

* ". . . there is little indication yet as to how well this potential for control will be exercised," says Epstein, one of the original authors of the Act (Epstein, 1978:373).

** Wynder became president and medical director of the American Health Foundation. He remained a consulting epidemiologist at MSKCC.

In the mid-1960s, for instance, Frank Horsfall, the director of Sloan-Kettering, was asked by a reporter if he thought that certain occupations were dangerous with respect to cancer. This was more than a decade after scientists had proven that bladder cancer could be caused by the chemical beta-naphthylamine. Many other industrial causes of cancer were either then known or strongly suspected. Horsfall's answer was a very qualified yes:

A farmer, for instance, who works in the sun all day, with the ultraviolet rays beating on his skin. This, plus the dirt that get in the crevices of the skin, may lead to skin cancer (*U.S. News and World Report*, April 19, 1965).

Granting that "certain petroleum products and such things" could contain "incitants," Horsfall cautioned his audience:

These should not be emphasized, because the frequency with which they lead to cancer is very low indeed, and industry has been particularly effective in detecting and getting rid of them. Industrial hazards of this kind are of progressively smaller importance (ibid.).

After Horsfall's death, Leo Wade, M.D., became acting director of the Institute. Wade had a long career in industry before coming to Sloan-Kettering as first vice-president. He was medical director of Standard Oil of New Jersey from 1951 to 1961, and was a member of the American Petroleum Institute, the Manufacturing Chemists Association, and the National Association of Manufacturers—organizations which have generally been unfriendly to stringent government health regulation.[*]

In 1964 Wade granted that some workers show an increased incidence of certain types of cancer. Nevertheless, he remained unconvinced that particular chemicals could actually *cause* that cancer:

Although some assume a true cause-and-effect relationship to have been established, I believe the relationship more properly considered as one of association. The common causes of cancer in man are still unknown (Wade, 1964).

The Sloan-Kettering leader considered the provisions of the Workmen's Compensation Act, which reimbursed workers for occupationally induced cancer, "a 'gold mine' for those willing to exploit medical ignorance" (ibid.). Efforts to control chemicals suspected of causing cancer were "both futile and suspect" (Wade, 1962). Far from being a problem created by industry, "cancer is now

---

[*] Wade's publications at Standard Oil included articles on "Why People Don't Work" and "Medical Public Relations for the Physician in Industry" (Wade, 1958, 1953). Biographical information on Wade from MSKCC press release, May 16, 1961, and obituary, in *The New York Times*, January 6, 1975.

widely believed to consist of a heritable, and therefore genetic" problem (Sloan-Kettering, 1969).

The ascension of Robert Good to the directorship of Sloan-Kettering in the early 1970s seemed to augur a new, more liberal approach to this question. The 1972 *Annual Report* (prepared in 1973) promised "the development and use of better laboratory techniques for determining which chemicals in our environment cause cancer" (MSKCC, 1972:9).

Even had he wanted to, Good could not change the composition of the body he reports to, the MSKCC board of overseers, which is made up predominantly of bankers and industrialists (see Appendix A). Nor could he alter the long-established relationships between scientists at Sloan-Kettering and big business.

In 1974, in the midst of the furor over the potential danger of pesticides, Memorial Sloan-Kettering pathologist Stephen Sternberg headed a Shell Chemical Company Ad Hoc Committee of Pathologists which claimed that aldrin and dieldrin were *not* carcinogenic (Epstein, 1978:261).

Few steps have been taken to make preventive medicine a major focus at the Center. One long-anticipated move was the establishment, in July 1976, of an Epidemiology and Preventive Medicine Service in the Department of Medicine. The first major study this group undertook was an investigation of cancer in petroleum workers, which was funded by the American Petroleum Institute, a trade association of the largest oil companies (MSKCC *Center News*, September 1975 and September 1978).

At Sloan-Kettering Institute, only a small percentage of the overall research effort is directed toward prevention. Of approximately 100 laboratories listed in the 1976 *Annual Report*, for instance, only one—Chemical Oncogenesis—is exclusively occupied with the question of cancer prevention. In a few other laboratories, researchers work on questions of prevention, but often on a part-time basis.

This situation is partially the result of a lack of funding for such studies from the National Cancer Institute, the American Cancer Society, and private donors, and partially the result of attitudes and policies at MSKCC itself. (The link between the directors of MSKCC and cancer-causing industry is further explored in Chapter 16 and in Appendix A.)

The American Cancer Society

In the public's mind, the American Cancer Society (ACS) is associated with the one really large-scale cancer-prevention project ever attempted in the United States: the campaign against cigarette smoking. In the 1950s and the 1960s, the Society carried out a massive and expensive study on the relationship between smoking and health. About one million people were questioned by ACS volunteers and the Society kept track of more than 90 percent of these people for a dozen years.

This ACS study provided much of the basis for the Surgeon General's report of 1964 which condemned smoking as a cause of lung cancer. It linked the number of cigarettes smoked to the dramatic increase in lung cancer in certain populations. Follow-up studies in this country, England, and Japan have confirmed the basic validity of the ACS work.

Nevertheless, the overall ACS record on prevention does not impress Samuel S. Epstein or other environmentalists.

Its approach to the antismoking campaign is said to be too conservative and too exclusively concerned with education, to the detriment of more effective programs.

The ACS itself has taken a hands-off attitude toward regulating industry. Its stance, expressed recently by ACS officials, is that the Society "had used [its] resources to uncover the health risks of smoking. Now it was up to the government to take a stand and respond accordingly" (cited in Epstein, 1978).

The Society was one of the first health groups to ask President John F. Kennedy to take action against tobacco in 1961. But when a consumer activist petitioned the Federal Communications Commission for equal time against tobacco ads in 1971, "the Society refused to support him, let alone defend the subsequent FCC ruling in his favor" (ibid.).

The ACS's antitobacco campaign is highly dependent on voluntary programs, rather than on stiff controls of the $16 billion a year tobacco industry. For example, once a year the Society sponsors "The Great American Smokeout" in which people are encouraged to stop smoking for a day (ACS, 1978:14). It also distributes "I Quit Kits" to help individuals give up cigarettes on their own.

It is questionable whether such measures are adequate to stop the continuing problem of cigarette smoking and the related diseases caused by this habit. The death rate from lung cancer in men has increased more than twenty-five times in forty-five years. It is going up steadily in women, and the incidence has more than doubled in both men and women, black and white (ACS, 1979:7). More alarming is the fact that cigarette smoking is increasing substantially among teen-agers: in 1976 it was found that 27 percent of girls thirteen through seventeen now smoke, and four out of ten of these smoke at least one pack a day (*New York Times*, February 12, 1976).

ACS propaganda obviously had little effect on these youngsters, who represent a future solid base for the tobacco industry, unless something radical is done to reverse the trend.

Because of the ineffectiveness of its programs, Epstein calls the Society's efforts against tobacco "weak and diffuse" (Epstein, 1978:424). He himself has helped form a Cancer Prevention Committee within the Illinois Division of the Society, to try to swing the ACS toward a more activist stand.

Obviously stung by this sort of criticism, in 1978 the Society initiated a National Commission on Smoking and Public Policy, which recommended the following strictures: prohibition of smoking in most public places, as well as in the working environment and in schools; phasing out the government tobacco price-support system; a Food and Drug Administration study of potentially harmful cigarette additives; reduction of insurance rates for nonsmokers; basing the cigarette tax on tar and nicotine content; adoption of quit-smoking programs by all hospitals and clinics; banning all advertising of high tar and nicotine cigarettes and curtailing use of models in ads; holding the tobacco industry accountable to the FDA or the Consumer Product Safety Commission for the safety of its products; and an HEW interagency council to coordinate antismoking activities of different departments (ACS, 1978:15).

While these are the strongest recommendations with which the ACS has ever associated itself, it remains to be seen how vigorously the Society will push for them in the years ahead.

While the fight against tobacco is important, it sometimes seems as if the ACS uses this fight as a "smokescreen" to hide its inaction in the overall field of environmental and occupational cancer. The Society's Board of Directors contains many business leaders and bankers. Science writer Peter Barry Chowka contends that many of the known carcinogens "are by-products of profitable industries in which its [ACS's] directors have financial interests" (Chowka, 1978b).°

During the public debate on the banning of saccharin, the American Cancer Society took the side of the manufacturers and the Calorie Control Council (a soft-drink lobbying group) to argue that this known animal carcinogen should be allowed in foods and drinks because it is of great medical benefit and safe. In effect, the Society came out against the Delaney Amendment, which states that no

---

° Dan Greenberg has called the ACS House of Delegates "a Who's Who of the American establishment." It includes eighteen officers or directors of banks, seven members of investment firms, thirteen business or industrial executives, with the remainder drawn from communications, advertising, media, manufacturing, insurance, and pharmaceuticals (cited in Chowka, 1978b).

substance known to cause cancer in animals may be added to the food or water supply. Although many experts question the value of saccharin even for diabetics, ACS official R. Lee Clark declared that "banning saccharin may cause great harm to many citizens while protecting a theoretical few" (*New York Times*, April 6, 1977).

"The ACS has done the American people a really great disservice," declared Nobel Prize–winner David Baltimore, an ACS-fund recipient whose picture had appeared on page one of the Society's 1975 *Annual Report*. He added, "ACS has been playing into the Calorie Control Council's hands" (Chowka, 1978b). The Council's members utilize 75 percent of the nation's saccharin supply.

A key member of the Calorie Control Council is the Coca-Cola Company, which manufactures the saccharin-sweetened diet soda Tab. In its 1976 *Annual Report,* the ACS acknowledges that "a generous grant from Coca-Cola supported transportation" for a large delegation of the Society's executives and volunteers who visited the Soviet Union in that year. In addition, a vice-president of Pepsico, another prominent Calorie Control Council member, is on the ACS Commission on Smoking and Public Policy (ibid.).

For an organization which claims to devote "considerable effort to studying the link between the environment and cancer," the ACS has taken a number of other questionable positions. For example, the synthetic hormone DES (diethylstilbestrol) is a known carcinogen.[*] It is given to livestock to fatten them up, on the assumption that the hormone itself does not enter the food supply. In 1972, however, residues of the hormone were discovered in beef, and public-interest groups demanded an immediate ban on the food additive. However, the American Cancer Society refused to take any position on the matter, and thereby deprived the consumer advocates of what could have been their most powerful support (Epstein, 1978:232).

Similarly, when the Food and Drug Administration suggested a patient package insert for Premarin and other hormone-containing drugs, saying that these may increase a woman's risk of cancer, the ACS opposed the move on the grounds that this would "interfere with the practice of medicine" and "discourage patients" from taking such drugs (ibid.:236).[**]

---

[*] "When DES was first synthesized in 1938, it was also found to be carcinogenic, inducing breast cancer in male mice. Subsequent studies showed that DES was approximately ten times more potent as a carcinogen than natural estrogens. . . . Administration of female sex hormones has been shown to induce cancer of the uterus, cervix, vagina, breast, and ovary in women, and of the breast in men" (Epstein, 1978:219–20).

[**] The wording is from a suit filed in the U.S. District Court in Delaware against the FDA by the Pharmaceutical Manufacturers Association, the drug industry's lobbying group, and the American College of Obstetricians and Gynecologists in September 1977. The ACS supported these groups in their protest.

It is difficult to summarize the ACS's overall stand on cancer prevention. On the one hand, it has done more than any other organization to establish the link between smoking and cancer, although its actual programs to stop smoking have fallen far short of the mark. It has given support to some researchers in the environmental field (see Chapter 15), yet the overwhelming share of research funds has gone to efforts to improve the three orthodox treatment methods. It speaks about cancer prevention, yet at critical junctures has taken public positions that have hindered the effort to control carcinogens.

As an institution dependent on small donations for its continued existence the ACS, in the words of Lane W. Adams, executive vice-president, must watch out for "disturbing signs of skepticism about the effectiveness of the struggle against cancer" (ACS, 1978:3). It therefore must acknowledge the widespread and growing conviction that industry is responsible for a good deal of the cancer in the United States, and that prevention may well be "the only cure." On the other hand, ACS ties to a treatment-oriented medical profession, and to big business, preclude it from taking any really strong measures to enforce prevention. Increasingly, the ACS sounds like the sophisticated corporate spokesman who grants a link between cancer and the environment with one hand—only to take it away with the other. According to the ACS's 1978 *Annual Report:*

we are steadily extending our knowledge of cancer-causing agents. However, some misunderstanding has grown up around the probable extent of "environmental" cancer—an unexamined assumption that a very high percentage of human cancer is caused by dangerous chemicals in our air, food, water and work places. . . .

While the evidence is mounting that substances we eat, breathe or contact are contributing causes of most cancer, only a minority of these are industrial "chemicals" or by-products (ACS, 1978:6).°

With such an attitude, it is unlikely that the American Cancer Society can play a very active role in the struggle against environmental carcinogens.

° "An informed consensus has gradually developed that most cancer is environmental in origin and is therefore preventable" (Epstein, 1978:23). Studies by R. Doll, B. Armstrong and other epidemiologists have established that from 70 to 90 percent is environmental in origin (ibid.:514). The lack of research on occupational cancer has hindered the effort to determine how much of this is due to "chemicals." But Epstein estimates that "30 to 40 percent of cancers in the general population" may be due to pollution just from the large petrochemical plants (ibid.:27).

The National Cancer Institute/National Cancer Program

The policy of the National Cancer Institute (NCI) toward prevention resembles that of the American Cancer Society. This is more than a coincidence. ACS was instrumental in the founding of the government's cancer institute in 1937, and in the passage of the National Cancer Act of 1971, which quickly quadrupled NCI's budget. ACS and NCI personnel interlock on many committees (see Chapter 16). Usually, it is the ACS which influences the larger, but more weak-willed NCI. An "ACS-controlled clique . . . dominates NCI policy and funding decisions," according to journalist Ruth Rosenbaum. "They've [ACS] turned it into a dollar pump," a House Appropriations committeeman added graphically (Rosenbaum, 1977).

From the 1940s to the 1960s, NCI's involvement with environmental and occupational carcinogens centered around one man, William C. Hueper. A German-born physician, Hueper came to the United States in 1923 and established himself as an expert on environmental causes of cancer.

Hueper predicted correctly that dye workers at E. I. Du Pont de Nemours & Co. would soon start succumbing to bladder cancer. When the prediction came true (such occupational cancers were already known in Europe), Hueper was hired by the company to "solve the puzzle" of this disease. He received little cooperation from the company. When he made an unauthorized visit to a Du Pont factory, he discovered large, uncontrolled amounts of carcinogenic chemicals. He reported this to the top management of the giant chemical company.

"The result of that letter," Hueper recalls, "was that I was never permitted to see the dye works again" (Agran, 1977:176). Restricted to the laboratory, Hueper demonstrated that one of the chemicals used in the dye works (beta-naphthylamine) produced bladder cancer in dogs. Eventually, 339 out of 2,000 workers at Du Pont exposed to this chemical died of bladder malignancies (ibid.).

In 1942, Hueper published *Occupational Tumors and Allied Diseases,* now considered a classic of the epidemiological approach to cancer ("a definitive summary," Shimkin, 1977:230). In 1948 he was appointed chief of the Environmental Cancer Section of the National Cancer Institute.

Hueper's job was carrying out field studies to determine which chemicals were causing cancer among workers and the general population, and laboratory studies to determine the effect of chemicals on animals. This ambitious program was hampered by the fact that Hueper's total budget for 1948 was $90,000—out of a $14.5 million allocation to NCI. In fact, when Hueper retired from the Institute sixteen years later, his budget was *still* about $90,000, although NCI's allocation had jumped by 1,000 percent (Epstein, 1978:321).

Hueper was also concerned with the danger of radiation, and he attempted to warn the Colorado Medical Society of the peril faced by uranium miners. Hueper's director at NCI refused to allow Hueper to do so, reportedly telling the scientist, "You shall omit that from your presentation" (Agran, 1977). Hueper responded, "I did not join the Public Health Service [of which NCI was a branch] to be made a liar!" (ibid.). Corroborating recent revelations about the suppression of information on radiation's dangers (see Chapter 4), Hueper explained, "You see, the AEC [Atomic Energy Commission] was afraid that publication of that kind of information might interfere with the continued production of atomic bombs" (ibid.).

Similarly, when Hueper was asked to testify before Congressman Delaney's (D.-N.Y.) Select Committee Investigating the Use of Chemicals in Food and Cosmetics, his supervisors at NCI refused to allow him to use much of his data on additives and even suggested that he refuse to testify. He therefore testified as a private citizen and contributed to the passage of the Delaney Amendment, which bans carcinogens from the food supply (ibid.).

For the second time in his career, Hueper was restricted to his laboratory and not allowed to contact state health departments or industrial concerns. He poured out a steady stream of articles and books, eventually totaling over 350, detailing the manner in which occupational and environmental factors cause cancer (ibid.).

Although of major theoretical importance, Hueper's discoveries did not have a significant impact on NCI policy or direction. With the passage of the National Cancer Act of 1971, NCI did not indicate any pressing interest in expanding work on the environmental causes of the disease (unless one defines putative cancer viruses as "environmental causes"—as NCI does). Instead, the emphasis was put on finding a cure. Reviewing the "war on cancer," British science writer Dr. Roger Lewin commented:

> The scientists have brought their own distortions . . . emphasizing the glamorous and exciting areas of research, such as virology and immunology, while ignoring to an unjustified extent topics such as epidemiology and environmental carcinogenesis *(New Scientist,* January 22, 1976:168).

NCI's record on tobacco is worse than that of the American Cancer Society. NCI's Smoking and Health Program, discontinued in 1977, was designed not to fight tobacco consumption, but solely to devise a so-called safe cigarette. The Tobacco Working Group, which NCI established to oversee the program, included vice-presidents and research directors of Liggett & Myers, the Brown and Williamson Tobacco Company, R. J. Reynolds Industries, Lorillard Research Center, and Philip Morris—all giant cigarette manufacturers.°

A critical role in the direction of NCI's research is played by the National Cancer Advisory Board (NCAB). The NCAB reviews the Institute's budget twice a year, considers all grant applications over $35,000 and makes recommendations on which are to be funded (NCI, 1975). To consider the validity of grant applications concerning the environmental causes of cancer, the NCAB established a Subcommittee on Environmental Carcinogenesis, chaired by Dr. Philippe Shubik.

For an expert on environmental cancer, Dr. Shubik took a surprisingly lax stand on the control of chemicals. For example, he attacked the "cancer principles" which would have allowed regulatory agencies to treat all carcinogens the same. This action led to the refusal by an Environmental Protection Agency administrative law judge to ban the carcinogenic pesticides chlordane and heptachlor (Epstein, 1978).

In November 1975 Shubik was successful in getting NCI to abandon its "Memoranda of Alert" in which it warned the public about early findings in its animal testing program. This action came shortly after NCI had issued a "Memorandum of Alert" on a chemical used by General Foods to decaffeinate coffee.

Shubik also testified against banning a proposed Procter and Gamble detergent which contained a potentially harmful chemical. So vehement was Shubik's defense of this detergent that Dr. Umberto Saffioti, associate director of NCI's Carcinogenesis Program, was compelled to ask: "Would you for the record identify what capacity you are here under?"

Shubik replied, "Procter and Gamble" (ibid.).

It turned out that Shubik, an NCAB official, was also a paid consultant to General Foods, Royal Crown Cola, Abbott Laboratories, Miles Laboratories, Colgate Palmolive, the Flavor and Extract Manufacturers Association, and the Calorie Control Council.

° Epstein presents evidence that it may be impossible to create a safe cigarette, since there are hundreds of potentially harmful chemicals in tobacco smoke. Carbon monoxide, the result of incomplete combustion, is itself a health hazard. The new flavor additives, which make low tar and nicotine cigarettes more appealing to smokers, may be carcinogenic. There is even evidence that people who smoke low tar and nicotine cigarettes may have a higher incidence of lung cancer, since they inhale more deeply and smoke more than those who smoke unfiltered high nicotine cigarettes (Epstein, 1978:163–65).

On the record, however, Shubik speaks like a good environmentalist. "It is the universal opinion that cancer can be attributed to environmental factors, in the main," he has said. "Cancer is largely a preventable disease." He has also expressed "general astonishment" that the National Cancer Program "does not appear to have accorded an adequate priority or sense of urgency to the field of environmental carcinogenesis" *(Science and Government Report,* April 1, 1975; *New Scientist,* January 22, 1976:168).*

Shubik does not appear to be alone in his connections to industry. According to the *Cancer Letter:*

> Why [Congressman David R.] Obey [D.-Wisc.] has singled out Shubik as a target for conflict of interest charges is a mystery. Nearly every scientific member of the Board, the President's Cancer Panel, and the various advisory committees could be subject to such charges (cited in Rosenbaum, 1977).

For example, the chairman of the NCAB turned out, under congressional inquiry, to be a director of Pennwalt Corporation, a conglomerate with both pharmaceutical and chemical interests. NCAB member Frank Dixon was a consultant to Eli Lilly Co. *(Cancer Letter,* June 11, 1976). The business connections of NCAB members Benno Schmidt and Laurance S. Rockefeller are dealt with elsewhere.

Under pressure from Congress and the public, NCI has claimed that a major portion of its work is relevant to environmental and occupational cancer. In 1976 Frank Rauscher, then National Cancer Institute director, told Congress that 20 percent of his agency's budget was devoted to the study of environmental carcinogens (Epstein, 1978:326 ff).

Rauscher's statement was based on the fact that the Division of Cancer Cause and Prevention commanded 18 percent of the Institute's budget. This division included most of the work on cancer viruses, which are, technically speaking, environmental factors. The virus program received approximately half of the division's yearly budget.

The departments which studied the chemical causes of cancer and tabulated the results of epidemiological surveys, Carcinogenesis Program and Field Studies and Statistics, together received only 12 percent of the Institute's budget—a vast improvement since Hueper's day but less than what was needed, according to many critics (ibid.).

---

* In 1978 Dr. Shubik came under Congressional scrutiny for possible conflicts of interest in relation to millions of dollars in NCI grants to the Eppley Cancer Research Institute, of which he is the director (Epstein, 1978).

More important than the number of dollars spent was the dearth of results. Under Rauscher's directorship, NCI's chemical-testing program achieved little. Most of the testing of chemicals for carcinogenicity was "farmed out" to an industrial contractor, Tracor Jitco, Inc. In 1973 about 100 new chemicals were tested each year. By 1976, however, the program appeared to be grinding to a halt. Only 30 compounds were tested in that year. (There are 4 million compounds listed in the Chemical Abstract Service computer registry, and over 30,000 of them are in *common* use in the United States [ibid.].)

Only five scientists were employed at NCI to test chemical compounds for their carcinogenic potential, and only half a dozen reports were issued.

Dissatisfaction increased, and in early 1976 Rauscher was directed by federal legislators to increase emphasis on prevention and was allocated the money to do so. He was told specifically to hire a staff of sixty new people for the Carcinogenesis Program and seventeen scientists for a newly created Epidemiology Branch (ibid.).

In April 1976, however, NCI was shaken by the resignation of Dr. Umberto Saffioti as associate director of the Carcinogenesis Program. In his letter of resignation, Saffioti complained of a lack of manpower for the program and a general lack of support for cancer prevention. Following his departure, the rest of the staff of the Carcinogenesis Program also resigned, leaving NCI with almost no cancer prevention program at all (ibid.:330).

"It had become clear," says Epstein, "that Rauscher was not only crippling any possibility for using the vast resources of the NCI to prevent cancer, but that he failed to understand why he should do so" (ibid.:331).

Rauscher's inaction on this politically sensitive issue had become a liability to the Ford administration, especially in an election year. On November 1, 1976, Rauscher resigned his NCI post and assumed his present position as vice-president for research at the American Cancer Society.[*]

In July 1977, Dr. Arthur Upton was appointed director of NCI by President Jimmy Carter. Many scientists, labor leaders, and public-interest groups supported his nomination because they considered Upton an expert on radiation as a cause of cancer, and he seemed to express many of the same concerns as Rauscher's critics.

Upton's personal attitude toward the carcinogen program seems far more supportive than Rauscher's. Nevertheless, he has inherited a situation which may well be beyond his capacity to change.

[*] Rauscher attributed his resignation to financial factors: his salary at ACS, $75,000, is more than double what it was in government (Epstein, 1978:331n).

Just when his administration had succeeded in clearing up a backlog of 207 unwritten technical reports on possible carcinogens, Upton was hit with a barrage of government criticism in mid-1979.

Investigations by the General Accounting Office (GAO), the government's financial watchdog, as well as by two Congressional committees, made the following charges about NCI's carcinogen testing program:

—As of June 1979, NCI was sitting on the results of 223 additional studies completed before 1977—this in addition to the 207 reports previously disclosed.

—The Institute had been financially manipulated by its largest contractors, and given shoddy work at exorbitant prices. For example, it had agreed to pay Litton Bionetics a total of $225 million for its management of the Frederick Cancer Research Center, at which much of the animal (bioassay) studies of carcinogens was conducted. Yet, according to the House Appropriations Committee, Litton "has muddled along from catastrophe to catastrophe in the animal colony" (*Science*, June 22, 1979). For example, gaps underneath the doors permitted test animals which got loose to roam from room to room, spreading disease. Outbreaks of pinworm, salmonella infection, hepatitis, and other infections led to the slaughter of over 100,000 carefully bred animals, at a cost of almost $500,000 to the taxpayer.

—The animal-testing facilities of another major contractor, Tracor Jitco, were similarly inadequate. A GAO investigator found "holes and cracks in the ceilings, walls and floor," inadequate air exchange, and other problems in their facilities. Yet NCI did nothing to penalize these companies, but gave them a "handsome profit" on a cost-plus basis, a profit which a House investigation called "probably exorbitant" (ibid.).

The result of these deals has not only been to shortchange the public, but virtually to cripple the already inadequate chemical testing program.

One reason for this, says *Science*, is that the top leaders of the cancer war have no enthusiasm for government testing of environmental carcinogens:

> Benno Schmidt, the chairman of the President's Cancer Panel, is on record as favoring chemical testing by industry, not NCI, and members of other NCI advisory groups have said the same thing. To some extent, the attitude persists even among NCI staff (ibid.).

Having industry supervise tests on its own chemicals is similar to appointing the wolf to guard the sheep. Because of NCI's neglect of the program, some important details of numerous studies on chemicals used in insecticides, drugs, food, and manufacturing remain in NCI files. And NCI, apparently, has little enthusiasm about ferreting them out (ibid.).

To a certain extent, a spirit of rebelliousness seems to be growing in Congress, as officials feel increasing pressure to show real progress in the cancer struggle. During a break in one of the 1979 congressional appropriations hearings, Dr. Upton said that he felt as if he were being "marched up to the scaffold" by the questioners (ibid.). And the chairmen of these committees hinted that NCI's budget might suffer as a result of these scandals.

The Food and Drug Administration

Any analysis of the cancer prevention problem must include a discussion of the Food and Drug Administration (FDA). This government agency has prime responsibility for keeping carcinogenic substances out of the public's food, beverages, cosmetics, and drugs.

Critics contend, however, that the FDA is too close to the industries it is supposed to regulate, is a cumbersome bureaucracy incapable of decisive action, and is financially incapable of doing the job it has been assigned.

Long delays have often accompanied FDA action against a carcinogen in the food supply. The synthetic hormone DES (diethylstilbestrol) was shown to be carcinogenic at the time it was discovered in the late 1930s. DES was widely used as a drug and as a growth-stimulant for poultry, hogs, and cattle because it makes animals grow fatter on less feed and come to market sooner. But problems soon came to light. Commercially raised minks became sterile after being fed the heads and necks of chickens which had received DES pellet implants as a growth-stimulant. Scientific tests showed residues of DES in the muscle meat and especially the livers of animals which had received such pellets. In 1959, for example, some poultry were found to contain *1,000 times* the amount of DES necessary to cause breast cancer in mice (Epstein, 1978).

Rather than lead the fight to have DES removed from the food supply, the Food and Drug Administration often appeared to be the protector of the pharmaceutical industry which produced the synthetic hormone, and of the food industries which used it. When Representative James Delaney (D.-N.Y.) questioned the cancer-causing potential of DES in the *Congressional Record* in 1957, the FDA immediately issued a counterstatement denying that the hormone was carcinogenic (ibid.).

After passage of the Delaney Amendment, the FDA argued that

the rule could not be applied retroactively: DES must stay because it had been introduced before passage in 1958 of Congressman Delaney's amendment to the 1938 Food, Drug, and Cosmetic Act.° For years, the FDA has sought to annul the Delaney anticancer clause (ibid.).

After extensive lobbying by the industries involved, DES was explicitly exempted from the Delaney Amendment. Manufacturers simply promised to monitor their own poultry and livestock for DES levels. The FDA was still supposed to monitor meat for residues, but rarely did. Even if the agency found excess DES residues, the results of its inspections were kept secret. In 1970, at the request of Eli Lilly Co., the principal manufacturer of the hormone, the FDA allowed an across-the-board doubling of the DES which could be given to livestock. Even the rather feeble limitations of the "DES clause" were thus superseded (ibid.).

In 1971 doctors at Massachusetts General Hospital discovered that the daughters of women who had taken DES to prevent miscarriages were succumbing to vaginal cancer a dozen or more years later. This created a furor, and the U.S. Department of Agriculture began a series of tests for DES residue in animals. They found such residues as high as 37 parts per billion—a seemingly minute amount, but six times the amount needed to cause breast cancer in mice (ibid.).

The USDA is said to have attempted to squelch these findings, but news leaked out. Congressional hearings were held in November 1971, at which it was pointed out that twenty foreign countries had already banned DES and many Europeans would not eat American beef—specifically because of its DES content (ibid.).

At the hearings, the commissioner of the FDA appeared on behalf of industry's position and spoke against the ban. Charles C. Edwards, the commissioner at the time, argued that the amount of DES found was insignificant and American industry would lose between $300 and $400 million a year if DES were banned.

The regulatory agencies opted for a seven-day waiting period between the last DES treatment and the slaughter of treated animals. How did they know that this waiting period was sufficient to rid the meat of DES residue? According to Epstein, the decision was apparently based on an FDA experiment involving *one cow* which received *one dose* of the hormone (ibid.).

As often happens, the FDA found itself pushed by the consumer

---

° The Delaney Amendment states that "no additive shall be claimed to be safe if it is found to induce cancer when ingested by man or animal, or if it is found after tests which are appropriate for the evaluation of safety of food additives to induce cancer in man or animal" (Public Law 85–929, September 6, 1958).

movement on the one hand, and powerful industries on the other. There was a temporary ban on the additive for the better part of 1973, during which industry switched to the more expensive synthetic hormones Ralgro and Zeranol.° At the present time, the fate of DES is in the courts, after a Federal District Judge ruled in January 1978 that industry has the right to use the additive as long as residues are kept at the lowest possible level at which the drug can be monitored.

Consumers, however, have begun to rebel against the use of this chemical and its manufacturers. Mothers who had taken DES to prevent miscarriages have now organized into "DES-Action" groups in New York, Washington, D.C., San Francisco, and other major cities. In July 1979 Joyce Bichler, a twenty-five-year-old social worker, was awarded $500,000 in a damage suit against Eli Lilly Co., after she had undergone a hysterectomy and a vaginectomy for cancer at the Albert Einstein College Hospital. Her mother had taken DES to prevent miscarriage (New York Times, July 17, 1979).

The story of DES—and particularly of the Food and Drug Administration's involvement—is not unique. It resembles FDA behavior toward most food additives and potential carcinogens.°° FDA laxity toward the nation's largest manufacturers stands in sharp contrast to its eagle-eyed stand toward small businessmen, scientific innovators, and nonconformists, as demonstrated in the previous chapters.

According to Omar V. Garrison, the FDA has a "double standard of enforcement": the agency is deferential to the big manufacturers and "grossly unfair to the small operator" (Garrison, 1970:63). While there are a variety of reasons for this discrimination,

they all add up to one overall purpose: they provide a smoke-screen for failure of FDA to protect the consumer against big food and drug monopolies and giant food-processing corporations (ibid.).

Conclusions

An increasing number of scientists now believe that most cancer is environmentally induced and can therefore be controlled. Cancer

---

° Ralgro and Zeranol are manufactured by Commercial Solvents. H. Virgil Sherrill, a director of the company, is an overseer of Memorial Sloan-Kettering Cancer Center.

°° See Epstein for numerous other examples. As a derivative of coal tar, the first known chemical carcinogen, Red Dye #2 should have been high on the FDA's suspect list. Instead, the agency took years before it banned the chemical, and has refused to move against other, similar, food dyes.

prevention not only spares the victim the agony of suffering from the disease, but is ultimately far cheaper than the enormous and ever-growing social cost of treating a major ailment after its occurrence.

In the case of cancer, prevention means regulating and controlling some of the largest and most lucrative industries in the country. Particular targets must include the petrochemical, food, drug, rubber, automotive, mining, and other giant companies.

Although prevention is certainly economical in the long run, it would probably cost a great deal in the short run, both in terms of lost profit opportunities and increased environmental controls. Industry has traditionally resisted such threats to its profits, shunning responsibility for its share of the cancer problem.

Large industry not only spends millions of dollars to argue against the need for stringent control of carcinogens, but appears to play a powerful role in shaping the direction of cancer research and management. The Board of Overseers of Memorial Sloan-Kettering Cancer Center is composed predominantly of men and women closely associated with the very industries under attack. The American Cancer Society is similarly tied to big business, and to the treatment-oriented medical profession. A crucial position at the government's National Cancer Institute is occupied by the National Cancer Advisory Board, which is dominated by big businessmen and investors such as Benno Schmidt and Laurance S. Rockefeller. The Food and Drug Administration, which has ultimate responsibility to keep carcinogens off the shelves of America's stores, appears to be biased in favor of industry and to consider the consumer's interest secondarily—if at all.

In short, the road toward prevention, although theoretically a bright and simple highway, is a tortuous path, filled with numerous roadblocks and dangerous pitfalls. The difficulty involved in establishing a substance as a cause of cancer and bringing that substance under control can be illustrated by the case of one such pollutant—asbestos.

15

Asbestos:
The Harvest of Death

Not long ago, "asbestos" was a reassuring word. Literally meaning "unquenched" or "unceasing," the name refers to a family of minerals which share the unique and useful quality of being unharmed by heat or fire. For all practical purposes, asbestos will not burn.

Some 4,500 years ago, Finnish potters incorporated asbestos into their cooking utensils to insulate them against heat and fire. By the twentieth century, asbestos had become a big industry. Mined mainly in upper Quebec, Canada, by the giant Johns-Manville Corporation, asbestos is manufactured into over a thousand different products, including such household items as aprons, floor tiles, mittens, potholders, stove linings and mats, and table padding. Around 75 percent of asbestos is used in construction. In all, 25 million tons of it surround us in the United States alone.

Asbestos is remarkable in other ways. It is a rock, a mineral which can be spun like a fabric. It is relatively inexpensive and abundant. It is truly a "magic mineral," as the asbestos manufacturers have always claimed.

There is only one problem: asbestos is also one of the most dangerous environmental pollutants ever discovered. Originally used to protect us from a major hazard—fire—it has now turned out to be a hazard of nightmarish proportions on its own.

Asbestos fibers are virtually indestructible. When they are released into the air, they take a long time to settle. People who work or live in the vicinity of loose asbestos breathe in the microscopic fibers. They often do not breathe them out, however, for 50 percent of the fibers are trapped by the membranes of the lungs and the lining of the lungs and other parts of the body. Once there, by mechanisms still not understood, the fibers irritate the delicate cells, creating "asbestos bodies"—harmful lesions which are visible only under the microscope.°

If exposure persists, scarring of the lungs takes place. This condition is known as asbestosis. Eventually, after many years, scar tissue replaces healthy lung tissue. The victim progresses from persistent coughing to difficulty in breathing. Finally he dies—from a lack of oxygen or from heart failure, caused by the strain of pumping blood through the scarred lung tissue. It's a terrible death.

But asbestosis is only one of the dangers. The main problem is cancer. Lung cancer forms within and around the scar tissue. Another form of cancer attacks the linings of the lungs (mesothelial tissue). This is called mesothelioma. Once a rare disease, it has now become common among asbestos workers. Other kinds of cancer are also typical results of asbestos exposure.

U.S. Department of Health, Education and Welfare statistics estimate that between 4 million and 8 million American workers may die of asbestos-related diseases. In fact, it was once thought that only asbestos workers were in danger of these diseases. It is now known, however, that people who have worked near asbestos, and even people who have lived in proximity to it, are also in danger. Since these diseases take a long time to reveal themselves, often as long as thirty years, the millions of workers exposed during and after World War II are only now beginning to show up in the cancer clinics.

"The harvest time of the disease has now arrived," said Dr. Philip Polakoff, a specialist in occupational medicine in Berkeley, California (cited in Weinstein, 1978). It is a harvest of death for thousands.

Equally frightening is the fact that almost all of us have now been exposed to asbestos to some significant degree. A high percentage of all urban dwellers have asbestos bodies in their lungs at autopsy—even if they never worked near asbestos (Brodeur, 1974). Government officials now state that 10 to 15 percent of *all* cancer deaths are due to asbestos alone.

Since the mid-1970s, government officials and scientists have begun to acknowledge the danger of asbestos and to warn those who were exposed to get medical checkups. These officials often add that science has only recently learned of this danger. This, however, is not true. The perils of asbestos have been known for many years. But few scientists spoke out on behalf of workers and the public, and

---

° Asbestos bodies are inhaled asbestos fibers that have been altered by the reaction of the lung tissue and coated with a substance rich in iron.

those who did were not listened to by the institutions which stood to gain from asbestos's continued use.

In 1900 a London physician first identified a new disease, which he called "asbestosis." The London doctor didn't even see fit to publish his findings in a scientific journal but simply passed his observations on to a government commission, where they lay buried for several decades (Kotelchuck, 1974).

The medical profession in the early part of this century may have been ignorant of this disease and the danger of asbestos. But the people most concerned with the production of asbestos were not unaware of its dangers. The records show that many workers quit their jobs in asbestos mining and manufacturing soon after being hired because they considered it dangerous. In 1918 U.S. and Canadian insurance companies stopped selling personal life insurance policies to asbestos workers—a clear indication that these companies were also well aware of the asbestos hazard. It is a fair assumption that the asbestos manufacturers also knew of the dangers (Brodeur, 1974).

In 1924 the medical profession rediscovered asbestosis, when Dr. W. E. Cooke reported in the *British Medical Journal* the untimely death of an asbestos worker. This thirty-three-year-old woman had been an asbestos factory worker since the age of thirteen. On autopsy, Cooke found massive amounts of asbestos in her scarred lungs. Eleven more cases of asbestosis were reported in Great Britain in the 1920s. American doctors at the Mayo Clinic and Yale University also reported cases of asbestosis among U.S. workers. In fact, by 1935, twenty-eight cases of asbestosis had been reported in the leading medical journals of Great Britain and the United States (Kotelchuck, 1974).

The British government responded by making asbestosis a compensable disease under their workmen's compensation acts and instituted safety rules. American asbestos manufacturers began a campaign to *prevent* the same thing from happening in the United States. Recently released internal documents show how the various giant manufacturers—especially Johns-Manville (J-M) and Raybestos-Manhattan—colluded to prevent the hazard of asbestos from being known.

In the early 1930s, for example, the editor of *Asbestos*, a trade magazine, wrote to Sumner Simpson, the president of Raybestos, asking if the time might not be ripe for an article on "dust control" in American factories.

The Raybestos president forwarded the letter to a top Johns-Manville attorney with the comment, "I think the less said about asbestos, the better off we are," a statement which neatly summarized the strategy and thinking of the entire industry in those years. He added, however:

At the same time we cannot lose track of the fact that there have been a number of articles on asbestos dust control and asbestosis in the British trade magazines. The magazine *Asbestos* is in business to publish articles affecting the trade and they have been very decent about not reprinting the English articles (Weinstein, 1978).

On the specific request of the Raybestos president himself, Johns-Manville's lawyer wrote back:

I quite agree with you that our interests are best served by having asbestosis receive the minimum of publicity. Even if we should eventually decide to raise no objection to the publication of an article on asbestosis in the magazine in question, I think we should warn the editors to use American data on the subject rather than English (ibid.).

"American data" on the subject was far less extensive than that of the British and, as shall be shown, much of it was paid for by the manufacturers and biased in favor of industry's position that asbestos was harmless.

In order to counter the anti-asbestos studies, Johns-Manville and Raybestos-Manhattan sponsored a study of asbestos workers carried out by doctors at a Metropolitan Life Insurance Company and the Department of Public Health at McGill University, Montreal. Although the study appeared to be an objective, academic report it was actually guided by the asbestos industry.

According to South Carolina Circuit Judge James Price, recently released internal documents show "written evidence that Raybestos-Manhattan and Johns-Manville exercised an editorial prerogative" over this Metropolitan Life study. In fact, Price has granted a new trial to the family of a dead asbestos worker after seeing these documents (ibid.).

Specifically, minutes of a meeting between a Metropolitan Life doctor—Anthony J. Lanza—and a Johns-Manville attorney and other industry officials on November 28, 1933, revealed that the attendees felt that Lanza's study "would be helpful to us, if favorable, in the event we should ever be involved in litigation" (ibid.).

Before Lanza finished his study, he dutifully sent it to industry officials for their comments before publication.

In a letter to Dr. Lanza in December 1934 the Johns-Manville attorney wrote:

I am sure you understand fully that no one in our organization is suggesting for a moment that you alter by one jot or title [sic] any scientific facts or inevitable conclusions revealed or justified by your preliminary survey. All we ask is that all of the favorable aspects of the survey be included and that none of the unfavorable be unintentionally pictured in darker tones than the circumstances justify.

I feel confident that we can depend upon you and Dr. McConnell to give us this "break" and mine and (others') suggestions are presented in this spirit (ibid.).

The Metropolitan Life study was conducted on Johns-Manville workers between 1929 and 1931, but was not published until 1935. ("The name of the game is not truth, of course, but delay," says David Kotelchuck, a student of the asbestos controversy [Kotelchuck, 1974].) A total of 126 workers in Canada and the United States were examined for signs of asbestosis. The authors did not conclude that there was any serious problem of asbestosis among J-M workers. In fact, they claimed that the workers appeared healthy and were not at all disabled.

So much for the conclusions. If one looks at the *actual data* in their report, however, it reveals that of the 126 workers examined, 67 definitely had asbestosis, 39 may have had it, and only 20 appeared free of the disease. Thus, 84 percent seemed to show signs of lung scarring (the positives plus the doubtful) and only 16 percent were definitely clear at the moment they were examined.

In addition, out of 121 physical examinations, 96 workers—or 79 percent—complained of persistent coughing and shortness of breath, the classic signs of early asbestosis. In response to this finding, the authors of the Metropolitan Life report state that "too much emphasis should not be placed on statements of subjective symptoms" (cited in ibid.).

This study was then quoted by the United States government as proof that asbestosis was *not* a serious health hazard. In fact, the U.S. Public Health Service published the Metropolitan Life study as an official government Public Health Report. "Few actions more clearly illustrate the interlock between industry and government," writes Kotelchuck (ibid.).

The asbestos companies were quite concerned that the United States would follow the example of Britain and make asbestosis a compensable disease under the Workman's Compensation Act. This had, in fact, been proposed in New Jersey. A J-M lawyer therefore wrote to Dr. Lanza:

As it is the policy of Johns-Manville to oppose any bill that attempted to include asbestosis as compensable, it would be very helpful to have an official report to show that there is a substantial difference between asbestosis and silicosis [a similar disease caused by inhalation of silica dust] and by the same token, it would be troublesome if an official report should appear from which the conclusion might be drawn that there is very little, if any, difference between the two diseases (Weinstein, 1978).

Dr. Lanza complied with these requests and never made any comparison between asbestosis and silicosis, which was recognized as a compensable disease. (Had asbestosis been recognized as compensable, the company might have been held liable for damages.) In fact, asbestosis did not become compensable in New Jersey until after World War II.°

But the problems of the asbestos workers were not over. In 1935 two doctors at the Medical College of South Carolina performed an autopsy on an asbestos worker and found lung cancer amid the scar tissue. By 1942 ten such reports had followed in the medical literature and it became known—at least among specialists—that asbestos also caused lung cancer in workers.

With this revelation the industry took a more aggressive policy. They commissioned a study in 1938 from scientists at Saranac Laboratory, an Adirondack tuberculosis sanatorium and research center with a long history of cooperating with industry. The asbestos manufacturers paid $15,000 to support the study, and the J-M attorney wrote to another industry official:

It would be a good thing to distribute the information among the medical fraternity[,] providing it is of the right type and would not injure our companies (Weinstein, 1978).

The Saranac study, conducted by Drs. Arthur Vorwald and John Karr, simply dismissed the asbestos-cancer link by commenting that the workers found to have lung cancer were not a random sample of asbestos workers. They also had asbestosis. Perhaps, the scientists argued, there was some special relationship between asbestosis victims and lung cancer. The only way the asbestos–lung cancer link could be definitely proven was by carrying out a cancer study among a large number of asbestos workers, irrespective of any other disease.

But industry controlled the medical records of the asbestos workers, and it was not about to open these records to inquisitive scientists. Thus, the entire matter lay dormant for many years. Kotelchuck remarks:

Scientists did not protest the industry's denial of access to this information or insist in their scientific papers that epidemiological studies be car-

---

° Dr. Lanza rose from assistant medical director at Metropolitan Life to chairman of the Institute of Industrial Medicine at New York University Medical School. He was the author of well-known textbooks on lung diseases, and remained a leading expert on asbestos until his death in the early 1960s (Kotelchuck, 1974).

ried out. True to their professional codes, they kept silent. So nothing happened—except 20 more years of growing profits for the asbestos industry (Kotelchuck, 1974).

And, it might be added, twenty more years of cancer for asbestos workers.

In 1956 the Quebec Asbestos Mining Association (QABA) commissioned a study from the Industrial Hygiene Foundation (IHF—now the Industrial Health Foundation). Based in Pittsburgh, the IHF performs research for industry and is basically pro-management.

The IHF study examined 6,000 Quebec asbestos miners' health records for evidence of lung cancer. They found none. However, they had ignored one of the cardinal principles of such studies: the twenty-year time lag between first exposure to an agent causing lung cancer and the clinical appearance of the disease. This is called the "twenty-year rule" for lung cancer. According to Dr. Irving Selikoff:

> For lung cancer the percentage of all deaths that occurred at 10 years or less was trivial; it was not until 25 years after onset of employment that deaths [from lung cancer] became common [among shipyard workers] (Selikoff, 1978).

These facts were certainly known to the authors of the QAMA report, for they themselves cite studies, by Hueper and others, which contain explicit reference to the "twenty-year rule." But by studying a relatively young group of workers, two-thirds of whom were between twenty and forty-four years of age, the industry-sponsored scientists were able to make the report come out favorable to the companies.

By the early 1960s, the asbestos health hazard began to receive increasing attention. A doctor in South Africa discovered a high incidence of mesothelioma among asbestos workers. This disease was once so rare that it was not even listed as a separate cause of death in the International Classification of Causes of Death. The best estimates, based on autopsy series, was that only one out of 10,000 people died of it.

But among asbestos workers it was soon found that 7 or 8 percent were dying of this cancer of the lining cells—somewhere around 1,000 times the number expected.

At about the same time, Dr. Irving Selikoff and his co-workers at Mount Sinai Medical Center in New York broke through industry's monopoly of health data on asbestos workers by going directly to the unions involved.

Selikoff's findings were a bombshell. He, too, found that among young workers there was little change in their X rays. "In the New

York area," he has said, "when we examined somewhat over a thousand asbestos insulation workers, we found that of the 725 with *less* than twenty years from onset of exposure, most had normal X rays." After twenty years, however, extensive disease began to appear with appalling frequency (ibid.).

In 1943 there were 632 men in a New York pipefitters union. All of them have been "followed" by Selikoff and his colleagues. By 1977, the outspoken physician told a medical meeting, "instead of the 330 anticipated deaths (given their ages in 1943) there were 478 deaths.

Why did some 150 people die who were not expected to die? Well, there should have been 56 deaths from cancer, and there were 210. Instead of 13 deaths from lung cancer there were 93. One out of every three asbestos workers dies of lung cancer. This is simply a disaster! (ibid.).

"Interestingly, too, instead of 15 deaths from cancer of the esophagus, colon, stomach and rectum there were 43—a modest increase," Selikoff adds ironically. "Obviously, anyone who inhales dust also tends to ingest it."

Selikoff next followed up this New York study with a more extensive report on thousands of asbestos pipefitters across the country.

On January 1, 1967 there were 17,800 men in the international union. By 1977, there were 2,270 deaths, instead of 1,661 expected. . . . Once again, instead of 320 deaths due to cancer there were 994 (ibid.).

Selikoff and his Mount Sinai colleagues were able to draw some lessons from these studies.

First, until this time it had been assumed that the main hazard of asbestos came from asbestosis. In fact, as late as 1968, government officials shrugged off suggestions of any other danger (Brodeur, 1974:23). But, says Selikoff, "the major excess [of deaths] was from cancer" (Selikoff, 1978).

So prevalent was cancer among asbestos workers, their family members, and even neighbors of asbestos plants that the Mount Sinai doctor remarks, ominously, "We're beginning to understand why one out of every four Americans—if things go as they are—will have cancer in his or her lifetime and why 20 percent of all deaths in this country are now due to cancer" (ibid.).

Second, not only workers are susceptible to the ravages of asbestos and other environmental hazards. *Consumers* of these products are also at danger, and with over 1,000 products made of or with asbestos, that includes almost everyone. In fact, says Selikoff, sometimes consumers are at greater risk than workers, since in a factory carcinogens may be totally enclosed. There are *some* health regulations for production, but consumption is largely uncontrolled and unregulated.

Third, other chemicals may interact with asbestos to incite an even greater risk of disease. For example, asbestos workers who also smoke have an even greater risk of contracting lung cancer (Fraumeni, 1975:468). "They are sitting targets," says Selikoff.

Fourth, although even a brief exposure to asbestos can be hazardous—even fatal—in general the chances of contracting the disease is related to the length of time and the extent of exposure. The risk is obviously higher for those most heavily involved in the production of asbestos, who can inhale up to 8 billion fibers and fibrils (submicroscopic fibers) of asbestos a day, 50 percent of which are retained in the lungs.

Nor have workers generally been told when their health was threatened by asbestos exposure.

For example, Dr. Kenneth Wallace Smith, medical director of Johns-Manville until 1966, testified in a lawsuit that he could see early X-ray changes in a patient perhaps ten, twelve, or fifteen years before he developed any clinical signs of disability.

But he did not tell the J-M workers they were coming down with asbestosis or cancer. In a 1949 confidential report to management he urged:

> As long as the man feels well, is happy at home and at work and his physical condition remains good he should be permitted to live and work in peace. . . . Should the man be told of his condition today, there is a very definite possibility that he would become mentally and physically ill, simply through the knowledge that he had asbestosis (cited in Weinstein, 1978).

Many experts believe, however, that "early detection of asbestosis is critical since it is irreversible when fully developed and gradually destroys the lungs." If, on the other hand, the disease is monitored closely, the patient's life can be prolonged (ibid.).

Theoretically, the government should be a watchdog and should prevent such abuses from occurring. In fact, however, government scientists have been among the most vocal advocates of industry's position. Lewis Cralley, a top official of the Public Health Service's Division of Occupational Health, carried out a study of health conditions in the asbestos industry. He "suppressed its findings for six years," says Kotelchuck, "until they were released by other . . . officials over his objections" (Kotelchuck, 1974).

Although the asbestos industry has largely blocked investigations of the asbestos peril, Cralley told reporter Paul Brodeur, "all I know is that the first real interest came from industry. They asked for our help back in 1964, and they have cooperated with us magnificently" (Brodeur, 1974).

During Cralley's tenure as head of Occupational Health, government investigators were not required to identify individual factories in their reports on hazards, forward interpretations of data to state agencies, or even make any recommendations to factory owners (ibid.). In fact, says Brodeur in his award-winning study *Expendable Americans,*

in order not to embarrass management or make workers apprehensive, the government engineers who took air samples during the environmental surveys not only were forbidden to discuss the nature of their activities with any workers they encountered but were also instructed not to wear respirators, which would have afforded them some protection against the hazard of inhaling asbestos dust (ibid.).

Through scientists such as Cralley, industry was afforded an entrée into the inner circles of the medical establishment, including such prestigious universities as New York University, McGill Medical School, Wayne State, the University of Pittsburgh, and Carnegie-Mellon and other groups such as the American Public Health Association, the International Union Against Cancer, and the American Academy of Occupational Medicine. In fact, Dr. Lee B. Grant, medical director of Pittsburgh Plate Glass Company—a major asbestos user—eventually became president of the American College of Preventive Medicine (ibid.).

Over the years, most cancer scientists have shown a lack of interest in the asbestos problem, just as they have failed to deal with environmental factors in general. For many years, in fact, Selikoff and his group were among the few asbestos labs in the United States.

Since the early 1970s, the American Cancer Society has given financial support to Selikoff, and a page and a half of its 1974 *Annual Report* is taken up with a description of its joint work with the Mount Sinai team. In that same year, the Society gave Selikoff about $150,000, two-thirds of which went for research on asbestos (Garfinkel, 1979). While this seems to be a large sum, it represents only a fraction of 1 percent of what ACS garnered from the public that year ($108 million). By 1978 support for the Mount Sinai group had risen to $286,000 for all of Selikoff's projects, including asbestos research, while public donations to ACS had risen to almost $140 million (ibid.; ACS, 1978). This increase is a modest recognition of the growing public awareness of the asbestos problem.

The record of Memorial Sloan-Kettering Cancer Center is even worse. The 386-page 1976 *Annual Report* of the Sloan-Kettering Institute, which details hundreds of research projects, contains no mention of studies on asbestos.

This lack of interest in asbestos (as in other environmental and occupational causes of cancer) has had some unfortunate consequences for MSKCC employees, as well as for the public, which might benefit from such investigations. In 1976 the Center's administration began renovating two of the older buildings in the complex. Dust flew in the corridors of the hospital that summer and fall, but no one outside of the administration knew that these clouds contained asbestos, which had accidentally been freed from old pipe-coverings by workmen.

Jane McGill, the head of the Employee Health Service, wrote in her 1976 annual report that there had been certain "environmental problems." One of these, she noted, was that "asbestos-containing pipe-covering had been removed by the contractors by dry technique and not according to OSHA [Occupational Safety and Health Administration] precautions."

"It was determined that one area was contaminated with asbestos fibers," she said (McGill, 1976). Later that year, *Second Opinion,* the "underground" employees' newsletter at MSKCC, obtained a copy of this report and publicized it *(Second Opinion,* June 1977). No official announcement was made that for several months employees, visitors, and possibly patients had been exposed to asbestos-laden dust.

Apparently, MSKCC did not have an expert sufficiently versed in the problems of asbestos to deal with the question, for Dr. Irving Selikoff and Dr. Arthur Rohl, both from Mount Sinai, and Dr. Robert Sawyer of Yale University were called in and asked to assess the extent of damages (McGill, 1976).

Although there is more public awareness of the asbestos peril today, real improvement may be slow in coming. The National Cancer Institute now has literature which it sends to those who fear they stand a risk of developing asbestos-related diseases. It also has designed posters to warn the public of the risks involved. Other government agencies have begun to provide information, chest X rays, or, occasionally, inspections of possibly contaminated areas.

Much effort has been expended in trying to limit the number of fibers permissible in the air. While such controls are important, it is necessary to point out that even if fibers are tightly regulated, the problem may not end. Each fiber can—and does—break up into a multitude of smaller fibrils, so small that 1 million of them, side by side, measure an inch (Brodeur, 1974).

These fibrils can be detected only by electron microscope, which few industrial hygiene laboratories possess. Little research has been done on the fibril problem, but it is known that an asbestos worker in a supposedly safe plant, whose air contains only two fibers per cubic centimeter, can still inhale from 800 million to 8 billion fibers and fibrils in an eight-hour day (ibid.:30).

For the consumer, the problem of controlling asbestos exposure may be even more difficult. Asbestos is in the environment—millions of indestructible tons of it.

Given the past history of underestimating the danger of asbestos, several important and disturbing questions remain. How much of this asbestos poses an immediate danger to the public? How much is a "time bomb" which will explode each time an old building is demolished or falls into disrepair? Does the asbestos have to be removed, or can it be contained? Who is going to pay for this cleanup? Are there any ways to remove asbestos once it is entrapped in the body? Are there any really safe substitutes for this "miracle fiber"?

Answering such questions will certainly take a great deal more research. But while the scientists deliberate, asbestos continues to pour into the environment virtually unchecked—over 750,000 short tons in 1976 alone (Standard and Poor's, 1977).

The asbestos industry has sidestepped its heavy responsibility for this situation. The companies have even requested the government to pay for whatever losses they incur in over $2 billion in lawsuits which asbestos workers have filed against them. This "bailout" was discussed at a meeting of Congressman George Miller's (D.-Calif.) House Committee on Education and Labor. There is a large Johns-Manville plant in Congressman Miller's Martinez district, according to the *Guardian*, a New York–based radical newspaper (*Guardian*, December 20, 1978).

An even more questionable plan involved the exporting of asbestos to populations either unaware of its danger, desperate for work, or unable to do anything about the threat because of political repression. As regulations have tightened in the United States, the asbestos industry has begun to move its factories abroad. It has generally chosen poor countries, such as Taiwan, South Korea, Brazil, and India (ibid.).

This migration of so-called runaway hazardous shops began in the late 1960s. Taiwan, South Korea, and Brazil are now all large exporters of asbestos products to the United States: actually, they themselves import the raw asbestos from American companies, such as Johns-Manville, and ship their finished products back to the United States and other industrialized countries. The favorite spot for such relocation has been Mexico.

In 1967, for example, Amatex, a Pennsylvania asbestos firm, closed its Milford Square plant, although it was quite new, and opened an asbestos yarn mill in Agua Prieta, a small town across the border from El Paso, Texas. It also operates a plant in Juarez, Mexico. According to Barry Castleman, a consultant to the Environmental Defense Fund and an expert on asbestos:

In December 1974 Amatex began to import asbestos textiles into the U.S. from the Juarez plant. Amatex "imported" about 2 million pounds of asbestos textiles from its Mexican border plants in 1975, about one-fourth of U.S. imports from the entire world that year (ibid.).

U.S. journalists who visited the two Amatex plants in 1977 found "clumps of asbestos clinging to nearby bushes and fences where neighborhood children play. Inside the plants, the air was filled with the deadly white fibers" (ibid.).

The U.S. government has aided the asbestos industry in moving its hazardous plants out of the country—in effect, exporting asbestosis and cancer to foreign workers. For example, most of the imports come from so-called beneficiary countries. These countries are allowed to export their goods duty-free to the United States.

Some foreign asbestos plants are even subsidized directly by the United States. According to Castleman, a plant in Madras, India, "was covered by $1 million in political risk insurance by the Overseas Private Investment Corporation," a U.S. government agency (ibid.).

As knowledge of the asbestos peril spreads, however, foreign workers are fighting back against the threat. In Cork, Ireland, for example, asbestos workers and the community delayed the opening of a newly completed asbestos manufacturing plant, owned and operated by Raybestos-Manhattan. The $8 million plant was unable to open for many months, and did so only at reduced capacity after the Irish people imposed safety regulations on the owners (ibid.).

In the United States a series of struggles has been waged over asbestos in schools and other public buildings. This began in April 1972 when an elementary school in Lander, Wyoming, was ordered closed after it was found that children were breathing, according to a government report, "an unhealthy mixture of air and asbestos dust" (Bourne, 1978).

According to a Public Interest Research Group study, the school librarian had become suspicious of a layer of dust covering furniture throughout the school. The dust turned out to be asbestos, falling from deteriorating ceilings which had been sprayed with an asbestos insulation eleven years before. Such sprayed-on insulation was common all over the country from the 1950s to the 1970s. The school had to be closed until the hazardous material could be replaced.

In January 1977 six elementary schools in Howell Township, New Jersey, were closed when excessive levels of asbestos were found there. One child appeared to be sick from an asbestos-related disease, and dozens of other children complained of unexplainable headaches, sore throats, and respiratory congestion. The problems of Howell Township may have been aggravated by children who scraped the ceilings with sticks and grabbed at the insulation. Children played with pieces of the insulation, which looked to them like cotton candy, and threw it in each others' faces (*New York Times,* January 4, 1977).

In late 1978 Harlem parents shut down two adjacent New York City schools, P.S. 208 and P.S. 185, when they discovered asbestos flaking from a fourth-floor ceiling. The Board of Education attempted a "cosmetic cover-up," Helene Brathwaite, head of the Parents' Association, has said (*Second Opinion*, December 1978). They tried to put up a new ceiling and leave the asbestos in place. In doing so, they raised such a storm of asbestos that the children, teachers, and parents could hardly see their hands in front of their faces. So the parents shut the schools down. In some places, such as the auditorium, the asbestos had been exposed, behind a grill, since the school opened in 1967.

The Harlem parents demanded—and got—a secret Board of Education report which showed that at least 189 of the City's 1,000 public schools were contaminated with asbestos. This figure was later revised to about 500, although no one knows for sure how bad the situation really is. Even some school officials seem to think the Board of Education is underestimating the numbers involved (ibid.).

Although using asbestos to insulate buildings has been banned since the mid 1970s, millions of office workers still work in asbestos-laden buildings, including Madison Square Garden, the World Trade Center, and about half of the country's skyscrapers. Fresh-air systems often circulate right over the sprayed-on asbestos, picking up fibers and fibrils into the air current. In the furor that followed the Harlem exposures, many workers in New York suspected that they, too, were working or living in asbestos-contaminated buildings. It is very difficult for them to find out if they are in danger. Mount Sinai maintains the only electron microscope in all of New York City which can detect asbestos in the air. Using this machine, it takes a full day to test one building. When the head of the laboratory was asked what was being done to uncover the asbestos hazard, he replied—with unusual directness—"Nothing" *(New York Post,* November 17, 1978).

In an interview at the school Helene Brathwaite voiced her frustration over this situation:

Industry has bombarded us with different kinds of substances that are harmful to our health, without asking us if we wanted them or not, without testing properly, and then telling us *we* have a problem. This has to do with capitalism and the Almighty Dollar. That's the basic problem *(Second Opinion,* December 1978).

PART FOUR

The Cancer Business

16

The Cancer Establishment

In the United States today, the direction of cancer management appears to be shaped by those forces financially interested in the outcome of the problem. Distinct circles of power have formed which, while differing among themselves on many issues, are sufficiently cohesive and interlocking to form a "cancer establishment." This establishment effectively controls the shape and direction of cancer prevention, diagnosis, and therapy in the United States.

There is a common belief that the doctors who administer cancer therapy and the scientists who perform laboratory research control the cancer field. It is understandable that the public believes this, since it is the surgeon, radiologist, and chemotherapist who give treatment, and who appear to pass judgment on new forms of therapy. Yet most doctors practice the kind of medicine they learned in medical school. There are numerous social and even legal restraints on the kind of medicine a physician can practice. At large institutions, for instance, experiments involving humans are "increasingly being restricted by regulations and decrees" (Jukes, 1976).

Peer review committees within hospitals or medical societies are taking an increasingly active role in determining the actual course of therapy a physician can prescribe. The role of the government is also clearly on the rise. Those who seek to use new forms of therapy must first gain the approval of the Food and Drug Administration. If they seek research funds, they must pass "site visits" and reviews by the National Institutes of Health and other funding agencies.

Many of these regulations were instituted to prevent real abuses, such as the wanton human experimentation practiced on cancer patients until the mid-1960s (Katz, 1972). A side effect of this legislation, however, appears to have been to speed the centralization of power in a few hands and a growing conservatism toward new therapies within the medical profession.

Within the cancer field, it appears that the major decisions are made at the top of four or five organizations. These organizations are controlled mainly by laymen, and if a doctor or scientist exercises real decision-making power, it appears to be as a result of his inclusion in one of these groups, rather than through his professional expertise per se.

Doctors who still believe they are free to give whatever treatment they consider best for a willing patient are, in fact, toying with "quackery," as it is defined by these leading bodies.

At the pinnacles of power, the scientists and physicians are usually subordinated to the control of laymen. For example, at Memorial Sloan-Kettering, "the control and management of the operations of [MSKCC] shall be vested in its board of trustees" and the scientific administrators are "subject . . . to the control and direction of the board." °

More often than not, these laymen are the very people with the greatest vested interest in the outcome of the cancer problem. How such individuals, as well as their banks and corporations, attained their power in the cancer field, and why they seek such control, will be examined in the case of four of the most powerful organizations.

Memorial Sloan-Kettering Cancer Center

In the nineteenth century, when the U.S. Congress took little or no interest in health or welfare, it was only natural that hospitals would be financed by the philanthropic activities of wealthy families. Often a personal tragedy would stimulate a large donation. Thus, the Astors (whose wealth was derived from fur trading and tenement properties) provided the initial funds for the New York Cancer Hospital in the 1880s. After them came other wealthy families, such as the Huntingtons (railroads) and the Douglases (copper).

With these large contributions came influence and even control of the recipient organizations. The Astors' lawyer became the first chairman of the board of the New York Cancer Hospital. The Douglases not only held leading positions on the board of directors, but had their personal physician, James Ewing, appointed medical director of the newly renamed Memorial Hospital.° °

° In 1978, the board of trustees became known as the board of overseers. This reorganization does not appear to have altered the relationship of the doctors or scientists to the board (see Appendix A).

° ° Mrs. Percy L. Douglas continues as an overseer of MSKCC (see Appendix A).

Until the beginning of the twentieth century, control of a hospital conveyed great prestige, but little else. Not surprisingly, wealthy families sometimes lost all interest in a particular charity with a change of their leading members. Younger members of the Astor family abandoned all interest in Memorial, and the Harrimans, once prominent in the cancer field, lost that interest and turned instead to politics (Sugiura, 1971).

James Douglas saw an opportunity to mingle his charitable and his business interests. A miner, Douglas undertook the large-scale extraction of radium from Colorado ore. For the first time, cancer had become a topic of importance to the business community.

In this respect, the Rockefeller family followed in Douglas's footsteps. Since the beginning of the century, however, this group had mingled personal, financial, and political goals under a single heading—philanthropy.

There is every indication that John D. Rockefeller's (JDR I) much-vaunted support of medical causes was the result of financial calculation as much as softheartedness toward suffering humanity (Brown, 1979). According to a biographical study, JDR I "really had no way of understanding value except in dollar terms. . . . Money was the philosophical center of his world throughout his long life" (Collier and Horowitz, 1976).

JDR I's chief adviser, Frederick T. Gates, presented the value of medical research in terms of its financial benefits:

I pointed to the Koch Institute in Berlin and at greater length to the Pasteur Institute in Paris. . . . I pointed out . . . that the results in dollars or francs of Pasteur's discoveries had saved for the French nation a sum far in excess of the entire cost of the Franco-Prussian war (ibid.).

JDR I and his son, "Junior," first showed an interest in the cancer field when they contributed to the formation of the American Society for the Control of Cancer, predecessor of the ACS (Considine, 1959). In 1927 they began systematic contributions to Memorial Hospital—cash donations which eventually totaled several million dollars, as well as a square block of land on which a new Memorial Hospital was built in the 1930s (ibid.).°

These contributions gave the Rockefellers influence at Memorial

---

° Actually, the Rockefeller family's involvement with cancer began in the mid-nineteenth century. JDR I's father, William Avery Rockefeller, was a celebrated, if uneducated, cancer "therapist" in Cayuga County, New York. According to a recent biographical study, "He found a more promising career in patent medicines. He journeyed for hundreds of miles to camp meetings, passing out handbills that read: 'Dr. William A. Rockefeller, the Celebrated Cancer Specialist, Here for One Day Only. All Cases of Cancer Cured unless too far gone and then they can be greatly benefitted.' " He sold his remedy for $25 a bottle, the equivalent of two months' wages (Collier and Horowitz, 1976:8).

greater than any other family—including the Douglases, who remained nominally in control for over a decade longer. The policy of the Rockefellers, as it had been of Douglas, was to "back Ewing" (ibid.). Backing Ewing primarily meant backing radiation therapy.

In 1927 the Rockefellers greatly expanded their interest in pharmaceuticals when Standard Oil of New Jersey (Esso), which was dominated by the Rockefeller family, signed an extensive cartel agreement with the German I. G. Farben company.

I. G. Farben was a huge trust which controlled almost the entire German chemical and drug industries. Until its dissolution by the Allies after World War II, I. G. Farben was a hated and feared part of the German war machine. It had produced poison gas for the German armies in World War I and was to produce the nerve poison Zyklon B for the concentration camps during World War II. In fact, the concentration camp at Auschwitz was built to accommodate a huge Farben synthetic rubber plant nearby (Ambruster, 1947).

Esso signed a wide-ranging cooperative agreement with I. G. Farben. Under the terms of the agreement, the Germans would not market gasoline or gasoline products outside of their own borders. In return, Esso would "stay out of the existing market in all other chemical fields" (DuBois, 1952:148). In addition, the two companies set up a new firm—the Joint American Study Corporation, or JASCO—to mutually develop new discoveries, such as in the field of synthetic rubber.*

The significance of this "marriage" or "general partnership" (as Esso executives called it) was that the Esso–Rockefeller empire suddenly inherited a great interest in the worldwide pharmaceutical business.

Farben's interest in drugs dated to the nineteenth century when one of its predecessor companies, Bayer, discovered aspirin. Another component of the trust, Hoechst, had produced Antipyrin, Pyramidon, Novocain, Salvarsan, and Dolantin (Bäumler, 1968:215). The shadowy company had branches all over the world, and appears to have had an interest in many foreign drug companies as well.

It is interesting to note that in 1926, one year before the Rockefellers began their systematic contributions to Memorial, Frank

---

* This agreement was greatly loaded in I. G. Farben's favor, which became apparent when the Japanese cut off the United States' supply of natural rubber after Pearl Harbor. The United States had no synthetic rubber, and most of the information on how to make it was locked in Esso's vaults. Only swift action by the U.S. government prevented a disaster. The one man most responsible for this problem was Frank Howard. "Perhaps Howard's previous blocking of crucial industrial developments in the United States was unwitting; now [1939] he deliberately accepted, in friendly trust, the power to prevent the United States from seizing the Farben patents" (DuBois, 1952:283). (For a fuller explanation of Howard's role see Borkin, 1978.)

Howard, a vice-president of Esso, paid his first visit to the I. G. Farben laboratories. He later said that he was "plunged into a world of research and development on a gigantic scale such as I had never seen" (cited in Borkin, 1978). He soon discovered that the Germans were already deeply involved in cancer research.

In the first part of this century, Germany was the undisputed leader in the drug industry. During a visit to one of the German research laboratories in 1927,° I was mystified to find an adjoining greenhouse full of plants, bearing the most horrible-looking tumors. It was a nightmare of nature gone mad! In these greenhouses and in the connected laboratories, the German scientists were making a concerted effort to find out all they could in plants and animals (Howard, 1955).

In the 1930s, Howard was invited to join Memorial Hospital's board of managers. The Standard Oil executive was made chairman of the newly organized Research Committee. By 1941 limited research on chemotherapy had begun at Memorial, but this was interrupted by the outbreak of World War II. Cornelius P. "Dusty" Rhoads, who had headed this nascent program, became chief of research for the Chemical Warfare Service of the United States.

The official purpose of this service was to carry out defensive studies on the effects of poison gas. It is somewhat surprising to learn that human experiments with poison gas-like substances were also being carried out on cancer patients. In 1976 National Cancer Institute officials revealed that

under the mantle of military secrecy, clinical trials were initiated with HN_2 . . . which became the most widely used nitrogen mustard. By the time military restrictions were removed in 1946, a total of 160 patients had been treated by several groups of investigators (Carter and Kershner, 1976).

The limited success with nitrogen mustard as a chemotherapeutic agent stimulated interest in wide-scale research. As the war neared its end, Frank Howard and a New York banker, Reginald Coombe, then president of Memorial Hospital, drew up a Post-War Development Plan which called for a vast expansion of the hospital into a combination treatment–research center (Howard, 1955).

Such a project was clearly too vast even for the Rockefellers. Howard therefore asked two prominent executives of General Motors to join the project and provide funds for the new center. Together Alfred P. Sloan (1875–1966) and Charles F. Kettering (1876–1958) contributed several million dollars, and the new research cen-

---

° The Howard document states that the visit occurred in 1927. Borkin speaks only of one visit by Howard to I. G. Farben's laboratories, in March 1926 (Borkin, 1978:47).

ter, the Sloan-Kettering Institute for Cancer Research, was named in their honor in August 1945.

Until that time, Memorial Hospital had been under the control of the Rockefellers and, to a lesser degree, the Douglases. With the inclusion of Sloan and Kettering in leadership positions, members of the Rockefellers' traditional rival, the Morgan banking interests, were allowed to share power.

Sloan was president of General Motors, long associated with Morgan interests, and was also a director of Du Pont and of the Morgan Guaranty Trust Company itself. Kettering, or "Boss Kett," as he was called, was vice-president of General Motors, and a large shareholder in that company.°

The composition of the board of trustees at that time reveals a kind of balance of power, with the Rockefellers and their allies in overall control, but with those representing the Morgan interests assuming many positions of power.

The actual personnel changed over the years, of course, and new financial and industrial groups assumed key positions, but from this period forward the world's largest private cancer center was ruled by what looks like a consortium of Wall Street's top banks and corporations.°°

By the mid-1960s, the MSKCC board had begun to take on a rather uniform appearance. What stood out was that many of its leading members were individuals whose corporations stood to lose or gain a great deal of money, depending on the outcome of the "cancer war."

Appendix A lists the current members of the MSKCC board, and provides the corporate affiliations of the most influential. It is immediately apparent that representatives of large and powerful companies are well represented. These companies exercise their influence not only through their personal presence, but through often-substantial gifts which they make to the Center.

For example, in June 1978, MSKCC announced that it had received $7 million toward a $65-million fund-raising goal from Exxon,

---

° In 1957 Sloan's net worth was established at $200–$400 million and Kettering's at $100–$200 million (*Fortune,* November 1957).

°° Some of the leading Rockefeller-affiliated trustees of the 1940s and 1950s were James Murphy, president of Rockefeller Institute, Lewis Strauss (see Chapter 4), and, of course, Coombe, Howard, and Laurance S. Rockefeller, JDR II's son, who assumed top leadership of the Center in 1949. Leading Morgan-affiliated trustees included Sloan, Kettering, George Whitney, the J. P. Morgan chairman, and a number of scientists affiliated with Morgan-influenced universities such as MIT and Johns Hopkins (Lundberg, 1937:374). Some of the other corporations or institutions which were also represented on the board were Lazard Frères (through André Meyer), Kidder, Peabody (Albert H. Gordon), Amerada Petroleum (Alfred Jacobsen), Dillon, Read (Arthur B. Treman, Jr.), and IBM (Thomas J. Watson).

formerly Esso ($1.5 million), General Motors ($1.5 million), IBM ($1 million), Mobil Oil ($350,000), Texaco ($300,000), Union Carbide ($200,000), Morgan Guaranty ($175,000), and others. Chairman of the fund-raising effort was Clifton C. Garvin, Jr., chairman of Exxon (MSKCC *Center News,* June 1978).

These corporations undoubtedly regard their donations as the height of philanthropy and would probably regard any questioning of their motives as unfair. However, the study *Economic Factors in the Growth of Corporation Giving* gave three reasons why corporations donate money to charitable organizations such as MSKCC.

The first is the "immediate and certain tax savings that accompany contributions." Second, "contributions serve to create a favorable public image of the corporation." The third factor may be the most important in this case: "to encourage a social and political environment conducive to [the corporation's] survival and prosperity" (Nelson, 1970).

If we look at this last-named criterion, we can see immediately that many of the corporations which are making donations, or whose members serve as leaders of MSKCC, have been mentioned before—as corporate polluters. The oil companies in particular, whose refineries are said by some scientists to cause 30 to 40 percent of *all* cancer (see Epstein, 1978), are conspicuous supporters of the current methods of cancer management.

A review of Appendix A will also reveal that many corporations which stand to profit from the cancer field are also deeply involved in making decisions about the direction of research and treatment at Memorial Sloan-Kettering.

The enormous influence and prestige of Memorial Sloan-Kettering serves as an amplification mechanism for this group, spreading their decisions, ripple-like, to cancer treatment centers around the world.

The American Cancer Society

The American Cancer Society (ACS) is the nation's largest private fund-raising organization. In 1978 the Society brought in almost $140 million in donations and bequests, putting it ahead of its older rivals, such as the American Heart Association, the National Foundation (the March of Dimes), or the American Lung Association.

What accounts for the ACS's phenomenal success? Obviously, the ACS benefits from the importance of cancer as a public-health problem. But there is more to it than that. Heart and circulatory disease is a far greater cause of death than cancer. Yet the American

Heart Association receives far less in donations or research funds than the cancer establishment.

The most important element in the ACS's "success story" is its own skillful and sophisticated appeal to the public. "Among the numerous accomplishments of the American Cancer Society," a sympathetic student of the Society wrote some years ago, "the most profoundly important is its cultivation of cancer consciousness, a national frame of mind" (Richard Carter, 1961:139).

American awareness of cancer sometimes strikes foreign visitors as almost pathological. Hardly a day goes by without a newspaper report on cancer—usually a scary account of some new environmental chemical believed to cause the disease. One cannot listen to the radio or television for long without hearing the word "cancer." The death from malignancy of a Hubert Humphrey or a John Wayne becomes a national drama, a struggle against seemingly invincible odds which the public follows with fascinated horror. As Susan Sontag has pointed out, cancer has become one of the favorite metaphors of our language (Sontag, 1977). Often the disease seems imbued with a personality of its own, like an alien creature from a horror movie.

How did this "cancerphobia" develop? Was it a spontaneous development? Not exactly. In part, at least, as Richard Carter suggests in the above quote, it was "cultivated" by the American Cancer Society and the other opinion-shapers in the cancer field. It has proven to be an excellent fund-raising device, although "development" experts understand it must be used sparingly or it will lose its effectiveness.

The ACS was originally founded as the American Society for the Control of Cancer (ASCC) at the New York Harvard Club in 1913. John D. Rockefeller, Jr., provided funds for its founding, and most of those present at the inception were close to the Rockefeller financial group, especially the law firm of Debevoise, Plimpton.°

For several decades the ASCC was kept small and elite, a vehicle for the charitable impulses of New York's wealthiest families. Membership rarely went above two thousand. Money for the Society's activities came from the wealthy. For example, in 1921 Laura Spelman Rockefeller donated $8,000 for the Society's first movie, *The Reward of Courage*. In the late 1920s, Edward H. Harkness, a Stan-

---

° For example, Thomas M. Debevoise was secretary of the ASCC and his close friend, George C. Clark, was the first president. Mrs. Robert G. Mead, described as a "one-woman gang in civic and philanthropic work" was another prominent member. She was married to a Debevoise partner. Her father, Dr. Clement Cleveland, was a surgeon prominent in the Society (Richard Carter, 1961:144).

dard Oil heir active in medical affairs, gave $100,000. J. P. Morgan and Co. contributed $50,000, and founders were expected to donate $1,000 each (Richard Carter, 1961).

From the start, the Society was conscious of its role as a shaper of public opinion. "There is beyond question a perfectly legitimate use, even for a medical man, of the publicity man and the press agent," said a founder of the organization, Dr. Howard C. Taylor. "He is constantly used in the political world and there is no reason why we should not also use him to accomplish medical ends" (ibid.).

The main goal was to urge the general public to consult their physician at the first suspicion of cancer. "What they need," said the Society's managing director, George A. Soper, Ph.D., speaking of the public, "is to see the necessity of prompt and capable medical attention" (ibid.). But how to accomplish that goal?

"From the beginning [the Society] vacillated between a fear technique and the dissemination of hope," wrote Carter (ibid.). The reason for this vacillation is fairly obvious. If the Society spoke only of the brilliant hope for cancer patients (which was far less realistic in the 1920s than it is even today) people would not feel compelled to consult their doctors. On the other hand, if the Society only stirred up fear, they would feed the fatalism that still hangs over the word "cancer" like a pall.

Typical of the Society's early propaganda efforts was a 1919 poster which proclaimed boldly: "One Out of Every Ten Persons Over Forty Dies of Cancer." A subtitle then hit the "hope" theme: "Cancer Is Curable If Treated Early." Then the placard ended on the fear motif, by listing four ominous "Danger Signals," forerunner of the "Seven Warning Signals" of today.°

The Society's campaign raised the ire of the organized medical profession, the American Medical Association (AMA), which accused the Society of causing mass cancerphobia. Its "signs of cancer," said the Association's *Journal*, "is so small a part of the whole truth that it is better left unsaid. . . ." (ibid.).

An inherent contradiction in the Society's educational campaign was that it could urge people to consult their physicians for annual checkups or therapy, but it could not expand the medical services or pay for people to have these examinations. Because of this contradiction, in the late 1920s and 1930s the Society began to take on a populist coloring.

° "Cancer's Seven Warning Signals: 1. Change in bowel or bladder habits. 2. A sore that does not heal. 3. Unusual bleeding or discharge. 4. Thickening or lump in breast or elsewhere. 5. Indigestion or difficulty in swallowing. 6. Obvious change in wart or mole. 7. Nagging cough or hoarseness. If you have a warning signal, see your doctor" (ACS, 1978).

For example, Dr. Soper "aroused the ready hostility of organized medicine by advocating a network of free cancer clinics, to eliminate the financial barrier to prompt diagnosis" (ibid.:147).

Soper did not last long after such remarks, and in 1929 he was replaced by Clarence Cook Little, D.Sc., former president of the University of Michigan and a well-known geneticist.

Little opposed publicizing cancer among laymen and instead placed his emphasis on building up cancer treatment *as a profession.* "Superficial programs of lay publicity when adequate facilities for diagnosis, treatment, and follow-up are wanting or are scattered or uncontrolled, will be of little value," he said. Both he and Soper were confronting the same problem. But while Soper advocated the rapid extension of *free* cancer centers that could have become truly popular and effective, Little advocated increasing the number of private practitioners interested in cancer. "Nothing will scare the profession back into hiding more successfully," he said, "than a noisy lay campaign. . . ." (ibid.:151).

Even at this early date, the leaders of the Society showed signs of intransigence toward unorthodox approaches to the cancer problem. In particular, Little pursued a vigorous and at times unreasonable attack on Maud Slye, a highly innovative geneticist at the University of Chicago (McCoy, 1977).

In the mid-1930s a spin-off organization to fight cancer was formed which almost superseded the Society itself. This was the Women's Field Army, a kind of ladies' auxiliary of the Society. In retrospect it appears as if the temper and tensions of the 1930s was about to create a new type of health organization in the United States—a grassroots organization, tapping the energy of millions of Americans.

The Women's Field Army was almost paramilitary in its approach. Its volunteers wore perky brown uniforms, insignia with quasi-military rank, and made sure that suspected cancer victims "reported" to their physicians for diagnosis and treatment (Richard Carter, 1961:153).

The Field Army was enormously successful. In 1939 it raised $171,000 for impoverished patients, in 1942, $269,000, and in 1943—in the midst of a world war—$356,270. By 1944, at a time when the American Society for the Control of Cancer itself had 986 members, the Women's Field Army had over a million members and was already "one of the most important health organizations in the history of the United States" (ibid.:154). The blue-blooded Society members fretted over this development.

At the same time, orthodox medicine appeared to be losing

ideological control of the cancer field. New and innovative treatments sprang up all over the country. Harry Hoxsey, with his "Hoxide" herbal cures, was drawing thousands to mass meetings across the Midwest, where he mingled unorthodox cancer theory with populist politics. Hoxsey even had his own daily radio program (ACS, 1971b).

Looking back on this period, Frank Howard of Esso complained that "the search for new cancer treatments . . . was in danger of becoming abandoned to quacks, and to pseudo-scientific frauds in the years just before the war" (Howard, 1955).

In the early 1940s a group of wealthy individuals, deeply distressed by the situation in the cancer field, began to plan a reorganization of the ASCC. The "benevolent plotters" as they sometimes called themselves, actually took control of the Society in 1944, changed its name to the catchier American Cancer Society, and set about restructuring the organization.

One of the first things they did was to abolish the Women's Field Army and institute top-down control of all branches of the Society from its New York headquarters. Clarence Cook Little was also forced out. He eventually wound up as scientific spokesman for the tobacco lobby (Little, 1957).

Key figures among the new ACS leaders were:

• Elmer Bobst, president of the American branch of Hoffmann–La Roche and, later, of the Warner-Lambert pharmaceutical company. Bobst was basically a drug salesman, with close connections to the medical profession and to politicians, such as Richard Nixon (Bobst, 1973).

• Albert and Mary Lasker, health philanthropists and originators of the Lasker Awards, an American version of the Nobel Prize. Albert Lasker was among the most prominent advertising men of his day. Both Laskers were, at times, Memorial Sloan-Kettering trustees.

Ironically, Lasker's greatest advertising coup was for the American Tobacco Company. His slogan—"Reach for a Lucky instead of a sweet"—convinced thousands of women to start smoking in the 1930s and 1940s.

If Bobst spoke for the Society in Republican administrations, Mrs. Lasker was familiar and at ease amid the heirs of the New Deal. She was on close terms with Hubert Humphrey and Lyndon Johnson and became a familiar figure on Capitol Hill. It has been said: "She is able to produce results for congressmen and they love it. . . . Health in the abstract is a popular ideal for politicians, ranking just behind motherhood and apple pie" (*Medical Dimensions*, March 1976). Mrs. Lasker was and remains a skilled broker; she brought the congressmen who control federal funds together with prestigious medical leaders.°

As opposed to the American Society for the Control of Cancer, the American Cancer Society was dominated by laymen and lay-women. "We realized that the Board should include the businessmen who had become interested in the Society," Mrs. Lasker later said in a statement on the Society's reorganization (ACS, 1965).

Bobst and Lasker introduced the most advanced Madison Ave-nue techniques into cancer fund raising. Bobst ran it "like a business with a well-planned 'sales' campaign" (Bobst, 1973). "Dollars flooded the treasurer's office," an ACS writer recollects, "finally to-taling more than $280,000" from a single story in *Reader's Digest* (ACS, 1965).

Initially, the ACS used the fear motif rather heavily. The theme of the 1945 fund-raising campaign was "cancer kills people." It fea-tured pictures of gravestones, coffins, and a terrifying "beware of cancer" message. Bobst would begin his fund-raising speeches with a dramatic "One in five of us here—every fifth person in the audience—will die of cancer" (Bobst, 1973).

Then would come the ray of hope: "We want to cure cancer in your lifetime," and an appeal for funds. Using such techniques, the ACS was not only able to raise hundreds of millions of dollars, but to enlist over 2 million people as unpaid volunteers in its fund-raising activities. April was officially declared "Cancer Month" by the presi-dent of the United States, and spring was ushered in with a shake of the fund raiser's can.

The press has been carefully cultivated, an art which Lasker practiced in the 1920s when he used his clients' clout to influence stories or even, it is said, "to suppress . . . newspaper material hostile to [Lasker's] aims" (Lundberg, 1937).

About three decades ago, Patrick McGrady, Sr., the Society's science editor, initiated national tours of cancer laboratories for sci-ence writers. When these became too crowded, he initiated in 1958 the annual Science Writers' Seminar. Originally a chance for leading

---

° Other members of the group which took over the Society in the 1940s were Emerson Foote, an advertising associate of Albert Lasker; James Adams, a partner in the investment banking house of Lazard Frères, a director of Standard Brands, Inc., which had drug and food interests, and a former official of the Johns-Manville asbestos company; General William J. Donovan, director of the U.S. government's intelligence agency (OSS) which evolved into the Central Intelligence Agency; Howard Pew, Sun Oil executive, well-known for his espousal of ultraconservative causes; Ralph Reed, president of American Express; Harry Van Elm, presi-dent of Manufacturers Trust Co; Florence Mahoney, a personal friend of Mrs. Lasker's and a newspaper heiress; and Eric Johnston, president of the Motion Picture Association of America (Richard Carter, 1961; ACS, 1965).

science writers to meet prominent researchers in a congenial setting, McGrady believes the seminars have become a "medium of self-serving propaganda" for the ACS (cited in Chowka, 1978c). In the eyes of critic Robert Houston:

Held at holiday resorts to lure and pacify reporters, it can usually be counted on to generate a barrage of breathless copy about how a mote in a scientist's lens spells imminent victory against the dread disease. Softened up by the exalted false hopes (most of which later turn out to be cul-de-sacs, or worse, bottomless pits), the public is an easy prey for the Society's volunteer army, 2.3 million strong. This year's Seminar was booked for March 25–28 at Florida's Daytona Hilton. The strike-force hits on April 1 (Houston, 1979a). °

So successful has been this media cultivation that the Associated Press recently ran an ACS publicity piece as a ten-part "objective" news series on cancer, without acknowledgment of its origin within the Society.

Asked about the propriety of this, a top Associated Press executive replied, "I never considered the ACS to be a political organization. . . . That's just like saying that God is political" (Bloom, 1979).

The Society is a power among researchers in the United States. Approximately one-quarter of its income is spent on research. As the number of applications has increased, the Society is able to pick and choose among those research projects submitted. For example, in 1978, 1,912 scientists requested over $160 million in funds from the ACS. The Society awarded about $40 million to 639 of them. Scientists thus must be responsive to the goals and thinking of the Society if they expect to be funded in this competitive situation. Conversely, although no strings are attached to these grants, ACS's wishes can often be translated into the direction of the research (ACS, 1979).

ACS grants go out to most of the major research institutions in the country, and many around the world. Some of the biggest recipients include the University of California, with 54 projects totaling almost $3 million; Sloan-Kettering, with 25 grants totaling over $1.5 million; Yale University, which received 18 grants worth $1.3 million; and Yeshiva University in New York, which was given 17 grants worth in excess of $1 million. Cancer research laboratories in Switzerland, England, Scotland, and Israel spread the Society's influence abroad. In addition, the Society spent $375,000 in 1978 to sup-

---

° Even some very established science writers have begun to question the usefulness of the Science Writers' Seminar. Writing in the newsletter of the National Association of Science Writers, Ed Edelson of the *New York Daily News* and Jerry Bishop of the *Wall Street Journal* raised questions about the Society's motives for holding the seminar and about the value of attending (see *NASW Newsletter,* September and December 1978).

port Eleanor Roosevelt–ACS International Cancer Fellowships (ibid.).

The ACS also spends over half a million dollars to support twenty prominent scientists around the country in what is known as its Research Professorship Program, a lifetime stipend which frees these individuals to spend their full time on cancer research (ibid.).

The Society has numerous committees and holds many seminars and panels. By incorporating leading cancer specialists into these bodies, the ACS has involved the medical profession in its administrative and fund-raising apparatus, and made many of them committed to the Society's success. Many of those who have served on ACS committees have also benefited—either personally or institutionally—from the Society's largess (Chowka, 1978c).

Mary Lasker, who continues as honorary chairman of the ACS, is considered by some the "most powerful person in modern medicine" (*Medical Dimensions,* March 1976). Veteran science writer Barbara J. Culliton has called the National Cancer Act "Mrs. Lasker's War" (*Harper's,* June 1976).

The days are gone when a cancer specialist would think of opposing the leadership of his field by businessmen, bankers, and advertising men. The Society now has tens of millions of dollars to distribute to those who favor its growing power, and many powerful connections to disconcert those who oppose it.

The National Cancer Institute

In terms of dollars, the most powerful force in the cancer field is the National Cancer Institute, which has primary responsibility for funding the "war on cancer." NCI's budget in 1978 was $910 million, most of which was spent in support of scientists at various institutions.

Although NCI is larger than either Memorial Sloan-Kettering or the American Cancer Society, it is not as powerful as either. In fact, the smaller private organizations interlock with the federal giant and guide its thinking on many matters.

ACS (especially its Women's Field Army) was influential in the founding of the NCI in 1937. In the 1940s, ACS lobbied for extending the appropriations for the Institute. Senator Claude Pepper (D.-Fla.) held hearings on a bill to make "a supreme endeavor to discover the means of curing and preventing cancer" (cited in Haught, 1962).

Pepper's bill did not pass into law, but Mary Lasker and her co-workers did manage to generate a great deal of favorable publicity for cancer research. NCI's budget skyrocketed from $600,000 per year in 1946 to $92 million in 1960. It was no secret that Mary Lasker and the ACS were largely responsible for this phenomenal growth (Strickland, 1971). ACS influence within NCI grew proportionally.

"The Cancer Society and the National Cancer Institute work as partners," Dr. John R. Heller, former director of NCI, declared in 1960. "The Director of the Institute is a member of the board of directors of the Cancer Society, and the scientific advisory committees of both organizations interlock" (Richard Carter, 1961:142).

Since the early 1970s, NCI's funds have quadrupled, as a result of the "war on cancer" legislation. Passage of the National Cancer Act of 1971 appears to have increased ACS (and MSKCC) influence over the Institute.

Groundwork for the National Cancer Act was laid in the late 1960s when Senator Ralph Yarborough (D.-Tex.) established a twenty-six-person National Panel of Consultants on the Conquest of Cancer. This committee ultimately recommended the "war on cancer" to Congress.

Chairman of the panel was Benno Schmidt, leader of the Memorial Sloan-Kettering Cancer Center (see Appendix A). Vice-chairman was Dr. Sidney Farber, a former president of the American Cancer Society and a leading cancer drug researcher.

Other scientists on the panel included two other former ACS presidents (Jonathan Rhoads, M.D., and Wendell Scott, M.D.) and a prospective president, R. Lee Clark, M.D. From MSKCC came Joseph Burchenal, M.D., a chemotherapist, and Mathilde Krim, Ph.D., a researcher whose husband is prominent in Democratic party politics (*Austin American-Statesman*, April 14, 1973).

Lay members of the panel included Laurance S. Rockefeller of MSKCC; Elmer Bobst of Warner-Lambert; Emerson Foote, a Lasker associate; G. Keith Funston, chairman of the Olin chemical company; and Mrs. Anna Rosenberg Hoffman, a colleague of Mrs. Lasker's. All of these individuals, with the exception of Rockefeller, were board members of the American Cancer Society. (Olin has held the patents on a number of anticancer drugs, including one for the purification of interferon.)

In addition, there appears to have been token representation from the labor movement and the press: I. W. Abel of the United Steelworkers, and Michael O'Neill from the *New York Daily News*.

Thus, of the twenty-six panel members who framed the "war on cancer," ten were officers of the American Cancer Society and four were affiliated with Memorial Sloan-Kettering. Mrs. Lasker, who was not on the panel itself, is said to have supervised the actual writing of the panel's report (*Harper's,* June 1976).

After passage of the National Cancer Act in 1971, two special committees were set up so that the administrators of the new program could bypass some of the red tape of the National Institutes of Health, to which the National Cancer Institute belongs. These committees were the National Cancer Advisory Board (NCAB) and the elite and powerful President's Cancer Panel.

Head of the President's Cancer Panel from its inception has been Benno Schmidt, the aptly named "cancer czar" of the United States (*Science,* April 16, 1976). His two companions on the panel are chosen from the scientific community. Its first scientific members were R. Lee Clark, president of the M. D. Anderson Tumor Institute and Hospital in Houston (and ACS leader), and Robert A. Good, Ph.D., M.D., the soon-to-be-appointed head of Sloan-Kettering Institute.

The larger NCAB also shows decisive ACS–MSKCC influence. Its members include Mary Lasker, Elmer Bobst, and Laurance S. Rockefeller.

The drug industry has also exerted its influence on NCI in a number of ways.

In the past, Dr. Richard S. Schreiber, vice-chairman of the Upjohn Company, manufacturer of anticancer drugs (see Table 2), was a member of the National Advisory Cancer Council, predecessor of the NCAB. Dr. Alexander M. Moore of the Parke-Davis company was made a member of the Chemistry Panel of NCI. Dr. Andrew C. Bratton, Jr., also of Parke-Davis, was a member of the Institute's Drug Evaluation Panel, as was Dr. Karl A. Folkes of Merck Sharpe & Dohme.

Today drug-company influence appears to be more subtle, but no less real. As mentioned earlier (see Chapter 14), quite a few of the members of the NCAB are affiliated with drug companies. If they do not consciously do industry's bidding, they still probably share many of the attitudes and prejudices of their employers.

The importance of this can be seen when one considers the manner in which NCI grants are approved. A grant application submitted to NCI is first subjected to a site visit by a team of outside experts appointed by the administrators. (The reader will recall that Lawrence Burton was visited by a Sloan-Kettering chemotherapist when he applied for an NCI grant.) Not all applicants are visited— according to the NCI *Fact Book,* only about 10 percent are (NCI, 1975). An established center, such as Memorial Sloan-Kettering, is far less likely to be visited than a new applicant or one suggesting a controversial research or therapy project.

After the experts have made a visit, they assign the project a priority rating. The NCAB then considers all major grants (over $35,000). Although the final determination is made by the NCI's Division of Cancer Research Resources and Centers, it is very rare for this division to overrule the powerhouses on the NCAB.

In conclusion: the National Cancer Institute is a massively funded government bureaucracy, staffed mainly by career civil servants. Not only has its current size and structure largely been determined by outside forces, but the American Cancer Society, Memorial Sloan-Kettering, and the large drug companies appear to exercise an important influence on the Institute's direction.

The Food and Drug Administration

Like the National Cancer Institute, the Food and Drug Administration (FDA) is a government agency, staffed by civil servants and political appointees. But whereas the NCI is a source of largess to scientists, the FDA is generally a source of aggravation. The FDA's role is to prevent harmful or useless methods of treating cancer from entering the marketplace.

How well or equitably the FDA succeeds is a matter of dispute.

On August 15, 1974, eleven FDA scientists appeared before Senator Edward Kennedy's (D.-Mass.) Subcommittee on Health and Scientific Research and charged their own agency with being a virtual pawn of the industries it is supposed to control. Appearing without the foreknowledge of the FDA commissioner, the eleven, "testified before the Senate that they were harassed by agency officials—allegedly pro-industry—whenever they recommended against approval of marketing some new drug" (*Science*, June 11, 1976).

Secretary of Health, Education and Welfare Caspar Weinberger announced that he was going to hold a public investigation of the matter. Weinberger then announced that the "open inquiry" would be headed by an aide to former FDA commissioner Charles C. Edwards. The eleven FDA dissidents refused to participate in this investigation (*Science and Government Report*, April 1, 1975).

Meanwhile, FDA commissioner Alexander M. Schmidt (no relation to Benno Schmidt) spent almost $200,000 preparing a 900-page report which vindicated him and the agency of any wrongdoing. The HEW chief simultaneously appointed a "blue-ribbon panel" to investigate the FDA investigation. They countered with a $140,000,

525-page "Assessment of the Commissioner's Report of October, 1975." Dan Greenberg characterized the latter group as "a bickering lot of hairsplitting metaphysicians." If the secretary of HEW chose "to sweep them all out," he added, "it [would] be no loss to the Republic or drug safety and efficacy" (*New England Journal of Medicine,* June 24, 1976).

The net result of these reports was to cover the original charges of "the eleven" with an avalanche of verbiage. *Science* wondered aloud:

Who is running the Food and Drug Administration? The agency [,] or the drug industry it is supposed to regulate? No one knows for sure, and if the latest in an endless series of FDA investigations is any indication, no one is going to find out very soon (*Science,* June 11, 1976).

However, these metaphysical exercises hardly succeeded in killing the issue. Soon afterward, the government's General Accounting Office (GAO) issued its own report, which found widespread conflict-of-interest within the FDA. In particular, the auditing arm of Congress found that 150 FDA employees were owners of stock in twenty-seven FDA-regulated companies. In addition, 203 FDA employees simply had not filed financial disclosure statements, while several had ignored FDA requests that they divest themselves of their personal investments in drug companies (*New York Times,* January 20, 1976).

Improper and illegal stockholding is one of the ways in which the drug industry may influence policy decision making at FDA. Another is the "revolving door"—the process by which government officials are recruited by industry or sent from industrial positions into regulatory posts. For example, Surgeon General of the United States Leonard Scheele became president of Warner-Lambert's research laboratories. FDA commissioner Charles C. Edwards later became senior vice-president for research at Becton Dickinson, a medical supply company. Another former FDA commissioner, James L. Goddard, became chairman of the board of Ormont Drug & Chemical Co. The FDA's top physician, Joseph Sawdusk, later became president of Parke-Davis.

The disorganization at this vital agency has been so great as to strain credulity. Yet according to testimony offered to an HEW panel by Dr. J. Richard Crout, director of the FDA's Bureau of Drugs, the agency has been crippled by "what some people called the worst personnel in government" (cited in Pharmaceutical Manufacturers' Association, 1976). Crout then added:

There was open drunkenness by several employees which went on for months. There was intimidation internally by people. . . . [In] '72, '73 going to certain kinds of meetings was an extraordinarily peculiar kind of exercise. People, I'm talking about division directors and their staff, would engage in a kind of behavior that invited . . . insubordination—people tittering in corners, throwing spitballs; I am describing physicians, people who would . . . slouch down in a chair, not respond to questions, moan and groan with sweeping gestures, a kind of behavior I have not seen in any other institution as a grown man (cited in *New England Journal of Medicine*, May 27, 1976).

This behavior seems more characteristic of an insane asylum than of a top government agency—yet we have the uncontradicted testimony of Dr. Crout that his bureau was "full of unhappy, uprooted people"—at least in the early 1970s.

This anarchy may help explain some of the more bizarre episodes in the treatment of unorthodox cancer therapies; for example, the FDA's approval of Andrew McNaughton's request for permission to test laetrile clinically on April 27, 1970, only to revoke this permission one day later (see Chapter 8). It also throws light on a previously described episode in which Dr. Linus Pauling was invited to Washington to discuss vitamin C with the FDA commissioner only to have that invitation abruptly withdrawn shortly thereafter (see Chapter 11).

Similarly, it may explain the failure of the agency to prevent some potentially harmful drugs from entering the medical marketplace.

In 1975, for example, government investigators found that two widely prescribed drugs, Aldactone and Flagyl, produced by G. D. Searle & Co., caused cancer in test animals. Searle was then the tenth-largest drug company in the nation; its sales of these two items alone totaled $17.3 million.

How was it possible that these commonly used items, employed in the treatment of high blood pressure and trichomonas infections, respectively, had been approved for sale by the FDA? Further investigation revealed that Searle had known about the tumor-producing potential of these items but had simply given the FDA fraudulent data. For example, the company destroyed the records of mice which developed tumors, or it operated on some mice to remove their tumors, and then reported them as cancer-free in the test records.

At a hearing of Senator Kennedy's subcommittee, FDA officials presented evidence that at least three other companies similarly withheld information on their products or fed the agency false data. These three were Ciba-Geigy, Ayerst Laboratories, and Lederle Laboratories. In these cases the FDA began an investigation, which could have ended in criminal prosecution or at least strong administrative sanctions against the companies. These investigations simply disappeared. "The cases somehow went into some mysterious bottomless pit that we have not been able to identify," FDA commissioner Alexander M. Schmidt told the senators (*New York Times*, July 10, 1976).

At the same time, the FDA bureaucracy has slowed the number of new drugs being introduced in the United States. In 1962 it cost an average of $1.2 million to develop a new drug in the United States (Walter S. Ross, 1973). By 1976, according to the Pharmaceutical Manufacturers' Association (PMA), it cost $11.5 million (*Nature*, March 11, 1976). By 1979 some business analysts claimed that it cost $50 million to develop a new drug (Standard and Poor's, 1979). The paperwork has increased proportionally. In 1948 Parke-Davis had to submit 73 pages of evidence to secure the licensing of a new drug. Twenty years later, it had to submit 72,200 pages of data in support of an anesthetic application. The documents had to be moved to the FDA by van (Ross, 1973).

While these hurdles apply equally to both big and small companies, it is obvious that the big companies are able to overcome them with greater ease. In fact, the entire bureaucratic maze at FDA greatly favors the largest companies, which are represented by the powerful Washington-based lobby, the Pharmaceutical Manufacturers' Association.

George Schwartz, a spokesman for the smaller drug companies, explained the situation succinctly: "These regulations favor companies with greater financial strength. They're eliminating competition" (*Business Week*, January 17, 1977). *Fortune* has called the FDA the drug industry's "unwitting ally" (*Fortune*, March 1976). Some critics would say it is not so unwitting.

The existence of a bureaucratic maze at FDA is consonant with the interests of the biggest food and drug manufacturers. The influence of these companies appears to be deep and to be exercised in many diverse ways. This may explain the agency's generally poor record in controlling environmental carcinogens, when their source is big business (see Chapter 14).

It may also explain some of the agency's intransigent hostility to unorthodox approaches to cancer, or even to innovations made within established cancer centers. Such innovators, mavericks, or small companies are the antitheses of the large firms which dominate the agency. Often there is a financial conflict between the plans of the small fry and the giant companies.

The principal role of the FDA in the cancer field has been to stifle such innovators by denying their investigative new drug applications (INDs), and harassing them when they attempt to depart from orthodox practice. In 1976 Dr. Crout told the agency's Oncology Drugs Advisory Committee, "The fact of life is, we get INDs. . . . These come from a variety of places, not just NCI or the top research institutions. For some places you want harsh regulations backed by the full weight of the law—[we] have had INDs for laetril[e], for example, and other hoax remedies. . . . Sometimes we say it is proper to hinder research" *(Cancer Letter,* March 12, 1976). At the same time, the FDA has approved over two dozen requests to market anticancer drugs from the largest companies, which have the greatest financial weight, influence at the agency, and support of other sections of the cancer establishment.

Conclusion: The Cancer Establishment

Is there really a cancer establishment? The term "establishment" was first used to describe the Church of England, and later the entire English upper class. If we understand the "cancer establishment" to mean some formally organized body, such as the hierarchy of a church, then clearly there is no such organization.

Nevertheless, the leaders of the top organizations discussed in this book are certainly familiar with each other and interlock on many committees, panels, and boards. Sometimes they are friendly, and sometimes they disagree. What holds them together, however, is a community of interests and ideas. The top leaders generally see eye-to-eye on the major questions concerning cancer. They favor cure over prevention. They emphasize the use of patentable and/or synthetic chemicals over readily available or natural methods. They set the trends in research, and are careful to stay within the bounds of what is acceptable and fashionable at the moment. They are also, generally speaking, socially homogeneous—older white males predominate here.°

A union-sponsored study of the oil industry discovered a similar establishment, that is

a structured pattern based on concentration of control, interlocking directorates, financial services, joint ventures, professional conformity, reciprocal

---

° The existence of a "cancer establishment" does not preclude the possibility of conflicts among its constituent parts. In 1976 the FDA refused to allow NCI to distribute experimental drugs to cancer centers for the treatment of terminal cancer patients *(Cancer Letter,* January 30, 1976). The FDA cited the Flagyl–Aldactone scandal as its rationale for doing so (ibid.). The following year, it refused to allow cancer centers to *combine* approved drugs for therapy, a situation which "could put us back in the Dark Ages," according to an MSKCC official *(Staten Island Advance,* January 19, 1977). The ACS has asked Congress to remove control over the testing of new anticancer drugs from the FDA to NCI (ibid.).

favors, commonality of interests . . . long-term friendships and, at its worst, greed and arrogance (Medvin, 1974).

Not everyone accepts the existence of such an establishment. Dr. Robert C. Eyerly, chairman of the Committee on Unproven Methods of Cancer Management of the American Cancer Society, ridicules this view:

We, the "medical monopoly," the "cancer establishment," are purportedly involved in the "cover-up" and "suppression" of material. . . . In this time of public suspicion, such accusations are unfortunately given attention. It is difficult to respond to such an irrational statement (Eyerly, 1976).

On the other hand, certain representatives of the far right, who tend to see conspiracy in many areas of American life, have claimed that there is a conscious conspiracy to suppress laetrile. At the July 1977 hearings of the Subcommittee on Health and Scientific Research, Senator Edward Kennedy asked Dr. John Richardson, a laetrile-using physician, "Do you really think there is a conspiracy?" Richardson answered:

Well, I've thought so for quite some time, Senator Kennedy. And it was always a ludicrous thought that while I was trying to tell people about a conspiracy, that I was caught up in a conspiracy indictment [to import laetrile] myself.

But I definitely feel that there is; yes. Conspiracy is not unusual in any time in history, and particularly in this time. And it may be unwitting on the part of many people (U.S. Senate, 1977).

"Who is involved in the conspiracy?" Kennedy asked, obviously sensing a weak spot. Richardson went on to name various organizations interested in the cancer field: the American Cancer Society, the Food and Drug Administration, the American Medical Association, and Sloan-Kettering Institute. The only major group which Richardson explicitly exempted from this conspiracy was Congress, to which, as he pointed out, his friend (and fellow John Birch Society member) Larry McDonald (D.-Ga.) belongs (ibid.).

In *World Without Cancer*, a two-volume work which Richardson cited in support of his position, G. Edward Griffin speaks of a "malicious conspiracy hiding behind the smiling mask of humanitarianism" and a "conscious direction behind the opposition to laetrile" (Griffin, 1975:501–02).

The dictionary defines "conspiracy" as a planning or acting together secretly for an unlawful or harmful purpose. Not only is there no hard evidence that such a conspiracy to suppress a known cure for cancer exists, but such a theory defies logic as well.

A conspiracy theory must take into account the fact that the leaders of the cancer establishment themselves die of cancer. Many prominent cancer scientists, administrators, and politicians have died of the disease, as have many wealthy people associated with the establishment, including members of the Rockefeller family. Did someone fail to tell them about the suppressed cure?

In addition, it is apparent that the cancer establishment, while hindering the development of unorthodox approaches to cancer, is strenuously attempting to develop the orthodox approaches. For example, $2 million was recently poured into clinical trials of interferon. An orthodox cure for cancer would be "worth a fortune," as a drug company executive has said (see Chapter 5).

The important point is that the suppression of unorthodox methods—and the promotion of the orthodox approach—takes place mainly at an objective, unconscious level. It is an outgrowth of underlying economic and social trends rather than of conscious design. This may explain the opposition of members of the establishment itself (such as Dr. Eyerly) to this explanation, since they swim in the sea of this establishment, and are rarely conscious of its pressure all around them. On the other hand, representatives of the far right may prefer a simple conspiracy theory since this targets only a few "malicious" people and spares the system itself from any fundamental criticism.

Yet the evidence points to the fact that it is the system itself, rather than any particular clique of individuals, which is really to blame for failure to make progress against the cancer problem. In particular, the fact that cancer management is itself a big business means that it must function according to the rules of profit-oriented institutions.

17

Cancer and the Suppression of Science

American business seems to be unreservedly in favor of science. Most American industries are founded upon great technological innovations, and could not function without a constant input of ideas by scientists and technicians. Especially since the end of World War II, American industry has spent billions of dollars on research and development.

It seems contradictory, and downright perverse, to say that American business *suppresses* scientific development, and that because of this an industry-led effort to find a cure for cancer has little chance of success. Yet there is another side to American science, which is little known but has great relevance to the current impasse in cancer management.

The purpose of research from the point of view of business is, and always has been, to facilitate profit making. The first capitalists to sponsor medical research—John D. Rockefeller and his colleagues—were conscious of the monetary value of science. The modern executive, although perhaps more subtle in his approach, is still aware that profit is the bottom line in all research endeavors. Science can do wonders for a corporation's balance sheet, as the histories of the aerospace, electronics, or plastics industries show. But perceptive businessmen are also aware that uncontrolled, unbridled, and unrestricted research has the potential to *destroy* industry.

"Bankers regard research as most dangerous and a thing that makes banking hazardous due to the rapid changes it brings about in industry," wrote no less an authority than Charles Kettering, cofounder of Sloan-Kettering Institute (quoted in Bernal, 1967).

Justice Louis Brandeis pointed out in the early part of this century that the gas companies tried to suppress the electric light, Western Union fought against the telephone, and then both Western

Union and the telephone companies opposed the coming of radio (ibid.).

Many other instances, can—and have—been given. A government study made in 1937 concluded that "a banker who finances a new development that will destroy his present investments is asleep at the switch" (National Resources Committee, 1937).

Some of the factors leading to the suppression of science by business, according to Dr. S. Lilley, include

the permanent difficulty that manufacturers found from the late nineteenth century on in selling their products, chronic unemployment, and the formation of cartels and monopolies . . . which act by restricting production; but that means less incentive to install the latest type of machinery, which in turn implies less encouragement to invent yet better. Sometimes they go further and actively discourage new invention (Lilley, 1965).

How can industry "actively discourage new invention"? According to the well-known British chemist J. D. Bernal, "the process can take two forms. The stifling of existing invention and the choking of new invention by restricting research" (Bernal, 1967). Obviously it is easier and neater to stop an unwanted scientific development by refusing to fund it adequately than it is to destroy it once it has taken root.

Research into the chemical causation of cancer, for example, has been suppressed more frequently by the simple expedient of not sponsoring research into this controversial topic. It is only in rare instances, as in Searle's experiments with Flagyl (see Chapter 16), that outright stifling of scientific results is employed.

David E. Lilienthal, first head of the Tennessee Valley Authority and later an atomic energy commissioner, explained how the growth of giant corporations facilitated this sort of suppression:

The most effective way to "suppress" new inventions or technical ideas is simply not to develop them. Only large enterprises are able to sink the formidable sums of money required to develop basic new departures; a small corporation is rarely able to risk those large sums, perhaps enough to wreck the company if the gamble fails, on the success or failure of a major new project (Lilienthal, 1953:69).

In the 1930s, when social and economic problems were sharpened, this question of technological suppression received a considerable amount of attention. Some of the best research on it was done by special U.S. government commissions. Even a big businessman of those times admitted:

I have even seen the lines of progress that were most promising for public benefit wholly neglected or positively forbidden just because they might revolutionize the industry. We have no right to expect a corporation to cut its own throat (quoted in Bernal, 1967).

After World War II, however, little more was said in public about the suppression of science. The very idea had become—in the words of the *Wall Street Journal*—an "old canard" (March 4, 1976).

This change in attitude and perception was due to a number of factors. First, the period immediately following the war was one of economic growth and expansion. Many new products were marketed, and others, which had been held back by the Depression and the war (television and inexpensive aluminum, to name only two), were made available to the general public. Government action, in some cases, had broken scientific logjams. For example, by breaking up the Standard Oil–I. G. Farben cartel and seizing foreign patents, the government was able to wrest the secrets of artificial rubber production from the monopolies (DuBois, 1952).

In recent years, with growing economic problems, and with a more open attitude in general on social ideas, there has been increasing attention paid to the problem of suppression.

According to "The Breakdown of U.S. Innovation," an informative article in *Business Week* several years ago, American industry now favors "a super-cautious, no-risk management less willing to gamble on anything short of a sure thing" *(Business Week,* February 16, 1976).

"In the long march of American technology, innovation has become a giant killer," the article noted.

By attaching a diesel engine to a generator on an electric locomotive, General Motors Corp. all but murdered the steam engine and derailed many of the old, traditional names in locomotive manufacturing. . . . In the same way, the telephone tore up the telegram, the trolley car fell victim to the automobile, and passenger trains yielded to buses and planes (ibid.).

The tiny transistor "shook the $45 billion electronics industry to its foundations" and wiped out many old, established businesses. The goal of corporate directors, *Business Week* continued, is "to get the risks of innovation under even tighter control."

"The main thing a fellow in my position can do is turn things off," an executive vice-president for research and development of a large corporation admitted. "The curse of R&D is letting things go on too long." Another executive complained, "We constantly run into the attitude of 'let somebody else go first' even for processes proven overseas" (ibid.). Since the reworking of an old idea has *a ten times greater chance* of financial success than a really new idea, according to prominent management consultants, really new ideas are either not funded, are dropped in the development stage, or are actively stifled (ibid.).

Although the news hasn't yet reached the popular media, the business and science press in the past few years have carried a number of similar stories such as "The Silent Crisis in R&D" *(Business Week,* March 8, 1976), "The State of American Science—A Touch of Anemia" *(New England Journal of Medicine,* March 25, 1976), and "Innovative Research Is Taking Back Seat as Chemical Firms Weigh Costs, Profits" *(Wall Street Journal,* June 2, 1976).

But what does this have to do with cancer research?

We tend to think of cancer researchers as inhabiting a different, more ethereal and idealistic world from the grubby world of Wall Street or the practical sphere of industrial research. In some senses they do, but it is clear that the ultimate power in the cancer field rests with the same gentlemen who run the major banks and corporations.

As a consumer of corporate goods and services, a repository of invested funds, and a producer of one of America's largest service industries—health care—the cancer world is in every sense part of the industrial structure. It is business, and therefore can be expected to operate under the same rules as the rest of business.

Cancer drugs are subject to the same criteria of profitability as other commodities. Given the integration of the cancer field into the corporate and banking establishments, it could not be otherwise. Depending on its nature, a new drug can be an economic boon or it can be a "giant killer."

As indicated previously, one critical question is patentability. Most of the currently available anticancer drugs are or have been patented. Others are monopolized in some other way. All of them are manufactured by the major pharmaceutical firms (see Table 2 in Chapter 5). The authoritative Standard and Poor's *Industry Survey* on pharmaceuticals makes this criterion quite clear:

The key to profitability in the [drug] industry lies in the development of patent-protected new drug products, an established marketing force, and a diverse position in the world markets.

Patent expirations will bring pressures on margins over the next few years, thus accentuating the need for patented new drugs (Standard and Poor's, 1977).

Any common off-the-shelf chemical is thus unacceptable from an economic point of view, since it offers no possibility of patent protection. Anyone with a pill-making machine could market such a substance. Hydrazine sulfate, vitamin C, and vitamin A all fall into this category. Some money can be made from marketing them, but hardly the kind of high profits customary (and the companies would say necessary) in the drug industry.°

One critic has put the situation succinctly:

The production of nonpatented drugs will give only moderate profits while the production of patented drugs will give abnormally high profits. Drug manufacturers have attempted, therefore, by every conceivable means to divert the market into the sale of high-profit patented drugs (Medical Committee for Human Rights, 1972).

Other substances mentioned in this book appear to be similarly handicapped. No patents now apply to the manufacture of laetrile, for instance, and this chemical is currently being extracted from apricot kernels and bitter almonds in small foreign factories. Since laetrile occurs naturally in approximately 1,200 different plants, it would be impossible for anyone to corner the market on laetrile-containing substances.

This seems to be contradicted by the high cost of laetrile on the current market. It has been said, for example, that a $1.25 laetrile pill costs only 2 cents to manufacture and that the rest constitutes exorbitant profits for the laetrile profiteers (Schultz and Lindeman, 1973). While the charge of profiteering may have some merit, the exorbitant price seems to be a function of government harassment. Illegal or semilegal drugs are always expensive. Thus, decriminalization of laetrile would probably bring the price down dramatically. Vitamin B-15 (pangamic acid), also pioneered by Ernst T. Krebs, Jr., is a legal substance and is currently priced at between 3 and 5 cents for a 100-milligram pill on the open market. The reason for this small markup is that vitamin B-15, like laetrile, is an unpatentable product derived from fruit kernels. Since laetrile still cannot be freely manufactured and shipped in the United States, it seems likely that laetrile will continue to be priced far above its actual value for some time to come.

Without entering into a discussion of other noncancer controversies, it is worth noting that similar disputes have broken out in other fields of medicine. For example, proponents of the use of dimethyl sulfoxide (DMSO) in a wide variety of ailments have claimed that it, too, has been held back by its very cheapness (McGrady, Sr., 1973). Lithium chloride, a treatment for manic-depressives, was not accepted for several decades. According to a recent book on this topic,

° The drug companies claim to have extraordinarily high research and development costs and thus to need extraordinarily high profits. For a critique of this argument see Klass, 1975.

lithium, being a natural element, could not be patented, and the American pharmaceutical industry thus could not see any commercial potential in the drug, unlike most other psychopharmaceuticals (Fieve, 1976).

The pattern in these and other such controversies is often remarkably similar to those in the cancer field, and may stem from the same underlying economic and social causes.

In some instances, an unorthodox method is patented, or can become so, but the rights and know-how are in the hands of uncooperative or independent entrepreneurs, who refuse to share their find with the dominant firms. This was a major charge in the Krebiozen affair (Bailey, 1958). Some aspects of Livingston's work have been patented, and Burton has taken out patents on his procedures.

Is there a conscious conspiracy by the "drug cartel" against unpatentable methods? Again, it is not necessary to postulate such a conspiracy in order to explain the suppression of cheap and readily available alternatives.

Leaving aside the fact that complicated chemicals are often more intriguing to scientists than simple ones, all researchers need money to carry out their work. Most of the funds for cancer research come from the National Cancer Institute or the American Cancer Society. But, as Laurance Rockefeller and Lewis Thomas, M.D., wrote in the 1977 MSKCC *Annual Report:*

there is an increasing tendency, understandable enough at a time of so much competition for a diminishing pool of federal funds, that favors the award of grant support to "safe and sound" research programs. This means that it will henceforth be much more difficult to obtain support for scientific "gambles" (MSKCC, 1977a).

Since, as they say, "major advances have been made, almost without exception, by what seemed at the time to be gambling on unlikely hypotheses," the provision of "venture capital" or "seed money" takes on a critical importance (ibid.).

Who else, besides the ACS or the NCI, provides the money to start a research project on a new compound, or a new avenue of attack on the cancer problem? Some may come from individual philanthropists, such as Laurance Rockefeller himself. But the Rockefeller Brothers Fund, which he chairs, is currently in the process of phasing out its support of Memorial Sloan-Kettering and other recipient institutions. This support is slated to end on December 31, 1986 (*New York Times*, May 27, 1979).

Thus, to an increasing degree, this crucial "seed money" is provided either by foundations associated with profit-making businesses, or directly by the drug companies.

This support can take many forms.

In 1975, for example, the giant chemical company Monsanto gave $23 million to Harvard University Medical School to support the work of various scientists, including some working on cancer (*Harvard University Gazette,* February 7, 1975).

Bristol-Myers has a $2.5 million grant program with five cancer research centers—at Baylor, Chicago, Johns Hopkins, Stanford, and Yale universities. The grants reputedly go for "unrestricted, innovative cancer research." In turn, grant recipients from these institutions give out the annual Bristol-Myers Award for Distinguished Achievement in Cancer Research, a $25,000 cash prize (*Immunology Tribune,* April 30, 1979).

To an outsider, this appears to be money well spent, even if it does not directly result in marketable commodities for Bristol-Myers. The company buys goodwill, displays its earnest interest in the cancer problem, and makes invaluable contacts with leading scientists.

Sometimes, the "seed money" is targeted toward a specific goal. Pharmaceutical companies routinely make what are called "restricted" contributions to medical centers, whose research goals are carefully pinpointed in advance. This is an ongoing practice: in May 1977, for example, Ortho Pharmaceutical Corp. gave Sloan-Kettering $25,000 in a restricted contribution, Burroughs Wellcome gave $15,000, and American Hoechst Corp., Pennwalt, and Eli Lilly donated smaller amounts. In the next month, Newport Pharmaceuticals International gave $19,804.95, Sandoz, a Swiss drug company, gave two gifts totaling $1,500, and Hoffmann–La Roche, Ives Lab, and E. R. Squibb & Sons all made smaller donations (MSKCC, 1977b).

The Sloan-Kettering documents do not state the purpose of these grants. It is a fair assumption that many go to further research projects in which these companies have a proprietary interest. Newport Pharmaceuticals International, for example, manufactures antiviral compounds which it has patented and "developed jointly with Sloan-Kettering" (*Wall Street Journal,* September 19, 1978).

Should a researcher want to investigate the anticancer potential of a readily available, nonpatentable, unprofitable compound, he will find great difficulty in getting such a project started, or in continuing it once it has begun. Thus the invisible hand of the marketplace is quite sufficient to prevent the development of many innovative research projects.

In addition, we must consider the so-called human factors which certainly play a real—although secondary—role in the suppression of new cancer therapies. A Columbia University sociologist found that "the mere assertion that scientists themselves sometimes resist scientific discovery clashes, of course, with the stereotype of the scientist as 'the open-minded man' " (Barber, 1961). Nevertheless, it is a fact.

From the earliest times, innovative scientists have faced opposition simply because their ideas have been daring and new. To chronicle all the scientists who have been unfairly opposed would require writing a history of science.

Sometimes the innovator has trampled on preexisting dogmas, religious or scientific. Anaxagoras was expelled from "enlightened" Athens in the middle of the fifth century B.C. because he maintained that the sun was a red-hot disc of stone and not a god (Farrington, 1965:74).

The discoverer of antiseptics, Ignaz Semmelweis, was expelled from his hospital position in Vienna because he dared to urge doctors to wash their hands before delivering babies. Lister, who had greater success in promoting similar ideas, later spoke of the blindness to new ideas in science which he also encountered (ibid.). Even ideas which in retrospect appear to have been readily accepted sometimes faced short but fierce seasons of opposition. Lord Kelvin regarded the announcement of Roentgen's discovery of X rays as a hoax (ibid.). Einstein faced hostile opposition to his theory of relativity. According to physicist A. M. Taylor, "Indeed, physicists were sharply divided into two camps, one enthusiastically supporting the theory, the other bitterly critical" (A. M. Taylor, 1970:32).

Almost without exception, innovators in medicine have faced opposition. The strength of the opposition often appears to be proportional to the freshness of their ideas. This does *not* prove that their ideas are correct. Orthodox science will also oppose incorrect, absurd, or harmful ideas—and there is no way to know, without a thorough investigation, whether a new concept is being opposed because it is threatening to the status quo or because it is dangerous and absurd.

The history of science does prove that a new concept should not automatically be rejected simply because it is attacked by the experts. Sometimes an attack or controversy is merely the birth cry of a great idea.

Right or wrong, the innovators in this book are all proposing concepts and methods which are at variance with current beliefs. For instance, it is not generally believed that cancer is a deficiency disease, and this idea is supposed to have been refuted in the 1940s. In fact, such commonly used drugs as methotrexate are literally *anti*vitamins (Shimkin, 1977:405).

Because the medical profession in general does not believe that cancer is caused by a lack of nutrients, one could predict serious difficulty for therapies such as laetrile, vitamin C, vitamin A, or abscisic acid which claim to restore some lost nutritional element.

Similarly, it is a dogma that cancer is not caused by a microbe. This, supposedly, was disproven many years ago. The fact that a scientist like Virginia Livingston claims to have new evidence makes little impression on doctors who were educated to believe that this is a passé theory.

Chemotherapy, after struggles of its own, has now been accepted as a third modality in cancer therapy. But it is generally believed that chemotherapy must be toxic in order to work. Specifically, it must interfere with the metabolism or replication of cells and kill them by direct poisoning. Gold's hydrazine sulfate, however, is relatively nontoxic, and appears to work in a different manner—by interrupting gluconeogenesis. This idea appears to be too new to gain ready acceptance by many oncologists.

It sometimes takes many years for the establishment to acknowledge that a pioneer was right and that it was wrong. Usually, all the contestants in the battle have passed away before that happens. Coley was generally ignored, and his method was cited in the ACS Unproven Methods list. Later Coley was hailed as a "cancer-immunology pioneer" (New York Times Magazine, April 2, 1978) and his name was quietly removed from the ACS list, even if his promising therapy is still not being used (see Chapter 7).

Coley did not know why the toxins had the effects he saw. In the intervening seventy-five years orthodox scientists discovered, by a circuitous route, that immune-stimulating products could indeed have a beneficial effect on some animal tumors. Coley's empirical observations were thus given what appears to be scientific justification.

Mainstream science may similarly find a new justification for Burton's vaccine in "normal human globulin," or for laetrile in the "synthetic mandelonitriles" supposedly being tested at Sloan-Kettering (Chowka, 1979).

New methods can also be suppressed through the normal day-to-day functioning of the funding mechanisms. Most of the research funds in the United States come from the federal government, specifically from the National Cancer Institute. The government might appear to be an ideal source of funds for an innovator; it does not have to satisfy stockholders with the profitability of a research venture.

In some instances, in fact, the government has sponsored cancer projects that would not be funded by drug companies. The National

Cancer Institute, for example, put up the money to gain FDA approval of the Italian anticancer agent Adriamycin (Applezweig, 1978). It did so at a time when no American drug company was willing to invest in this effective but highly toxic product (see Chapter 5). In other cases, NCI has undertaken in-house research into rather unusual compounds, such as maytansine, an agent derived from an African plant *(Science,* September 19, 1975).

In general, however, it is very difficult for new ideas to survive the funding mechanism. For one thing, for years NCI spent only about half of its appropriation on grants to outside researchers. The remainder went to contracts whose topics had been chosen at NCI itself, or to in-house research (NCI, 1975).

For a grant to be approved it has to follow a complicated maze laid down by the National Cancer Act of 1971 (see Figure 3). This involves assignment to an institute by a National Institutes of Health division; review and evaluation by members of the Initial Review Group; a site visit from scientists chosen by NIH administrators; a meeting of the review group to vote and assign the project a priority number; consideration of the application by the NCAB, with its recommendations; a funding determination by the Division of Cancer Research Resources and Centers of NCI; and negotiations and final review (NCI, 1975).

All along the line, bureaucrats and outside advisers of the agency are called upon to pass judgment upon the application, and a strong negative opinion at several important junctures can severely damage the chances of success. To win a grant, an applicant must please the "experts" in his field, and almost by definition must be working within the accepted definitions of that field.

To a certain degree, each person who approves an application has put his own reputation on the line in doing so. The safest and most politic thing to do is to give priority to those applications coming from the more conventional and established researchers at well-known institutions. As a sign of the faith placed in them by NCI, such institutions receive site visits less frequently. Should anything go wrong, the grant giver can justify his decision by the prestige of the recipient institution and the high probability of success.

To approve the grant application of a small research center (such as the Syracuse Cancer Research Institute or the Immunology Researching Centre) is a difficult and dangerous undertaking for any bureaucrat or adviser. It is fraught with peril; if the project becomes an embarrassment, there inevitably will be inquiries to find out who approved the application in the first place.

A new grant request must therefore be approved by a wide variety of scientists, bureaucrats, and businessmen. It must be the result

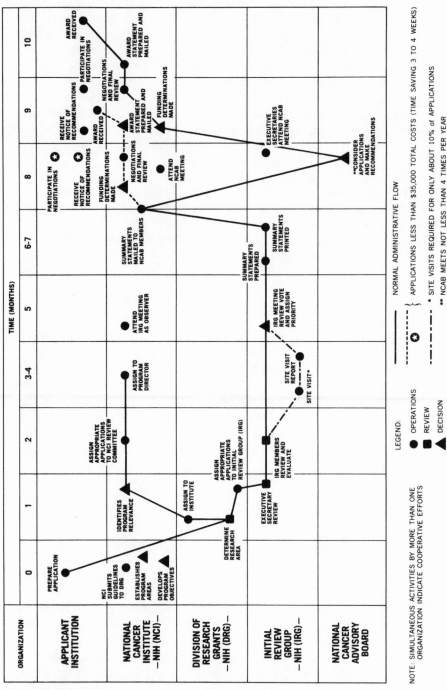

Source: 1975 NCI Fact Book

of a *consensus* of opinion among these many individuals. Almost by definition, however, such an application must be well within the bounds of conventional science. These "cumbersome constraints" make it difficult, if not impossible for radically new ideas to be approved by the NCI.[*]

Another factor which leads to the suppression of many new ideas is the mentality of those who lead the cancer establishment. These are powerful individuals, with long lists of achievements and publications. Some of them flatfootedly and categorically lay down the law in their particular field and do not appreciate being contradicted. Some also dream of Nobel Prizes or even of being immortalized for finding a cure for mankind's most dreaded disease. "Dusty" Rhoads was "absolutely determined that the cure for cancer was going to be found in his institute and nowhere else," reporter Bernard Glemser wrote admiringly. Those around Rhoads fed his ego. When the reporter suggested a book about Sloan-Kettering in general, an aide took him aside and said, "You don't want to write a book about all this. Do a book about the director. *He's* what counts here" (Glemser, 1969:35).

Robert A. Good, the current director of Sloan-Kettering, has been called "a scientific Sammy Glick who occasionally lets his ego get in the way of his intellect. . . ." (*Time*, March 19, 1973).

Time's reporter comments:

> Good, who often acts as if he is running for the Nobel Prize, does not deny their charges. "Of course, I'm an operator," he admits. "I'm the most self-centered person in the world. I'll use whatever there is to get things done the way I want them done. I hope I can become an effective operator when it comes to cancer" (ibid.:69).

Livingston attributed Rhoads's long-term opposition to her work to the fact that she was an "upstart" in the cancer field. Hostility to "upstarts" can apply not only to complete unknowns but also to well-known scientists who wander into someone else's preserve.

For example, Linus Pauling was not greeted with open arms by the medical establishment when he put forward his theories on vitamin C. Dr. H. L. Newbold was asked why he thought Pauling was repeatedly turned down by the National Cancer Institute:

> They're jealous of him because he's too famous. Things are done through personalities. You think of scientists as being objective, but science is full of little men doing their own little things. This is true of people who grant research funds (Newbold, 1979).

---

[*] The phrase "cumbersome constraints" is from the 1978 report of Lane W. Adams, executive vice-president of the ACS. In November 1978 the ACS voted to decline future federal aid in order to maintain its independence of the government bureaucracy (ACS, 1978:3).

Another factor promoting closed-mindedness toward new ideas is social prejudice. For example, many of geneticist Maud Slye's problems in the 1920s and 1930s appear to have been related to the fact that she was a woman—and a single woman at that—almost fanatically devoted to her work.

Even scientists who were supposed to be objective were prejudiced when it came to women in the scientific establishment. A number of them were quick to dismiss the work and findings of the few women scientists who were able to get their research published in the medical and scientific journals (McCoy, 1977).

Although discrimination in science today is not nearly as prevalent as it was in the 1920s, women are still not fully integrated into the cancer establishment.° One wonders how much of the resistance to the bacterial theory is due to the fact that many of its advocates in this country have been women? °°

Predictably, spokesmen for the cancer establishment deny that the suppression of new ideas even takes place. "As a result of the medical profession's insistence upon reliable standards of proof of cure," according to the American Cancer Society's book *Unproven Methods,* "the proponents of unproven remedies are prone to charge that they are being persecuted by the 'medical trust' or 'organized medicine' " (ACS, 1971b:18).

"A look at two of many well-known facts will serve to answer this charge," the ACS book states, and goes on to cite two of the triumphs of modern medicine: the discovery of penicillin and the polio vaccine. According to the Society,

when Sir Alexander Fleming discovered penicillin, all that was demanded was that the new "medicine" measure up to rigid scientific and clinical tests, to determine its efficacy and its adverse effects, if any. The tests were met. Penicillin was adopted for medical use, and today is widely accepted as one of the most important means of treating infection (ibid.).

The example is poorly chosen, from the point of view of orthodox medicine, for Fleming's discovery was ridiculed and ignored for over a dozen years after his initial publication in 1928. Typical was the reaction of a distinguished colleague of the Scottish bacteriologist, who wrote in 1929:

° As of 1978 at Memorial Sloan-Kettering Cancer Center no woman held a major administrative post. The Committee on Scientific Policy was all male, the board of overseers was four-fifths male, less than 10 percent of the medical board was female, and only five out of forty-nine members of Sloan-Kettering Institute were women (MSKCC, 1978).

°° Virginia Livingston-Wheeler, Eleanor Alexander-Jackson, Irene Cory Diller, Eva Bordkin, and Camille Mermod.

The penicillium moulds are pleasant enough and we are content to use them to bring our Camembert and Roquefort cheeses into a pleasant condition of ripeness, and in that respect I would not like to miss them. But beyond that, and especially with a view to therapy in medicine, these moulds are completely useless (Böttcher, 1964).

It was only with the approach of World War II, when huge casualties loomed and the Allies faced the loss of German sulfa drugs, that some British scientists began a campaign to develop penicillin commercially (Bäumler, 1968). Two British scientists were brought to the United States in 1941, under the auspices of the Office of Scientific Research and Development (OSRD), to try to get private pharmaceutical companies interested in working on the project. "They had almost no luck," Richard Harris wrote in *The Real Voice*, summarizing the results of an investigation by Senator Estes Kefauver's staff (Richard Harris, 1964).

A few weeks after the Japanese attacked Pearl Harbor, Dr. Vannevar Bush, director of OSRD, personally brought a number of drug companies into the research effort. A year and a half later, he wrote:

Now, the pharmaceutical companies have cooperated in this affair after a fashion. They have not made their experimental results and their development of manufacturing processes generally available, however (cited in ibid.).

The problem, Harris remarks, "was that most firms were too busy trying to corner patents on various processes in the production of penicillin to produce much of it. . . ." (ibid.). On January 19, 1944, the coordinator of the penicillin program of the War Production Board wrote that he could not "with a clear conscience assume the responsibility for coordinating this program," because of the refusal of the drug companies to exchange information, a refusal which was costing thousands of lives on the battlefield.

The deadlock was broken only when an obscure outpost of a government agency, the Department of Agriculture's laboratory in Peoria, Illinois, figured out how to mass-produce penicillin, took out a patent on the method and then made "all of its patents . . . available to any producer without charge" (ibid.).

Even so, the drug companies never showed much enthusiasm for penicillin. "The synthesis of penicillin brought laurels to the scientists," wrote *Fortune* (March 1976), "but precious little else." For this reason, John McKeen, the president of Pfizer, said in 1950, "if you want to lose your shirt in a hurry, start making penicillin and streptomycin" (quoted in Rozental, 1961). Economics professor Alek A. Rozental commented further:

Pfizer announced that it would henceforth concentrate on the development of new and exclusive antibiotic specialties. Other firms had the same idea. Today the few that control production of the broad-spectrum antibiotics (Achromycin, Terramycin, Aureomycin, and tetracyclines) have managed to avoid repetition of the "unhappy" penicillin experience (ibid.).

The ACS's second "well-known fact" concerns the polio vaccine:

When Dr. Salk discovered his polio vaccine, again it was only required that he provide clear proof that his vaccine was safe and effective. He did so under the most rigid rules, and the result was that the Salk vaccine shots became an accepted prophylactic measure against poliomyelitis (ACS, 1971b:18).

The Salk vaccine is certainly a triumph of modern medicine. But it is simply not true that it was required only that Salk prove his vaccine safe and effective for it to be automatically snapped up by the medical profession or the pharmaceutical industry.

The vaccine was the result of efforts by the National Foundation, whose relations with the medical profession were often strained. Salk's intention of making a *killed* virus vaccine instead of a live one made him something of a maverick within the establishment. When the National Foundation announced the development of Salk's vaccine, the American Medical Association responded:

Whereas . . . the American medical profession was surprised and put in a difficult situation, so far as public relations were concerned in recent months, when a national health organization, without any official consultation with any qualified council or group of the American Medical Association, launched a nationwide comprehensive program for the use of a new vaccine which gives great theoretical promise of success in combatting a dread disease and yet which admittedly had been used a few months without sufficient time to evaluate the safety as well as the efficacy of the vaccine. . . . (cited in Wayne Martin, 1977:63).

When in May 1955 Cutter Laboratories sold batches of vaccine which accidentally included some live virus, and 204 cases of polio resulted, orthodox medicine attempted to stop all production of the Salk vaccine for two years. In fact, the Surgeon General of the United States withdrew the vaccine from use, until a public uproar made him restore the program (ibid.:67).[*]

There is no doubt that the Salk vaccine was highly effective: it reduced the incidence of polio from 28,985 cases in 1955, to 3,190 in

---

[*] The hostility of the American medical profession also stemmed from the fact that the chairman of the National Foundation, Basil O'Connor, sought to raise $15 million to pay for *free* public vaccination of children in the United States. "The American Medical Association resisted the idea as being a step toward socialized medicine" (Wayne Martin, 1977).

1960, and 910 in 1962. The remaining cases were almost entirely among poor people who could not afford the cost of a private-doctor visit to obtain the vaccine (ibid.). Moreover, the Salk vaccine was quite safe when produced correctly. It was the responsibility of the U.S. government—not Salk—to make sure the drug companies complied with good production standards. Yet the "government remained passive during the massive field trials of 1954," which led to the debacle of 1955 (ibid.:68).

On the other hand, the Sabin vaccine, while effective, was potentially dangerous because it was made from live vaccine. In 1964, for example, the Surgeon General warned of a very small risk involved in taking this vaccine. Yet the American Medical Association, on the basis of Russian trials, endorsed the Sabin vaccine. The Salk vaccine was pushed into near oblivion by the force of medical orthodoxy. "A vaccine which had come within 98 percent of eradicating polio and which would not cause polio," said Basil O'Connor, "was replaced with a new vaccine that could cause polio" (cited in ibid.:69).

Nor was the pharmaceutical industry's role in the Salk vaccine one that is likely to be pointed to with pride. The drug companies contributed very little to polio research—the American people did that by contributing $500 million to the March of Dimes, the National Foundation's fund-raising appeal. When a Winthrop Laboratories executive was asked by the National Foundation to participate in the development of the Salk vaccine, he declined, saying, "We felt it would be a socialized rat race" (quoted in Rozental, 1961). "This premonition," says Rozental, "seems to have been unwarranted."

When the Justice Department indicted the makers of the vaccine for criminal conspiracy and demanded to see their books in the pre-trial examination, the manufacturers opposed the request on the grounds that disclosure of their high profits might prejudice the jury (ibid.).

These are the *best* examples the American Cancer Society spokesman can come up with as proof that there is no suppression of innovations by the medical establishment! Nothing in the history of these innovations or of any of the other examples cited in this book contradicts the idea that new ideas often have a difficult time getting established, and must face the indifference and even the hostility of vested interests.

As people become aware of this suppression, however, they are increasingly thrown into action against it. Millions of people no longer automatically believe what the leaders of the cancer establishment tell them. They are resisting the introduction of carcinogens into the environment; demanding alternate forms of therapy; suing companies; signing petitions; writing, picketing, and protesting. Scientists and doctors are pursuing independent avenues of research.

There is no need to exaggerate the scope of this rebellion: it is still embryonic. But given the current impasse in the war on cancer, it is most likely that it will gain strength and spread. Eventually it may play a decisive role in bringing the war on cancer to a successful conclusion.

Appendix A

STRUCTURE AND AFFILIATION OF THE MEMORIAL SLOAN-KETTERING CANCER CENTER LEADERSHIP

An analysis of the leadership of the world's largest private cancer center shows that those men and women with a vested interest in the cancer problem control the direction of research.

The board of overseers, reorganized in 1978, is composed of fifty individuals. Only five of these are medical doctors and four others are Ph.D.s. Most of these serve ex officio as executives of MSKCC itself or of affiliated institutions.

Board of Overseers

David M. Baldwin
Edward J. Beattie, Jr., M.D.
Mrs. Elmer H. Bobst
Mrs. H. Lawrence Bogert
Mrs. Neville H. Brown
Mrs. J. Frederic Byers III
Robert G. Chollar
Theodore Cooper, M.D.
Dale R. Corson, Ph.D.
Peter O. Crisp
Mrs. Percy L. Douglas
Harold W. Fisher
James B. Fisk, Ph.D.
Richard M. Furlaud
Clifton C. Garvin, Jr.
Louis V. Gerstner, Jr.

The full board of overseers has responsibility for "overseeing the direction of the Center" (MSKCC, 1978). It meets three times a year. This plenum group elects, in turn, a board of managers which "sets policies" and "monitors the activities of the corporations" (ibid.). Actually, it elects three boards, virtually identical in membership, for the three corporations—Memorial Sloan-Kettering, Memorial Hospital, and Sloan-Kettering Institute.

° Died on September 10, 1979.

The more select board of managers consists of twenty-five individuals, plus the president of the Society, MSKCC's fund-raising auxiliary.

Board of Managers

Edward J. Beattie, Jr., M.D.
Peter O. Crisp
Clifton C. Garvin, Jr.
Louis V. Gerstner, Jr.
Robert A. Good, Ph.D., M.D.
Albert H. Gordon
Mrs. Virginia S. Hutton °
James D. Landauer
Richard D. Lombard
Mrs. George G. Montgomery, Jr.
Alfred Ogden
Ellmore C. Patterson
John S. Reed
James D. Robinson III
Laurance S. Rockefeller
William Rockefeller
Robert V. Roosa
Benno C. Schmidt
Frederick Seitz, Ph.D.
H. Virgil Sherrill
William S. Sneath
J. McLain Stewart
Lewis Thomas, M.D.
John D. White
James H. Wickersham, Jr.
Harper Woodward

In addition, there are a number of other committees, appointed by these boards, which deal with particular aspects of managing the Center. The most significant, from the point of view of direction of research, appears to be the Institutional Policy Committee, composed of nine overseers.

The two primary interests of the banking and business community in cancer are the *causation* of cancer and the profitable *cure* of the disease. Thus, it is instructive to look at who these individuals

---

° Ex officio as president of the Society.

are, and what their connections are with polluting industries or with companies interested in profiting from a solution.

Much environmentally induced cancer comes from the petro-chemical industry, the automobile industry, and various other major industries and companies. At least a dozen of the overseers are affiliated with such companies:

Peter O. Crisp	Rockefeller Family & Associates, associate
Harold W. Fisher	Exxon, chairman of the board
James B. Fisk, Ph.D.	American Cyanamid, director
Richard M. Furlaud	Olin, director
Clifton C. Garvin, Jr.	Exxon, president
James D. Landauer	Consolidated Oil and Gas, director
Thomas A. Murphy	General Motors, chairman of the board
Ellmore C. Patterson	Atlantic-Richfield, director
John S. Reed	Philip Morris, director
Laurance S. Rockefeller	Exxon, Mobil, Standard Oil of Indiana, Standard Oil of California, etc., major shareholder
Robert V. Roosa	Texaco, director
Benno C. Schmidt	San Jacinto Petroleum, Transcontinental Gas Pipe Line Corporation, Freeport Minerals, director
° Arnold Schwartz	Texaco, vice-president
Frederick Seitz	Organon, director
H. Virgil Sherrill	Commercial Solvents, director
William S. Sneath	Union Carbide, president
T. F. Walkowicz	Rockefeller Family & Associates, associate
Harper Woodward	Rockefeller Family & Associates, associate

Thus eighteen overseers—or 36 percent—are rather closely tied to large polluting industries, especially those connected to oil, chemicals, and automobiles. This follows the traditional affiliation of both Memorial Hospital and Sloan-Kettering Institute, which have been dominated by oil and automotive fortunes, respectively.

The interest of these individuals on the board is greater than may appear at first sight. For fully half (eleven out of twenty-two) of the *outside* board of managers are on this list (excluding ex officio and inside members), including the chairmen of all the Center's boards.

Their corporations produce a wide panoply of known or suspected carcinogens. Exxon is one of the world's major producers of benzene. Many of the products of the petroleum industry are prime

---

° Died on September 10, 1979.

suspects in the hunt for industrial carcinogens (Epstein, 1978). According to Ralph Nader, General Motors alone is responsible "for about a third of the nation's air pollution by tonnage" (Esposito and Silverman, 1970). American Cyanamid produces acrylonitrile, which, a government official claims, "can pose a life-threatening danger in a very brief period of exposure" (Epstein, 1978:211).°

Union Carbide has had a long history of environmental pollution. Commercial Solvents produces the carcinogenic feed supplements and implants Ralgro and Zeranol (ibid.:233).

And these are only the direct corporate links. If one looks at interlocks (boards on which MSKCC directors serve with other polluters) the list becomes far longer. For example, the Rockefeller-dominated Chase Manhattan Bank has a director on the board of Raybestos-Manhattan, the asbestos manufacturer. Ellmore C. Patterson's Morgan Guaranty Trust Co. has a director on the board of Johns-Manville. General Motors president Thomas A. Murphy sits on the GM board with the chairman of Allied Chemical, manufacturer of Red Dyes #2 and #40.

If one asks, like the Romans, *"Cui bono?"* (Who stands to gain?), it is immediately apparent that the overseers and managers of Memorial Sloan-Kettering have a large stake in the outcome of the cancer problem.

The other main vested interest of the overseers is in corporate investments. Many of these men and women are bankers, stockbrokers, and "venture capitalists." Again, looking at the MSKCC board of overseers, one finds:

Peter O. Crisp	Rockefeller Family & Associates, manager of investments
Albert H. Gordon	Kidder Peabody, chairman of the board (investment bank)
Richard D. Lombard	Lombard, Nelson & McKenna, chairman, ret. (investment bank)
Mrs. George G. Montgomery (née Elinor White)	wife of George Montgomery, Jr., vice-president, White, Weld (investment bank)
Ellmore C. Patterson	Morgan Guaranty Trust Co., chairman of the executive committee
John S. Reed	Citibank, executive vice-president

° In fact, a 1979 strike at American Cyanamid's organic chemicals division in Bound Brook, New Jersey, centered largely around workers' concern about the possible cancer-causing hazard of the company's products *(New York Times,* January 14, 1979).

James D. Robinson	American Express, chairman; former investment banker with Morgan Guaranty and with White, Weld
Laurance S. Rockefeller	Rockefeller Brothers Fund, chairman
William Rockefeller	Shearman and Sterling, partner (law firm closely associated with Citibank)
Robert V. Roosa	Brown Brothers, Harriman, partner (investment bank)
Benno C. Schmidt	J. H. Whitney & Co., managing partner (investment bank)
H. Virgil Sherrill	Bache Halsey Stuart Shields, president (investment bank, stock brokerage)
James H. Wickersham, Jr.	Morgan Guaranty Trust Co., vice-president
Harper Woodward	Rockefeller Family & Associates, associate

In other words, fourteen out of fifty—or 28 percent—of the board of overseers is composed of professional investors, or closely associated with such investors (e.g., William Rockefeller, James D. Robinson). More significant is the manner in which these investors dominate the select board of managers. Fully fourteen out of twenty-two of the outside managers, or 64 percent, are investors by profession or closely involved with such investors.

Why would investors be attracted to these positions? Part of the reason seems to be the need of investors to understand the latest scientific and technological developments before they become generally available.

The career of the chairman of the board, Laurance S. Rockefeller, can be taken as a paradigm for the rest. He is a self-described venture capitalist who has made a career of turning science into money. "In venture capital investments," reads his official biographical handout, "the main line of Mr. Rockefeller's activities has involved new or young enterprises operating on the 'frontiers of technology' . . . with his risk capital keeping pace with scientific developments and changing technology. ("Laurance S. Rockefeller," 1971).

Since MSKCC is on the "frontiers of technology," this puts Rockefeller and his colleagues in a good position to pursue business, as well as philanthropic, interests.

Although it would be illegal for an overseer to personally sell products or services to the Center, it is not illegal for a public company with which he or she is associated to do so. In fact, according to the by-laws of the Center,

no Trustee or other officer of the Corporation [i.e., MSKCC] shall be deemed to be personally interested, directly or indirectly, and no personal interest shall be presumed or inferred, solely because of his ownership of shares in any publicly owned corporation or solely because of his being an officer or director of any corporation which has any such contract with the Corporation (MSKCC, 1960).

There are a number of instances in which directors' companies appear to have benefited from their association with the Center or with other such research facilities.

Two companies in which Laurance S. Rockefeller is a major shareholder, Standard Oil of California and Standard Oil of Indiana, own 25 percent and 22 percent respectively of Cetus; this corporation, valued at $100 million, specializes in recombinant DNA techniques. The president of Rockefeller University, which is headed by Laurance's brother David, is chairman of Cetus's board of scientific advisers *(Science,* November 9, 1979). Since 1976, Sloan-Kettering has been deeply involved in such research as well.

An associate of Rockefeller's, M. Frederick Smith, is director of Mallinckrodt, a drug and chemical company which does extensive business with MSKCC and other cancer centers.° Such an affiliation would imply a substantial investment on Rockefeller's part (Collier and Horowitz, 1976:296). Rockefeller was an early investor in Airborne Instruments Laboratories, which produced one of the first automated cell analyzers *(New York Times,* August 23, 1954). Nationwide, the automated clinical laboratory instruments industry has grown to over half a billion dollars a year *(Business Week,* May 10, 1976).

Connections of this sort are difficult to discover, since the laws on disclosure of corporation ownership are more lax than an investigator might wish. Sometimes these links are made through interlocking board membership. Thus biographical information on Benno Schmidt does not reveal any financial interest in the cancer field. Yet Don E. Ackerman, one of his partners at J. H. Whitney & Co., is a director of Worthington Biochemical Corporation, which has advertised its PHI monitoring system for cancer therapy in the medical journals *(Cancer,* April 1973).

° Mallinckrodt is a producer of radioactive tests and medicines. Since the 1950s, it has been considered a leader in attempting to develop anticancer drugs in conjunction with Sloan-Kettering *(Chemical Week,* July 24, 1954).

The industry which stands to gain the most from cancer research is the pharmaceutical business. This industry in particular has great influence on the MSKCC board, especially on the select Institutional Policy Committee of MSKCC. Influencing institutional policy toward a chemotherapeutic approach to cancer is certainly a key objective of the drug companies. The committee is composed of nine members, listed below with their pharmaceutical affiliations:

Lewis Thomas, M.D., chairman	Squibb, director
Benno C. Schmidt, vice-chairman	Worthington Biochemical (interlock)
Edward J. Beattie, Jr., M.D.	[none known]
Richard M. Furlaud	Squibb, chairman and chief executive officer
Louis V. Gerstner, Jr.	[none known]
Robert A. Good, Ph.D., M.D.	Merck Sharpe & Dohme, consultant
Laurance S. Rockefeller	Mallinckrodt (interlock)
Frederick Seitz, Ph.D.	Organon, director
William S. Sneath	Union Carbide, chairman of the board °

Thus, seven out of nine—or 78 percent—of the members of the Institutional Policy Committee are affiliated (or interlocked) with companies with a direct interest in the cancer drug (or diagnostics) market.

In 1954 Sloan-Kettering director C. P. Rhoads declared that future gains in cancer research would depend largely upon the pharmaceutical industry, and that without close cooperation between cancer researchers and industry "we can see no possibility of achieving our goal. . . ." (Drug Trade News, October 25, 1954).

At the time, the drug industry needed prodding to get involved in a serious way in the cancer field. Twenty-five years later, the industry appears not only to have become involved but also to have gained a decisive voice in the direction of research at MSKCC.

The members of the MSKCC board represent many industrial interests, and not all of them are associated with the cancer field. Nor is it necessary to postulate a conspiracy to direct cancer re-

° Union Carbide, although not thought of as a drug company, has had an interest in cancer-related pharmaceuticals since the early 1950s (Chemical Week, July 24, 1954). In 1977, attempting to diversify, Union Carbide bought Cleon Corp., maker of a medical diagnostic machine, and signed a $10-million agreement to distribute a breast X-ray machine (Business Week, January 24, 1977). William Sneath joined the MSKCC board in the same year.

search. There are many reasons why a corporate investor would serve on the MSKCC board, not all of them suspect.

Nevertheless, it is clear that these directors can—and must—bring to their jobs as MSKCC officials the same general philosophy and interests which guide their business and financial activities. The result is the direction of research away from prevention, away from radical solutions and inexpensive remedies, and toward more profitable avenues.

In effect, the MSKCC board is a very private and exclusive club which meets regularly to discuss and take actions which have great repercussions for the majority of Americans. Meeting in private, keeping a low profile, they are accountable to no one but themselves for the policy decisions they make.

Appendix B

SOURCES OF INFORMATION ON
ALTERNATE APPROACHES TO CANCER

1. Arlin J. Brown Information Center
   P.O. Box 251
   Fort Belvoir, VA 22060
   (703) 451-8638

   "A clearinghouse for information on constructive natural and nutritional health modalities."

2. Cancer Control Society
   2043 North Berendo Street
   Los Angeles, CA 90027
   (213) 663-7801

   The CCS publishes a magazine—*Cancer Control Journal*—with news and features on alternate therapies. It maintains the Cancer Book House with "books and reprints on nutrition, cancer and other. . . related diseases." Price list available on request.

   The CCS "reviews and reports on all of the aspects of cancer and other. . . related diseases . . . and especially cancer therapies and tests of great promise, which have been arbitrarily suppressed."

3. Committee for Freedom of Choice in Cancer Therapy, Inc.
   146 Main Street, Suite 408
   Los Altos, CA 94022
   (415) 948-9475

   "The Committee for Freedom of Choice in Cancer Therapy, Inc., is a nonprofit organization, subsisting on contributions from its committees and friends." The Committee's main activity has been to lobby for the legalization of laetrile. Publishes *The Choice.*

4. International Association of Cancer Victims and Friends
   7740 Manchester Avenue, Suite 110
   Playa del Rey, CA 90291
   (213) 822-5032

Publishers of the *Cancer News Journal,* "a layman's journal for laymen and professionals." The IACVF describes itself as a "charitable, educational, nonprofit organization that serves as a clearinghouse for the accumulation of material on nontoxic cancer therapies and other related topics for laymen and professionals. As a lay organization we cannot prescribe, only provide enlightenment on the current status of various cancer therapies, approaches to prevention, and research achievements."

5. National Health Federation
   P.O. Box 688
   212 West Foothill Boulevard
   Monrovia, CA 91016
   (213) 357-2181

"The National Health Federation is America's largest organized noncommercial health consumer group. It is a nonprofit corporation founded in 1955. Its members believe that health freedoms are inherently guaranteed to us as human beings, and our right to them as Americans is implied in the words 'life, liberty and the pursuit of happiness.' . . . The NHF opposes monopoly and compulsion in things related to health where the safety and welfare of others are not concerned. . . ."

The NHF publishes the *National Health Federation Bulletin* and *Public Scrutiny.*

6. Second Opinion
   P.O. Box 548
   Bronx, NY 10468

"Second Opinion is the voice of rank-and-file employees of Memorial Sloan-Kettering Cancer Center. It presents news and opinions of the Center and the cancer field from the employees' point of view. . . . In cancer, we believe in putting prevention first; making research relevant to human diseases; an open-minded policy toward new and unorthodox methods; making the best treatment available to all people; taking the profits out of cancer."

Has published bimonthly newsletter for employees as well as Second

Opinion's *Special Report: Laetrile at Sloan-Kettering*, which is available from the above address (price on request).

The following sources of information are generally hostile to unorthodox treatments:

7. American Cancer Society
   777 Third Avenue
   New York, NY 10017
   (212) 371-2900

8. American Medical Association
   535 North Dearborn Street
   Chicago, IL 60610
   (312) 751-6000

9. Food and Drug Administration
   5600 Fishers Lane
   Rockville, MD 20852
   (202) 245-1144

10. Memorial Sloan-Kettering
    Cancer Center
    1275 York Avenue
    New York, NY 10021
    (212) 794-7000

11. National Cancer Institute
    9000 Rockville Pike
    Bethesda, MD 20014
    (301) 496-6641

A Note on the References

This list contains all the books and some of the magazine and newspaper articles cited in the text. Wherever possible, however, the latter items have been referenced in the text itself.

Some of the items (marked with + below) are from the author's files or are not readily available at research libraries. A portfolio of these items has been deposited with the University of California, San Diego Biomedical Library, whose director, Robert F. Lewis, has kindly agreed to make these items part of the library's permanent Special Collection on Laetriles. The collection is available for scholars or the general public.

Items marked with ° are excellent material for a further study of this subject. In addition, annotations have been added for some of the entries.

References

Acevedo, Hernan F. "Immunohistochemical Localization of a Choriogonado-trophin-like Protein in Bacteria Isolated from Cancer Patients." *Cancer* 41:1217–29, 1978.

° Agran, Larry. *The Cancer Connection—And What We Can Do About It.* Boston: Houghton Mifflin Company, 1977. [Interesting investigation of the chemical causes of cancer. Especially valuable for its interview with Dr. William C. Hueper.]

Ambruster, Howard Watson. *Treason's Peace: German Dyes and American Dupes.* New York: Beechhurst Press, 1947.

American Cancer Society. "A Twentieth Anniversary." In *Annual Report.* New York, 1965.

———. *Cancer Facts and Figures.* New York, 1971a.

———. *Unproven Methods of Cancer Management.* New York, 1971b. [Updated periodically. Indispensable guide to orthodox thinking on the question of "quackery." Not to be confused with a small pamphlet of the same name.]

———. *Annual Report.* New York, 1972.

———. *Cancer Facts and Figures.* New York, 1974.

———. "Plants That Cure and Cause Cancer." *Cancer News* 29(2), Fall 1975.

———. "Hydrazine Sulfate." *CA—A Cancer Journal for Clinicians* 26(2), March–April 1976.

———. *Annual Report.* New York, 1978. [N.B.: Annual reports are routinely published in the year following the date in their title. To avoid confusion, all such reports are listed by the year which they describe.]

———. *Cancer Facts and Figures.* New York, 1979. [ACS's *Cancer Facts and Figures* is routinely published in the year *before* the cover date; e.g., the above volume was actually published in 1978. To avoid confusion, the fact books are listed according to the year to which they refer on the cover.]

Anderson, Alan, Jr. "The Politics of Cancer: How Do You Get the Medical Establishment to Listen?" *New York,* July 29, 1974.

Applezweig, Norman. "Cancer and the Drug Industry: The Business of Cancer Chemotherapy." *Medical Marketing and Media* 13(1), January 1978.

Bailey, Herbert. *A Matter of Life and Death: The Incredible Story of Krebiozen.* New York: G.P. Putnam's Sons, 1958.

――――. *Vitamin E, Your Key to a Healthy Heart*. New York: Arco Books, 1971.

――――. *The Vitamin Pioneers*. New York: Pyramid Publications, 1972.

Barber, Bernard. "Resistance by Scientists to Scientific Discovery." *Science* 134:596–602, September 1, 1961.

Bard, Morton. "The Price of Survival for Cancer Victims." In *Where Medicine Fails*, edited by Anselm Strauss. New Brunswick, N.J.: Transaction Books, 1973.

Bäumler, Ernst. *A Century of Chemistry*. Translated by David Goodman. Düsseldorf: Econ Verlag, 1968.

Beard, H. H. *A New Approach to the Conquest of Cancer, Rheumatic and Heart Diseases*. Los Angeles: Cancer Book House, 1962.

Beard, John. *The Enzyme Treatment of Cancer and Its Scientific Basis*. London: Chatto and Windus, 1911. [Provides the theoretical underpinnings for much of the laetrile movement.]

Bernal, J. D. *The Social Function of Science*. Cambridge, Mass.: MIT Press, 1967.

――――. *Science in History*. Cambridge, Mass.: MIT Press, 1971.

Bernheim, Bertram M. *The Story of the Johns Hopkins*. New York: Whittlesey House, 1948.

Bloom, Mark. "AP Syndicates Blakeslee Cancer Series." *National Association of Science Writers Newsletter* 8(3), August 1979.

° Bobst, Elmer H. *Bobst: Autobiography of a Pharmaceutical Pioneer*. New York: David McKay Company, 1973. [Unwitting self-revelations from a key member of the cancer establishment.]

Boesch, Mark. *The Long Search for the Truth About Cancer*. New York: G. P. Putnam's Sons, 1960.

Bohanon, Luther. *Opinion in the Case of Glen L. Rutherford vs. U.S.A. in the U.S. District Court for the Western Region*. No. CIV-75-0218-B, filed December 5, 1977.

Borkin, Joseph. *The Crime and Punishment of I. G. Farben*. New York: Free Press, 1978.

Böttcher, Helmuth M. *Wonder Drugs—A History of Antibiotics*. Translated by Einhart Kawerau. Philadelphia: J.B. Lippincott Company, 1964.

Bourne, Gaylord. *Asbestos Contamination in School Buildings*. Washington, D.C.: Public Interest Research Group, 1978.

° Brodeur, Paul. *Expendable Americans*. New York: Viking Press, 1974. [Excellent study of the asbestos problem by a *New Yorker* reporter.]

Brody, Jane, and Holleb, Arthur. *You Can Fight Cancer and Win*. New York: Times Books, 1977.

+ Bross, Irwin. Personal communication. June 15, 1979.

Brothwell, Don, and Brothwell, Patricia. *Food in Antiquity*. New York: Praeger Publishers, 1969.

Brown, E. Richard. *Rockefeller Medicine Men: Medicine and Capitalism in America*. Berkeley: University of California Press, 1979.

Brown University News Service. "One of Oldest Medicines May Assist Cancer Fight." Providence, R.I., February 10, 1976.

Burdick, Carl G. "William Bradley Coley, 1862–1936" (memoir). *Annals of Surgery* 105:152–155, January 1937.

Burk, Dean. "On the Cancer Metabolism of Minimal Deviation Hepatomas."

Proceedings of the American Association for Cancer Research 6(9), 1965.

——. "New Approaches to Cancer Therapy." *New England Natural Food Association Bulletin,* Spring 1974a.

——. "See How They Lie, See How They Lie." *Cancer News Journal* 9(3), 1974b.

——. *A Brief on Foods and Vitamins.* Sausalito, Calif.: McNaughton Foundation, 1975.

+ ——. Personal communication. December 13, 1977.

Burnet, Frank MacFarlane. *Immunological Surveillance.* Oxford: Pergamon Press, 1970.

+ Burton, Lawrence. Personal communication. November 18, 1978.

Burton, Lawrence, et al. "The Purification and Action of Tumor Factor Extracted from Mouse and Human Neoplastic Tissue." *Transactions of the New York Academy of Sciences* 21:700–707, June 1959.

Burton, Lawrence, and Friedman, Frank. "Detection of Tumor-Inducing Factors in *Drosophila.*" *Science* 124:220–21, August 3, 1956.

California Cancer Commission. "The Treatment of Cancer with 'Laetriles.' " *California Medicine* 78(4), April 1953.

Cameron/Friedlander, Inc. *Immunology Center—Cancer Release.* Fort Lauderdale, Fla., 1979.

Cancer Care, Inc. *The Impact, Costs and Consequences of Catastrophic Illness on Patients and Families.* New York, 1973.

Cancer Information Service. *National Cancer Institute Statement on Mammography.* New York: Memorial Sloan-Kettering Cancer Center, November 1977.

——. *National Cancer Institute Statement on Vitamin C.* New York: Memorial Sloan-Kettering Cancer Center, April 12, 1978.

Cancer Research Institute. *A Review of Progress and Hope.* New York, 1976.

Cantor, Robert Chernin. *And a Time to Live.* New York: Harper and Row, 1978.

Cantwell, Alan R., and Kelso, Dan W. "Acid-Fast Bacteria in Scleroderma and Morphea." *Archives of Dermatology* 4, June 1971.

Carter, Richard. *The Gentle Legions.* New York: Doubleday and Company, 1961.

+ Carter, Stephen. "Meeting on Amygdalin" (photocopy). Bethesda, Md., March 4, 1975. [Minutes by co-chairman and deputy director of Division of Cancer Treatment, National Cancer Institute. Obtained under the Freedom of Information Act.]

Carter, Stephen, and Kershner, Lorraine M. "Cancer Chemotherapy: What Drugs Are Available." *Medical Times,* February 1976.

Chowka, Peter Barry. "An Interview with Dr. Gio Gori." *East West Journal,* January 1978a.

° ——. "The National Cancer Institute and the Fifty-Year Cover-Up." *East West Journal,* January 1978b.[One in a series of provocative essays by a bright young critic of establishment medicine.]

° ——. "The Cancer Charity Rip-Off." *East West Journal,* July 1978c.

———. "U.S. to Test Laetrile." *New Age,* February 1979.

Clark, Sir George. *A History of the Royal College of Physicians of London.* Vol. I. Oxford: Oxford University Press, 1964.

+ Clement, R.J. Personal communication. November 18, 1978.

Cohen, Herman, and Strampp, Alice. "Bacterial Synthesis of a Substance Similar to Human Chorionic Gonadotrophin." *Proceedings of the Society for Experimental Biology and Medicines* 152(3), July 1976.

Coley, William B. "A Preliminary Note on the Treatment of Inoperable Sarcoma by the Toxic Product of Erysipelas." *Post-graduate* 8:278–86, 1893.

° ———. "The Cancer Symposium at Lake Mohonk." *American Journal of Surgery* (New Series) 1:222–25, October 1926. [Coley's call for an open-minded attitude on all unorthodox approaches to the cancer problem.]

Collier, Peter, and Horowitz, David. *The Rockefellers: An American Dynasty.* New York: Holt, Rinehart and Winston, 1976.

Collins, Vincent J. *Principles of Anesthesiology.* Philadelphia: Lea and Febiger, 1966.

Committee for Freedom of Choice in Cancer Therapy, Inc. *Anatomy of a Cover-Up: Successful Sloan-Kettering Amygdalin (Laetrile) Animal Studies.* Los Altos, Calif., 1975.

° Considine, Bob. *That Many May Live.* New York: Memorial Center for Cancer and Allied Diseases, 1959. [Informative, but one-sided, history of Memorial Hospital from 1880s to 1950s.]

Creagan, Edward T.; Moertel, Charles G.; et al. "Failure of High-Dose Vitamin C (Ascorbic Acid) Therapy to Benefit Patients with Advanced Cancer." *New England Journal of Medicine* 301:687–90, September 27, 1979.

° Crile, George, Jr. *What Women Should Know About the Breast Cancer Controversy.* New York: Pocket Books, 1974. [Simply written but powerful argument against radical mastectomy, by a leading surgeon.]

Culbert, Michael L. *Freedom from Cancer.* Seal Beach, Calif.: '76 Press, 1976.

Curie, Eve. *Madame Curie.* Translated by Vincent Sheean. Garden City, N.Y.: Doubleday and Company, 1943.

D'Angio, Giulio J. "Pediatric Cancer in Perspective: Cure Is Not Enough." *Cancer* 35(3), March 1975.

Danova, L. A., et al. "Results of Administration of Hydrazine Sulfate to Patients with Hodgkin's Disease." *Therapeutics Archives: Questions in Hematology* (Moscow) 49:45–47, 1977.

+ Delaney, T. Gerald. "An Update on Laetrile" (memo). New York: MSKCC Department of Public Affairs, January 26, 1977a.

+ ———. "Statement on Laetrile" (memo). New York: MSKCC Department of Public Affairs, February 1, 1977b.

de Haen, Paul. "New Drug Introduction 1973–74." *Journal of the American Medical Association* 234(7), November 17, 1975.

Delmotte, N., and Meiren, L. van der. "Recherches Bactériologiques et

Histologiques Concernant la Sclérodermie." *International Journal of Dermatology* (Basel) 107(3), 1953.

DuBois, Josiah E., Jr. *The Devil's Chemists*. Boston: Beacon Press, 1952.

Edson, Lee. "The Cancer Rip-Off." *Science Digest*, September 1974.

Ehrenreich, Barbara, and English, Deirdre. *Complaints and Disorders: The Sexual Politics of Sickness*. Old Westbury, N.Y.: Feminist Press, 1973.

Ellison, N.M. "Special Report on Laetrile: The NCI Laetrile Review—Results of the National Cancer Institute's Retrospective Laetrile Analysis." *New England Journal of Medicine* 299:549–52, September 7, 1978.

° Epstein, Samuel S. *The Politics of Cancer*. San Francisco: Sierra Club Books, 1978 (rev. ed. Garden City, N.Y.: Anchor Press/Doubleday, 1979). [Exhaustive study of environmental carcinogens. Inadequate treatment, however, of cancer establishment.]

Esposito, John C., and Silverman, Larry J., eds. *Vanishing Air: The Ralph Nader Study Group Report on Air Pollution*. Foreword by Ralph Nader. New York: Grossman Publishers, 1970.

Everson, T. C., and Cole, W. H. *Spontaneous Regression of Cancer*. Philadelphia: W. B. Saunders Company, 1966.

Ewing, James. *Neoplastic Diseases*. 2nd ed. Philadelphia: W. B. Saunders and Company, 1922.

———. *Neoplastic Diseases*. 4th ed. Philadelphia: W. B. Saunders and Company, 1940.

Eyerly, Robert. "Laetrile: Focus on the Facts" (interview). *CA—A Cancer Journal for Clinicians* 26(1), January–February 1976.

Farrington, Benjamin. *Science and Politics in the Ancient World*. London: Unwin University Press, 1965.

Fieve, Ronald R. *Moodswing: The Third Revolution in Psychiatry*. New York: Bantam Books, 1976.

Fisher, Bernard, et al. "Surgical Adjuvant Chemotherapy in Cancer of the Breast." *Annals of Surgery* 161:339–56, 1968.

Fogg, Susan. "Laetrile Tests on Cancer Patients Delayed." *Mobile* [Ala.] *Press,* March 21, 1979.

+ Fogh, Jørgen. Personal communication. January 3, 1979.

+ Food and Drug Administration. "Meeting on Laetrile" (photocopy). Beltsville, Md., July 2, 1974. [Part of these minutes, obtained under the Freedom of Information Act, are signed by H. L. Walker, M.D.]

———. *Consumer Memo: Laetrile*. DHEW Publ. No. (FDA) 75–3007. Beltsville, Md., 1975.

Frank, Mark D. "A Drug to Fight Cancer's Starvation Effects." United Press International feature. New York, January 26, 1979.

Fraumeni, Joseph F., Jr., ed. *Persons at High Risk of Cancer*. New York: Academic Press, 1975.

+ Fredericks, Carleton. Personal communication. November 25, 1978.

+ Garfinkel, Lawrence. Personal communication. October 2, 1979. [Garfinkel is vice-president for epidemiology and statistics at the American Cancer Society.]

Garrison, Omar. *Dictocrats: Our Unelected Rulers.* Chicago: Books for Today, 1970.

° Gerson, Max. *A Cancer Therapy—Results of Fifty Cases.* New York: Whittier Books, 1958. [Documented presentation of Gerson's theories and cases.]

Glasser, Ronald. *The Greatest Battle.* New York: Random House, 1979.

Glemser, Bernard. *Man Against Cancer.* New York: Funk and Wagnalls, 1969.

Gold, Joseph. "Proposed Treatment of Cancer by Inhibition of Gluconeogenesis." *Oncology* 22:185–207, 1968.

———. "Inhibition of Walker 256 Intramuscular Carcinoma in Rats by Administration of Hydrazine Sulfate." *Oncology* 25:66–71, 1971a.

———. "Combination Therapy of Hydrazine with Cytoxan and Mitomycin C on Walker 256 Intramuscular Carcinoma in Rats." *Proceedings of the American Association for Cancer Research* 12(9), 1971b.

———. "Inhibition by Hydrazine Sulfate and Various Hydrazides of In-Vivo Growth of Walker 256 Intramuscular Carcinoma, B-16 Melanoma, Murphy-Sturm Lymphosarcoma, and L-1210 Solid Leukemia." *Oncology* 27:69–80, 1973.

+ ———. Letter to Manuel Ochoa, M.D. April 3, 1974.

———. "Enhancement by Hydrazine Sulfate of Anti-Tumor Effectiveness of Cytoxan, Mitomycin C, Methotrexate, and Bleomycin in Walker 256 Carcinosarcoma in Rats." *Oncology* 31:44–53, 1975a.

+ ———. Personal communication. June 16, 1975b.

———. "Use of Hydrazine Sulfate in Terminal or Preterminal Cancer Patients: Results of Investigational New Drug (IND) Study in 84 Evaluable Patients." *Oncology* 32:1–10, 1975c.

+ ———. Personal communication. June 21, 1979.

+ Grauer, Marshall Jay. Letter to Dr. Lewis Thomas. November 24, 1975.

Green, Thomas. *Gynecology.* Boston: Little, Brown and Company, 1971.

Greenberg, Daniel S. "A Critical Look at Cancer Coverage." *Columbia Journalism Review.* January–February 1975.

Greenberg, David M. "The Vitamin Fraud in Cancer Quackery." *The Western Journal of Medicine* 122:345–48, April 1975.

Griffin, G. Edward. *World Without Cancer: The Story of Vitamin B-17.* Thousand Oaks, Calif.: American Media, 1975.

Gunther, John. *Death Be Not Proud: A Memoir.* New York: Harper and Brothers, 1949.

Halstead, Bruce. *Amygdalin (Laetrile) Therapy.* Los Altos, Calif.: Committee for Freedom of Choice in Cancer Therapy, 1977.

Harper, Harold W. and Culbert, Michael L. *How You Can Beat the Killer Diseases.* New Rochelle, N.Y.: Arlington House, 1977.

+ Harris, Mrs. Bertha. Personal communication. November 4, 1979.

Harris, Richard. *The Real Voice.* New York: Macmillan Publishing Company, 1964.

Harris, Seale. *Woman's Surgeon: The Life Story of J. Marion Sims.* New York: Macmillan Publishing Company, 1950.

Haught, S. J. *Has Max Gerson a True Cancer Cure?* Canoga Park, Calif.: Major Books, 1962.

Hixson, Joseph. *The Patchwork Mouse.* Garden City, N.Y.: Doubleday and Company, 1976a.

———. "Vitamin A and the Forces That Be." *Harper's,* June 1976b.

Hoefer-Amidei Public Relations. "Linus Pauling Rebuts New Mayo Study on Vitamin C" (press release). San Francisco, September 28, 1979.

Hoffman, Frederick L. *Cancer and Diet.* Baltimore: Williams and Wilkins Company, 1937.

Holleb, Arthur I. "Risks vs. Benefits in Breast Cancer Diagnosis" (editorial). *CA—A Cancer Journal for Clinicians* 26(1), January–February 1976.

Houston, Robert. "Dietary Nitriloside and Sickle Cell Anemia in Africa." *American Journal of Clinical Nutrition* 27:766, August 1974.

° ———. "Food for Peace?" *Our Town,* December 24, 1978. [One in a series of iconoclastic pieces on cancer in a New York community newspaper.]

° ———. "Contributing to Cancer." *Our Town,* April 1, 1979a.

° ———. "The Burton Syndrome." *Our Town,* April 22, 1979b.

———. "Reply to Letter." *Our Town,* June 24, 1979c.

Houston, Robert, and Null, Gary. "War on Cancer: A Long Day's Dying." *Our Town,* October 29, 1978.

+ Howard, Frank. Speech at Sloan-Kettering Institute dinner. New York, October 18, 1955.

+ ———. "Organizing for Technical Progress" (privately printed). Speech delivered in the Engineering Administration Program of George Washington University. Washington, D.C., December 5, 1956.

+ ———. "Industrial Cooperation in Cancer Chemotherapy Research" (privately printed). Paper delivered at the 8th International Cancer Congress, Moscow, July 25, 1962.

Huffman, J. D. *Gynecology and Obstetrics.* Philadelphia: W. B. Saunders Company, 1962.

° Hunter, Donald. *The Diseases of Occupations.* 6th ed. Boston: Little, Brown and Company, 1978.

Immunology Researching Centre, Ltd. "Current Fee Schedule." Freeport, Bahamas, 1979.

Inosemtzeff, F. J. "Histoire de Deux Cas de Fongus Médullaire, Traités avec Succès par l'Emploi des Narcotiques." *Gazette Medicale de Paris* 37:577–82, 1845.

International Workshop on Interferon in the Treatment of Cancer. *Report.* New York: Memorial Sloan-Kettering Cancer Center, March 31, April 1, and April 2, 1975.

Israël, Lucien. *Conquering Cancer.* New York: Random House, 1978.

Issels, J. *Cancer: A Second Opinion.* London: Hodder and Stoughton, 1975.

° Johnston, Barbara. "Clinical Effects of Coley's Toxin. 1. A Controlled Study. 2. A Seven-Year Study." *Cancer Chemotherapy Reports* 21:19–68,

August 1962. [One of the few controlled double-blind studies ever conducted on an "unproven method of cancer management." Remarkable photographs of regressions.]

+ ——. Personal communication. December 27. 1976.

Jones, Hardin B. "A Report on Cancer." Speech delivered to the ACS 11th Annual Science Writers' Conference. New Orleans, La., March 7, 1969.

Jukes, Thomas H. "Human Testing." *Nature* 261:451, June 10, 1976.

Karnofsky, David A. "Cancer Quackery: Its Causes, Recognition and Prevention." *The American Journal of Nursing*, April 1959.

Kassel, Robert, et al. "Complement in Cancer." In *Biological Amplification Systems in Immunology*, edited by Noorbibi K. Day and Robert A. Good. New York: Plenum Publishing Corporation, 1977.

Kassel, Robert; Burton, Lawrence; and Friedman, Frank. "Utilization of an Induced *Drosophila* Melanoma in the Study of Mammalian Neoplasms." *Annals of the New York Academy of Sciences* 100:791–816, February 15, 1963.

Kassel, Robert; Burton, Lawrence; Friedman, Frank; and Harris, J. J. "Synergistic Action of Two Refined Leukemic Tissue Extracts in Oncolysis of Spontaneous Tumors." *Transactions of the New York Academy of Sciences* 25:39–44, November 1962.

Katz, Jay. *Experimentation with Human Beings.* New York: Russell Sage Foundation, 1972.

+ Kisner, Daniel L. Letter to Joseph Gold. November 7, 1978.

Klass, Alan. *There's Gold in Them Thar Pills.* Baltimore: Penguin Books, 1975.

+ Kline, Tim. Personal communication. November 7, 1979.

+ Koide, Samuel. Personal communication. July 20, 1979.

° Kotelchuck, David. "Asbestos Research: Winning the Battle But Losing the War." *Health/PAC Bulletin* 61, November–December 1974. [Thorough investigation of the role of the scientific profession in the asbestos problem.]

Krebs, Ernst T., Jr. "The Nitrilosides (Vitamin B-17): Their Nature, Occurrence, and Metabolic Significance." *Journal of Applied Nutrition* 22:3–4, 1970.

——. *The Extraction, Identification, and Packaging of Therapeutically Effective Amygdalin.* Redwood City, Calif.: Nutrisearch Foundation, 1979.

Kreig, Margaret. *Green Medicine: The Search for Plants That Heal.* Chicago: Rand McNally, 1964.

Kushner, Rose. *Breast Cancer: A Personal History and an Investigative Report.* New York: Harcourt Brace Jovanovich, 1975.

Langton, H. H. *James Douglas: A Memoir.* Toronto: Privately printed, 1940.

+ "Laurance S. Rockefeller" (biographical sketch, official handout). New York, June 1971.

Leaf, Alexander, and Launois, John. *Youth in Old Age.* New York: McGraw-Hill, 1975.

Lerner, Harvey J., and Regelson, William. "Clinical Trial of Hydrazine Sulfate in Solid Tumors." *Cancer Treatment Reports* 60:959–60, July 1976.

Lilienthal, David E. *Big Business: A New Era.* New York: Harper and Row, 1953.

Lilley, S. *Men, Machines and History—The Story of Tools and Machines in Relation to Social Progress.* London: Cobbett Press, 1965.

Little, Clarence Cook. *Report of the Scientific Director.* New York: Tobacco Industry Research Committee, 1957.

° Livingston, Virginia. *Cancer: A New Breakthrough.* San Diego: Production House, 1972. [Autobiography which describes the search for *Progenitor cryptocides.*]

Livingston, Virginia Wuerthele-Caspe, and Livingston, Afton M. "Some Cultural, Immunological, and Biochemical Properties of *Progenitor Cryptocides.*" *Transactions of the New York Academy of Sciences* (Series 2) 36:569–82, June 1974.

Livingston–Wheeler, Virginia, and Wheeler, Owen Webster. *The Microbiology of Cancer: Compendium.* San Diego: Livingston–Wheeler Clinic, 1977a. [Collection of Livingston's articles in the field, plus confirmatory papers.]

————. *Food Alive.* San Diego: Livingston–Wheeler Clinic, 1977b.

+ ————. Personal communication. June 26, 1979.

Lundberg, Ferdinand. *America's Sixty Families.* New York: Vanguard Press, 1937.

McCarty, Mark. "Burying Caesar: An Analysis of the Laetrile Problem." *Triton Times* (University of California, San Diego), November 29, 1975.

° McCoy, J. J. *The Cancer Lady: Maud Slye and Her Hereditary Studies.* New York: Elsevier/Nelson Books, 1977. [A revealing look at the cancer establishment in the period between the two world wars.]

+ McGill, Jane. *Annual Report.* New York: Employee Health Service, Memorial Sloan-Kettering Cancer Center, 1976.

° McGrady, Pat, Sr. *The Savage Cell.* New York: Basic Books, 1964. [A still-useful study of cancer research from a man who has been called "just about the best science public relations person there ever was."]

° ————. *The Persecuted Drug: The Story of DMSO.* Garden City, N.Y.: Doubleday and Company, 1973. [How suppression may work in fields other than that of cancer research.]

° ————. *The New Immunology.* Ardsley, N.Y.: Independent Citizens' Research Foundation, 1975. [Unconventional approaches to cancer immunotherapy.]

+ ————. Personal communication. January 4, 1979.

McGrady, Pat, Jr. "The American Cancer Society Means Well, But the Janker Clinic Means Better." *Esquire*, April 1976.

NcNaughton Foundation. *The Laetriles—Nitrilosides—in the Prevention and Control of Cancer.* Sausalito, Calif., 1967.

Mallinckrodt, Inc. *Annual Report.* St. Louis, 1975.

Manner, Harold, et al. *The Death of Cancer.* Chicago: Advanced Century Publishing Corporation, 1978a.

————. "Amygdalin, Vitamin A, and Enzyme-Induced Regression of Murine Mammary Adenocarcinomas." *Journal of Manipulative and Physiological Therapeutics* (Chicago), December, 1978b.

Markle, Gerald E., and Petersen, James C. *Laetrile and Cancer: The Limits of Science*. Presented at the annual meeting of the Midwest Sociological Society. Kalamazoo, Mich.: Center for Sociological Research, Western Michigan University, 1977.

Martin, Daniel S. "Laetrile—A Dangerous Drug." *CA—A Cancer Journal for Clinicians*. September–October 1977.

Martin, Daniel S., et al. "Solid Tumor Animal Model Therapeutically Predictive for Human Breast Cancer." *Cancer Chemotherapy Reports* (Part 2) 5(1), December 1975.

Martin, Wayne. *Medical Heroes and Heretics*. Old Greenwich, Conn.: Devin-Adair Company, 1977.

Maugh, Thomas H., and Marx, Jean L. *Seeds of Destruction: The* Science *Report on Cancer Research*. New York: Plenum Publishing Corporation, 1975.

Medawar, Sir Peter B. "The Strange Case of the Spotted Mice." *New York Review of Books*, April 15, 1976.

Medical Committee for Human Rights. *Billions for Band-Aids*. San Francisco, 1972.

Medvin, Norman. *The Energy Cartel: Who Runs the American Oil Industry*. New York: Vintage Books, 1974.

Memorial Hospital. *Annual Report*. New York, 1924.

————. *Annual Report*. New York, 1934.

+ ————. "Dependence of Medicine on Industrial Invention and Research" (press release). New York, March 8, 1940.

+ Memorial Sloan-Kettering Cancer Center. "By-Laws of Memorial Sloan-Kettering Cancer Center (A New York Membership Corporation), as Amended Through September 20, 1960." New York, 1960.

————. *Annual Report*. New York, 1972.

+ ————. "Official Laetrile Statement." New York, Fall 1973.

————. *Annual Report*. New York, 1976.

————. *Annual Report*. New York, 1977a.

+ ————. "Contributions, Bequests, and Grants Received in Cash by Division of Support Activities." New York, May–June 1977b. [MSKCC internal memoranda.]

+ ————. Taped laetrile press conference. New York, June 15, 1977c.

+ ————. Statement on the firing of Ralph W. Moss. New York, November 21, 1977d.

+ ————. "Statement on the Second Opinion Report on Laetrile." New York, November 30, 1977e.

————. *Annual Report*. New York, 1978.

Moertel, Charles. "A Trial of Laetrile Now" (editorial). *New England Journal of Medicine* 298:218–19, January 26, 1978.

° Morris, Nat. *The Cancer Blackout*. Los Angeles: Regent House, 1977. [A history of unorthodox approaches to cancer.]

Morrone, John A. "Chemotherapy of Inoperable Cancer." *Experimental Medicine and Surgery* 4, 1962. [Preliminary report of ten cases treated with laetrile.]

+ Moss, Ralph W. "Hydrazine Sulfate" (memo). New York: MSKCC Department of Public Affairs, July 25, 1974. [Co-signed by Manuel Ochoa, M.D.]
+ ——. "Subject: Laetrile" (memo). New York: MSKCC Department of Public Affairs, July 30, 1976. [Confidential report to T. Gerald Delaney.]
——. "Newly Found Tumor Necrosis Factor Under Study by Institute." MSKCC Center News, March 1977.

National Cancer Institute. Fact Book. DHEW Publication No. (NIH) 75–512. Bethesda, Md., 1975.
——. Special Communication: Accomplishments of Benefit to People Since 1971. Bethesda, Md.: National Cancer Program, June 9, 1976a.
——. Cancer Patient Survival, Report No. 5. Bethesda, Md., 1976b. [A report from the Cancer Surveillance, Epidemiology and End Results (SEER) Program.]
——. Statement on Dr. Lawrence Burton/Immunology Research Foundation. Bethesda, Md., April 1978.
National Institutes of Health. Guide for Grants and Contracts. Bethesda, Md., September 25, 1978.
——. NIH Public Advisory Groups. DHEW Publication No. (NIH) 79–11. Washington, D.C., January 1, 1979.
National Resources Committee. Technology and Planning. Washington, D.C., 1937.
Nauts, Helen Coley. "Immunotherapy of Cancer by Bacterial Vaccines." Paper read at International Symposium on Detection and Prevention of Cancer. New York, April 25–May 1; 1976a.
+ ——. Personal communication. December 20, 1976b.
° Nauts, Helen Coley, et al. "A Review of the Influence of Bacterial Infection and Bacterial Products (Coley's Toxins) on Malignant Tumors in Man." Acta Medica Scandinavica 145 (Suppl. 276), April 1953. [First in Mrs. Nauts's series of monographs on Coley's work.]
Nelson, Ralph L. Economic Factors in the Growth of Corporation Giving. National Bureau of Economic Research Occasional Paper No. 111. New York: Russell Sage Foundation, 1970.
Newbold, H. L. "Design for Living." Interview by Carleton Fredericks, Ph.D. WOR-AM. New York, May 9, 1978.
+ ——. Personal communication. January 22, 1979.
Nieper, Hans. "Problems of Early Cancer Diagnosis and Therapy. 1. Nitrilosides, Particularly Amygdalin in Cancer Prophylaxis and Therapy." Agressologie (Paris) 11(1), 1970.
Nobile, David F. "The Chemistry of Risk." Seven Days, June 5, 1979.
Null, Gary. "This Man Could Save Your Life, But He Can't Get the Money to Do It." Our Town. May 13–19, 1979.

Ochoa, Manuel. "Trial of Hydrazine Sulfate in Patients with Cancer." Cancer Chemotherapy Reports 59:1151–54, 1975.
Old, Lloyd J., and Boyse, Edward A. Current Enigmas in Cancer Research. The Harvey Lectures, Series 67. New York: Academic Press, 1973. [The lecture was delivered on April 20, 1972.]

Passwater, Richard A. "In Defense of Laetrile." *Let's Live*, June 1977.

———. *Cancer and Its Nutritional Therapies.* New Canaan, Conn.: Keats Publishing, 1978.

Pauling, Linus. *No More War!* New York: Dodd, Mead and Company, 1958.

———. *Vitamin C and the Common Cold.* New York: Bantam Books, 1971.

———. *Vitamin C, the Common Cold, and the Flu.* San Francisco: W.H. Freeman and Company, 1976.

+ ———. Personal communication. June 18, 1979.

Pauling, Linus, and Cameron, Ewan. "Supplemental Ascorbate in the Supportive Treatment of Cancer: Prolongation of Survival Times in Terminal Human Cancer." *Proceedings of the National Academy of Sciences,* 73:3685–89, October 1976.

Pharmaceutical Manufacturers' Association. *Newsletter.* Washington, D.C., April 26, 1976.

Physicians' Desk Reference. Oradell, N.J.: Medical Economics, 1978.

Prescott, Eleanor. "Mary Lasker: The Most Powerful Person in Modern Medicine." *Medical Dimensions,* March 1976.

Pressman, Gabe. Program on laetrile (in series on cancer), WNEW-TV. New York, May 16, 1979.

Reitnauer, P. G. "Prolonged Survival of Tumor-Bearing Mice Following Feeding Bitter Almonds." *Archiv Geschwulstforschung* (Dresden) 42:135, 1973.

° Richards, Victor. *Cancer, the Wayward Cell: Its Origins, Nature, and Treatment.* Berkeley: University of California Press, 1972. [Despite stereotyped view of unorthodox therapies, a useful account of the cancer problem for laymen.]

Richardson, John, and Griffin, Patricia. *Laetrile Case Histories.* New York: Bantam Books, 1977.

Robertson, Wyndham. "Merck Strains to Keep the Pots Aboiling." *Fortune,* March 1976.

° Rosenbaum, Ruth. "Cancer, Inc." *New Times,* November 25, 1977. [Acerbic critique of cancer establishment, especially the ACS.]

Ross, Joseph P. "Laetriles—Not a Vitamin and Not a Treatment" (editorial). *Western Journal of Medicine,* April 1975.

Ross, Walter S. "The Medicines We Need—But Can't Have." *Reader's Digest,* October 1973.

Rossi, B., Guidetti, E., et al. "Clinical Trial of Chemotherapeutic Treatment of Advanced Cancers with L-Mandelonitrile-Beta-Diglucoside." In *Proceedings of the Ninth International Cancer Congress,* 1966. (Reprinted by the McNaughton Foundation, 1967, see above.)

Rorvik, David M. "Who Wrote the American Cancer Society's Denunciation of Hydrazine Sulfate?" *Alicia Patterson Foundation Newsletter* (New York), November 29, 1976.

+ Rottino, Antonio. Personal communication. December 18, 1978.

Rozental, Alek A. "The Strange Ethics of the Ethical Drug Industry." In *Crisis in American Medicine,* edited by Marion K. Sanders. New York: Harper & Row, 1961.

Rubin, Philip. *Clinical Oncology for Medical Students and Physicians.* New York and Rochester: American Cancer Society and University of Rochester School of Medicine, 1971.

+ Schloen, Lloyd H. "Notes from First Annual Convention of the International Association of Cancer Victims and Friends, Inc." New York, April 15, 1973. [Prepared for MSKCC administration.]

Schmidt, E. S., et al. "Laetrile Toxicity Studies in Dogs." *Journal of the American Medical Association* 239: 943–947, 1978.

Schultz, Terri, and Lindeman, Bard. "The Victimization of Desperate Cancer Patients." *Today's Health,* November 1973.

+ Second International Workshop on Interferons in the Treatment of Cancer. *Report.* New York: Memorial Sloan-Kettering Cancer Center, et al., April 22–24, 1979.

Second Opinion. *Special Report: Laetrile at Sloan-Kettering.* Bronx, N.Y., 1977.

Seits, I. F., et al. "Experimental and Clinical Data of Antitumor Action of Hydrazine Sulfate." *Problems of Oncology* (Leningrad) 21:45–52, 1975.

Selikoff, Irving. Speech to the Society for Clinical Ecology. Key Biscayne, Fla., November 19, 1978.

Shimkin, Michael B. *Science and Cancer.* DHEW Pub. No. (NIH) 74–568. Bethesda, Md.: National Institutes of Health, 1973.

° ———. *Contrary to Nature.* DHEW Pub. No. (NIH) 76–720. Bethesda, Md.: National Institutes of Health, 1977. [Readable, profusely illustrated account of cancer history.]

Shryock, Richard Harrison. *Medicine and Society in America: 1660–1860.* Ithaca, N.Y.: Cornell University Press, 1962.

Simonton, Carl, and Matthews-Simonton, Stephanie. *Getting Well Again.* Los Angeles: J. P. Tarcher, 1978.

Sloan-Kettering Institute. "Carcinogens . . . Internally Manufactured?" *Report.* New York, 1969.

+ ———. "Meeting on Amygdalin" (minutes). New York, July 10, 1973.

———. *Annual Report.* New York, 1974.

Smith, Richard D. "The Laetrile Papers." *The Sciences,* January 1978.

Sontag, Susan. *Illness as Metaphor.* New York: Farrar, Straus and Giroux, 1977.

Standard and Poor's. *Industry Survey.* New York, 1977.

———. *Industry Survey.* New York, July 1979.

+ Stock, C. Chester. "A Second and Low Opinion of Second Opinion's Special Report: Laetrile at Sloan-Kettering." New York: Sloan-Kettering Institute, November 21, 1977. [Internal memorandum.]

Stock, C. Chester, et al. "Antitumor Tests of Amygdalin in Spontaneous Animal Tumor Systems." *Journal of Surgical Oncology* 10:81–88, 1978.

Stone, Irwin. *The Healing Factor, Vitamin C Against Disease.* New York: Grosset & Dunlap, 1972.

Strickland, Stephen P. "Integration of Medical Research and Health Policies." *Science,* September 17, 1971.

° ———. *Politics, Science and Dread Disease.* Cambridge, Mass.: Harvard University Press, 1972. [History of United States medical research policy.]

Sugiura, Kanematsu. *The Publications of Kanematsu Sugiura: Memorial Edition.* 4 vols. Foreword by C. Chester Stock. New York: Sloan-Kettering Institute, 1965.

° ———. "Reminiscence and Experience in Experimental Chemotherapy of Cancer." *Medical Clinics of North America* 55(3), May 1971. [Charming account of early cancer research.]

+ ———. Unpublished taped interview. July 1974.

+ ———. Personal communication. August 5, 1975.

+ ———. Personal communication. February 10, 1976a.

+ ———. Personal communication. July 29, 1976b.

+ ———. Personal communication. September 9, 1976c.

+ ———. Personal communication. December 20, 1976d.

+ ———. Personal communication. January 17, 1977a.

+ ———. Letter to Alec Pruchnicki. November 22, 1977b. [Pruchnicki is chairman of Second Opinion.]

+ ———. Personal communication. March 23, 1979.

Summa, Herbert M. "Amygdalin, a Physiologically Active Therapeutic Agent in Malignancies" (in German). *Krebsgeschehen Schriftenreihe* (Heidelberg) 4, 1972.

Syracuse Cancer Research Institute. Informational brochure. Syracuse, N.Y., July 1979.

Taylor, A. M. *Imagination and the Growth of Science.* New York: Schocken Books, 1970.

Taylor, Renée. *Hunza Health Secrets.* New York: Award Books, 1960.

Thomas, Lewis. "Disease, Cancer and the Progress of Science" (interview). MSKCC *Center News,* March 1975.

Thompson, Morton. *The Cry and the Covenant.* New York: New American Library, 1949. [Fictional account of the life of Ignaz Semmelweis.]

United States Department of Commerce, Bureau of the Census. *Current Industrial Reports: Pharmaceutical Preparations, Except Biologicals.* Washington, D.C., 1977.

United States Senate. "Breast Cancer—1976." Hearing Before the Subcommittee on Health and Scientific Research, Committee on Human Resources. Washington, D.C., May 4, 1976.

———. "Banning of the Drug Laetrile from Interstate Commerce by FDA." Hearing Before the Subcommittee on Health and Scientific Research, Committee on Human Resources. Washington, D.C., July 12, 1977.

Upton, Arthur C. Letter to Lawrence Burton. August 11, 1978. [Letter in possession of Dr. Burton. Authenticity confirmed by Dr. Upton in following entry.]

+ ———. Personal communication. July 26, 1979.

Vallery-Radot, René. *The Life of Pasteur.* Translated by R. L. Devonshire. Garden City, N.Y.: Garden City Publishing Company, 1924.

Vogel, Virgil J. *American Indian Medicine.* Norman, Okla.: University of Oklahoma Press, 1970.

Von Hoffman, Nicholas. "Fund Shortage Hurts Pauling Cancer Project." Syndicated column, *Lawton* [Okla.] *Constitution*, November 17, 1976.

Wade, Leo. "Medical Public Relations for the Physician in Industry." *New York Medicine* 9:686–88, September 20, 1953.

———. "Why People Don't Work." *Texas State Journal of Medicine*, July 1958.

+ ———. "The Environment in Relation to Cancer" (mimeographed). New York, December 1962.

+ ———. "Occupation and Cancer: The George Gehrmann Memorial Lecture" (mimeographed). New York, February 6, 1964.

Warburg, Otto. *The Metabolism of Tumors*. London: Constable and Company, 1930.

° Weinstein, Henry. "Did Industry Suppress Asbestos Data?" *Los Angeles Times*, October 23, 1978. [Incisive investigative journalism based on documents unearthed in the course of asbestos-related law suits.]

Williams, Roger J. *Nutrition Against Disease: Environmental Protection*. New York: Plenum Publishing Corporation, 1971.

Wolf, Max, and Ransberger, Karl. *Enzyme Therapy*. Los Angeles: Regent House, 1972.

Wuerthele-Caspe, Virginia [now Virginia Livingston-Wheeler], et al. "Etiology of Scleroderma—A Preliminary Clinical Report." *Journal of the Medical Society of New Jersey* 44:256, July 1947.

Yarborough, Ralph. "Foreword" in *Report of the National Panel of Consultants on the Conquest of Cancer*. Prepared for the Committee on Labor and Public Welfare, U.S. Senate. Washington, D.C. 1970.

Yasgur, Steven S. "Can Cancer Be Destroyed by the Body's Own Agents?" *Modern Medicine,* January 1, 1975.

Young, James H. *The Medical Messiahs*. Princeton: Princeton University Press, 1967.

Zimmermann, Caroline A. *Laetrile: Hope—or Hoax?* New York: Zebra Books, 1977.

Index